Specific Learning Disabilities

Yitzchak Frank, MD

Clinical Professor of Pediatrics, Neurology, and Psychiatry
Icahn School of Medicine at Mount Sinai

OXFORD
UNIVERSITY PRESS

OXFORD

UNIVERSITY PRESS

Oxford University Press is a department of the University of
Oxford. It furthers the University's objective of excellence in research,
scholarship, and education by publishing worldwide.

Oxford   New York
Auckland   Cape Town   Dar es Salaam   Hong Kong   Karachi
Kuala Lumpur   Madrid   Melbourne   Mexico City   Nairobi
New Delhi   Shanghai   Taipei   Toronto

With offices in
Argentina   Austria   Brazil   Chile   Czech Republic   France   Greece
Guatemala   Hungary   Italy   Japan   Poland   Portugal   Singapore
South Korea   Switzerland   Thailand   Turkey   Ukraine   Vietnam

Oxford is a registered trademark of Oxford University Press
in the UK and certain other countries.

Published in the United States of America by
Oxford University Press
198 Madison Avenue, New York, NY 10016

Library of Congress Cataloging-in-Publication Data
Frank, Yitzchak, author.
Specific learning disabilities / Yitzchak Frank.
    p. ; cm.
ISBN 978–0–19–986295–5 (alk. paper)
I. Title.
[DNLM: 1. Learning Disorders.   2. Adolescent.   3. Brain—abnormalities.
4. Brain—anatomy & histology.   5. Child.   6. Neuropsychology—methods. WS 110]
RC394.L37
616.85′889—dc23
2013051029

Medicine is a rapidly changing field. As new research and clinical experience broaden our
knowledge, changes in treatment and drug therapy occur. The author and publisher of this
work have checked with sources believed to be reliable in their efforts to provide information
that is accurate and complete, and in accordance with the standards accepted at the time of
publication. However, in light of the possibility of human error or changes in the practice of
medicine, neither the author, nor the publisher, nor any other party who has been involved in
the preparation or publication of this work warrants that the information contained herein
is in every respect accurate or complete. Readers are encouraged to confirm the information
contained herein with other reliable sources, and are strongly advised to check the product
information sheet provided by the pharmaceutical company for each drug they plan to
administer.

9 8 7 6 5 4 3 2 1
Printed in the United States of America
on acid-free paper

This book is dedicated to my wife Claudia Oberweger Frank

CONTENTS

INTRODUCTION

Specific learning disabilities (SLD) are among the most common medical conditions of children and adolescents. Studies place the prevalence of SLD at 5% or more of school age children.

SLD may have a very significant effect on children's academic performance in school and also affect other aspects of their lives including social skills, family relationships, and emotional well being.

There are a number of reasons why SLD can have such enormous effects. First, SLD are developmental conditions that affect children during the first years of life. These are the years of formal learning, when the child's life evolves mostly around school, and academic achievements are most important. Second, although it is a developmental condition, SLD is present throughout life and continues to have adverse effects on adolescents and adults. Third, SLD is not only a problem of academic achievements, but has other inherent deficits, including motor coordination deficits and behavioral comorbidities, which interfere with the child's abilities and success. And last, SLD is not adequately recognized by parents, teachers, and physicians, and therefore there are usually long delays in diagnosis, giving rise to severe behavioral and emotional consequences that continue into adolescence and adulthood.

This book describes the primary and secondary manifestations of these very heterogeneous conditions, and the different therapies advocated for SLD, but is mostly dedicated to the neurological basis of SLD. It summarizes the evidence for brain-based abnormalities underlying SLD, suggesting that those are mostly a result of genetic abnormalities that affect brain systems, changing cognitive networks and, thus, interfering with academic school learning and with other perceptual and motor functions, and having, in addition, primary and secondary effects on behavior and emotions. It outlines the brain structures responsible for normal learning and the brain changes that are associated with SLD. Other chapters of the book, including chapters on the neuropsychology of SLD, provide the essential information needed for the understanding of the neurology of SLD.

The first part of the book includes a short historical review of SLD (Chapter 1), clinical aspects of SLD (Chapter 2), and some theories of the pathophysiology of SLD (Chapter 3). The second part has a short review of brain correlations of learning (Chapter 4) followed by the anatomy (Chapters 5–9), physiology (Chapter 10), and genetics (Chapter 11) of SLD. Separate chapters are dedicated to cognitive and anatomical abnormalities of dyscalculia (Chapter 12) and (a short chapter) to nonverbal learning disabilities (Chapter 13). The third part includes a chapter on the on the behavioral and emotional abnormalities associated with SLD (Chapter 14), a chapter on the clinical evaluation of SLD (Chapter 15), and a chapter on treatment and prognosis of SLD (Chapter 16). A multifaceted approach to the treatment of SLD, which includes educational and psychological components, is suggested. Although there is no clear pharmacological therapy for SLD, medications are at times indicated for the treatment of behavioral comorbidities. Chapter 17, the conclusions, summarizes the information put forward in this book and defines goals for future research and therapy.

The coverage of the various aspects of SLD in this book is not even. While an attempt is made to discuss the biological aspects of SLD and the underlying brain abnormalities in more detail, the discussion of other parts, including neuropsychological evaluation, aims to provide the knowledge necessary to understand the biology but does not constitute a comprehensive review.

CHAPTER 1

Specific Learning Disabilities

Definitions and Facts

INTRODUCTION

The *Shorter Oxford English Dictionary* (1959) defines the act of learning as "to get knowledge of a subject or skill, by study, experience, or teaching." According to this definition, learning is an ongoing process that continues throughout life. We learn something new almost every day: new methods or regulations related to our work or profession, new applications for our computer, or how to use a new electronic device, to mention but a few. We meet new people, learn to recognize their faces and voices, remember their names, and form social associations with them.

If we limit the discussion to earlier life and school years, a very important, and perhaps very demanding type of learning that goes on is the academic learning: the learning of reading, arithmetic, writing, and, subsequently, more sophisticated school courses based on these abilities. Students attending school or college need to learn and retain a large body of new material daily, complete complex projects, and successfully negotiate tests.

People have different learning aptitudes. The capacity for academic learning differs in the same way as the abilities to run, throw a ball, or create art differ. Some people learn some subjects faster than others. Some individuals may be able to learn historical facts, stories, or poems more efficiently than mathematical concepts whereas others may excel in acquiring mathematical or geometrical knowledge. This normal diversity of academic learning ability is probably determined by a variety of factors including developmental, genetic, and cultural, which influence our cognitive systems—these intricate, complex networks in the brain that carry out perception, language, information processing, and memory, thereby facilitating learning.

Why do some children fail academically? There are reasons for academic failure which do not relate to the child's ability to learn. We can refer to those as external reasons. Some children simply do not attend school or attend schools with inadequate teaching resources. Some have a chaotic home environment with absence of parental guidance. In many countries around the world, children do not get to attend school, working instead to put bread on their family table. These children grow up illiterate, may never learn to read or write, and are thus unable to achieve academic success. There are many schools, in poor regions, that lack teachers and teaching equipment. Reading and mathematics achievements of the students of these schools are low. In families with a low socioeconomic status, students may not have the motivation and close supervision needed to get through school. Many of them will be low achievers. Similarly, children with chronic debilitating diseases who miss many school days, those with abnormal sensory organs, mostly the hearing and visually impaired, frequently fail to achieve normal academic milestones. They cannot learn and achieve adequately, especially under conventional teaching methods. Significant behavioral and emotional problems can also seriously interfere with normal learning, causing low academic achievements. Another group of youngsters with low academic achievements are those with deficient intelligence (intellectual disability). They may have a "ceiling" to their academic abilities. Some of them, with borderline intelligence or mild intellectual disability, may learn to read but usually do not have normal academic achievements. They have pervasive difficulties in obtaining and retaining information, and are slow to acquire any kind of knowledge. Thus, their problems will not be confined to academic learning.

Although those groups of students discussed above have low academic achievements, none of them are defined as having a "Specific Learning Disability" (SLD). This term is reserved for children who are intellectually normal, who have normal vision and hearing, who do not have any chronic medical or mental disease, and who receive adequate education—but still do not succeed academically. The reason for the failure to learn and achieve adequately in these subjects is a neurologically based learning problem. These children and adolescents are the subject of this book.

The question that obviously arises is what differentiates a normal learner who is on the slower range of normal from a learning disabled person. In other words, if it is claimed that children with SLD are a specific group, further specification and characterization are necessary. Indeed, many cases of SLD can be characterized by specific brain-based cognitive abnormalities that are not pervasive, as in a generalized intellectual disability or in some cases of brain damage, but rather confined to certain cognitive domains (e.g., language processing), leaving other cognitive domains intact. Ideally, identifying specific biological abnormalities in subjects with SLD will further characterize this group. Such biological abnormalities have already been found in research studies, in particular for reading disability but have not had the specificity and reliability needed for a biological diagnosis of SLD.

Reading disability, more commonly known as "dyslexia," and the best known type of an SLD, manifests itself through variable levels of reading and spelling difficulty. A lesser known type of SLD is impaired mathematical ability, or dyscalculia. Combined types of SLD, with difficulties in both reading and mathematics, are frequently present. Other types of SLD include those involving writing and those involving social skills.

It needs to be stated from the onset that apart from the obvious effects on academic abilities, SLDs also have significant social and psychological effects, both on children and on their families. School is the place where children spend the majority of their time outside of home and is comparable to the adults' workplace. The consequences of failure in school on the child's self-esteem and social standing are comparable to the consequences of failure in the workplace. This makes SLD not just an academic problem but a condition with possible profound effects on these children and their families.

A significant number of school children have SLDs. These conditions are present in all societies and cultures (Yamadan, 1995). The educational system in the United States is mandated by law to provide special education services to children who cannot learn because of physical or mental problems. Half the recipients of special education are children with learning disabilities, and the price of special education for them places a tremendous burden on the financial resources of school systems. Therefore, defining what constitutes specific learning disabilities and the eligibility criteria for special education services for these children is also a very important financial issue, and at times a source of contention between administrators and parents.

WHAT ARE SPECIFIC LEARNING DISABILITIES (SLDs)?

As a student in grade school and in high school I had no knowledge of the existence of SLD. In my memory, though, I can divide the students in my school into different groups. There were the "A" students, always in tight competition with each other, for whom a score of A-minus was a failure. Another group was the "troublemakers" group—disruptive during class, getting into fights during recess, eager parties to any mischievous ideas, whose parents could be frequent seen in school waiting by the principal's office. And there were, of course, the rest of us, going about our business, studying for tests, sitting through the usual school ceremonies, involved with our social groups, doing our homework, and finally graduating high school on our way to college.

In hindsight, I can remember yet another group of students. Usually quiet, sometimes sad-looking, frequently not part of any of the class' social groups. They were immature, sometimes acting as class clowns. Academically they were always struggling, achieving only "C" and "D" grades. Teachers frequently lost patience with their inability to grasp or retain simple academic concepts, occasionally referring to them as "lazy," "slow," "dumb," or "stupid." For some of these students, life during recess or sport activities was no better. They were clumsy, especially in team sports, missing clues as to the whereabouts of the ball, trying but not succeeding to catch, hit, or throw. Strangely, when I met some of them out of school they appeared different—clever, much more sure of themselves, and paradoxically knowledgeable about worldly affairs and nonacademic facts of life. Some of them have gone on to a very productive life, frequently to our surprise. It occurs to me now, many years later, that these students could have been those with Specific Learning Disabilities—intelligent and sometimes very perceptive, but academically unsuccessful.

The ability to detect and diagnose children with SLD has consistently improved over the last decades. Much has been learned about the natural history of the condition, about its different symptoms and manifestations, and about early signs and risk factors. This knowledge, though, is not shared by all who encounter children with SLD. Many professionals and parents are not sufficiently informed of the condition, some have misconceptions of its origin, and some simply refuse to recognize it, adversely affecting these children and adolescents.

Why is it difficult to recognize SLD? Because the learning abnormalities at the core of this condition are neither absolute, nor uniform, but rather "focal" and variable. What does this mean? Unlike intellectual disability, where learning abnormalities are global and affect academic as well as nonacademic domains, the learning difficulties of SLD are much more circumscribed. Many children with SLD are very capable in various ways except academically. Their academic disability may relate to only one type of academic learning (e.g., reading, calculation, writing), and may depend on the complexity of the material learned. Although some encounter difficulties from the onset, learning how to read single words, others may not have problems early in the first year of school but may have difficulties later when they have to read and comprehend paragraphs or an entire book. Children with SLD may be able to answer simple question but may not able to prepare a complex project; they may do well on oral tests but not on a written essay. I have frequently heard parents say in disbelief: "My son does not have a reading disability. I gave him a book and he could read for me," without realizing that their son indeed reads, but well below grade level or not sufficiently fast for the regular class work. Another common scenario with SLD children is an ability to learn the material (e.g., words for a spelling test), but only after additional instructions and tutoring to an extent not given in a regular classroom. In other words, SLD is rarely an absolute disability and may become more or less evident depending on the novelty and the complexity of the learned material, and on the chance for training and repetition. Because of these, it is sometimes hard for a lay person to comprehend it, even after an attempt of explanation.

The first step on the way to recognition and understanding of SLD, as well as to the development of clinical expertise and of remedies, is the exchange of knowledge between clinicians and researchers working on SLD. Such exchange of knowledge demands a clear definition and classification of these conditions. Indeed, the lack of an acceptable definition and classification of SLD has been a significant obstacle to advances in diagnosis, treatment, and research, and in particular to a wider recognition of the condition (Hastings et al., 1993). A formal, generally accepted definition of SLD also has important legal implications. Federal laws mandate education to all handicapped children. Under these laws, the children defined as "learning disabled" are entitled to special education and other services. The definition of learning disabilities determines which students are entitled to special education help. Because SLD is a common condition, its definition has great financial implications on school systems, states, and parents.

A universally agreed upon definition will advance knowledge and research, and enable many children with SLD to receive the educational and other special services they need.

DEFINITIONS OF SPECIFIC LEARNING DISABILITIES

Historically, the conditions recognized today as "Specific Learning Disabilities (SLD)" has undergone a succession of frequently changing names reflecting the lack of understanding of the pathophysiology of these conditions. The names used included "word blindness," "minimal brain damage," and "minimal brain dysfunction," reflecting the various theories of the underlying pathology causing these conditions, as well as the absence of consensus. For the last 30 years there has been an ongoing effort to obtain a clear definition, a task made difficult by the fact that SLDs are complex disorders, and a simple definition is difficult and may minimize the different aspects of these conditions (Critchley, 1978; Hammil et al., 1987, 1990; Shaywitz et al., 1995).

A definition by the National Joint Committee on Learning Disabilities (NJCLD, 1987) states:

> Learning disabilities is a general term that refers to a heterogeneous group of disorders manifested by significant difficulties in the acquisition and use of listening, speaking, reading, writing, reasoning or mathematical abilities. These disorders are intrinsic to the individual, presumed to be due to central

nervous system dysfunction, and may occur across the life span. Problems in self-regulatory behavior, social perception, and social interaction may exist with learning disabilities but do not by themselves constitute a learning disability.

An important part of this definition is the notion that these disorders are intrinsic neurological disorders, resulting from a central nervous system dysfunction. The definition recognizes that there may be comorbidity with other conditions or influences—cultural, economic, and environmental.

The Diagnostic and Statistical Manual of Mental Disorders (DSM), in its previous editions, III and III-R, includes Learning Disabilities in the section of Specific Developmental Disorders, along with Language and Speech Disorders and Motor Skill Disorders, using the heading of Academic Skills Disorders. Specifically stated exclusions are demonstrable physical or neurological disorder, pervasive developmental disorder, mental retardation, or deficient educational opportunity (American Psychiatric Association, 1987).

The Diagnostic and Statistical Manual of Mental Disorders, fourth edition (DSM IV) defines learning disorders as follows:

> Learning disorders are diagnosed when the individual's achievement on individually administered, standardized tests in reading, mathematics, or written expression is substantially below that excepted for age, schooling, and level of intelligence. This group of disorders, usually named Learning Disabilities, need to be differentiated from learning disorders resulting from impaired vision or hearing, social or emotional disturbance, cultural differences, insufficient or inappropriate instruction. In addition, the concept of LD does not apply to inability to learn as a result of mental retardation or communication disorders. Underlying abnormalities of cognitive processing are frequently present, including language procession abnormalities, visual perception or memory abnormalities. Though these cognitive abnormalities underlying LD are frequently present from birth, the disorder is usually detected in school.
>
> (American Psychiatric Association, 1994)

The DSM-IV definition is a well-formulated, concise statement summarizing the essential criteria for learning disabilities (or "Specific Learning Disabilities"—the name used in this book), as currently understood. It defines learning disabilities as specific entities, clearly distinct from academic difficulties caused by failure of "peripheral" sensory organs like hearing or vision, by social and emotional problems, or by poor teaching. It excludes learning abnormalities that are a part of a global intellectual deficiency (mental retardation) or of a communication disorder (for example, autism). The definition also states that cognitive abnormalities, probably present from birth, are the underlying abnormalities in learning disabilities.

Other specific developmental disorders, including Motor Skills Disorder, Communications Disorders, Pervasive Developmental Disorders, and Attention Deficit and Disruptive Behavior Disorders, are listed in the DSM-IV under separate headings. These disorders may interfere with a student's performance in school, although not necessarily through a direct effect on academic achievements. Because the current concept of learning disabilities includes only disorders with deficient academic learning, manifested as abnormal scoring on academic achievement tests, these disorders are not listed as learning disabilities. In effect it may be appropriate to look at these groups of disorders as being forms of learning disabilities that involve non academic types of learning—for instance the learning of motor skills or of social skills. In the future we may classify learning disabilities in a more comprehensive way to better reflect all the various types of neurologically based learning deficiencies.

HISTORICAL NOTES

Gall's studies of adults with brain damage written in about 1800 recorded that brain abnormalities can impair the ability to learn (Wiederholt, 1974; Hammill, 1993). Dejerine, in 1891, reported that adults with (acquired) damage to the left inferior parietal-occipital region had an impairment of reading and writing, and suggested that this region plays a role in the processing of the "optic images of letters" (Dejerine, 1891; Habib, 2000). Descriptions of children with learning disabilities date back at least a century. In 1895 James Hinshelwood, an ophthalmologist, described patients with inability to read. He designated this difficulty as "congenital word blindness," a designation that was probably derived from cases of reading loss in adults with acquired brain damage in whom the abnormality involved damage to visual pathways. He noted also the more frequent occurrence of reading disability in boys and the presence of similar difficulties in other family members (Hinshelwood, 1917). He also urged that these children not be punished because of this deficit for which they were in no way responsible, and recommended using didactic efforts to help them learn to read. Hinshelwood's correct perception of the "organic" nature of reading disabilities 100 years ago is surprising. He probably erred in regard to the pathophysiology of reading disabilities, which in most, although not all, affected children is not related to abnormalities of visual perception. Another case, of a 14-year-old boy incapable of learning to read, was reported in 1896 by Pringle Morgan, an English general practitioner (Pringle Morgan, 1896). Samuel T. Orton, director of a mental health clinic in Iowa, described children with reading and writing difficulties who had reversals of letters, spelling errors, omissions, substitutions, and mirror writing. He, like Hinshelwood, described their problem as "word blindness" (Orton, 1925). He believed that these children had an abnormal pattern of brain development, "ambiguous occipital dominance," or mixed cerebral dominance, causing their inability to read, as well as the frequent occurrence of left-handedness and mirror reading. He also noted that many of the children with academic skill deficiencies had abnormal disorganized behavior. Other authors believed that the reading difficulties are aphasic in nature, whereas many considered it a psychological problem.

A theory that brain injury or damage caused learning disabilities developed during the 1940s and 1950s. The sources of this theory were reports that children who, during the influenza endemic at the end of World War I, had sustained encephalitis and resultant brain damage; had abnormal behaviors and educational problems along with cognitive, auditory, and visual problems; and were treated with special education (Strauss & Lehtinen, 1947). It was postulated that because cognitive functions are localized in the brain, early injury to specific brain areas can cause specific learning disabilities. There was, though, a major difficulty in using brain damage as a model for children with learning disabilities. Children with learning difficulties following encephalitis or head trauma had other significant neurological abnormalities, whereas most children with developmental learning disabilities had no gross neurological abnormalities to indicate brain damage. The term "minimal brain damage" was, therefore, introduced, but this term was frightening and offensive to the families of learning disabled children. More so, it was unjustified because in most children with learning disabilities there was no pathologic or neurologic evidence of brain damage. Consequently, in 1962 the Oxford International Study Group on Child Neurology and a National Institute of Child Health task force recommended discarding the term "Minimal Brain Damage" and replacing it with "Minimal Brain Dysfunction." This term remained in use for some time, serving as a catch all for a variety of developmental learning, and attentional and behavioral problems.

By the late 1960s the focus shifted from an attempt to define learning disabilities through the presumed etiology or pathophysiology, toward a clinical descriptive definition. In 1968, the World Federation of Neurology defined specific developmental dyslexia as "a disorder manifested by difficulty in learning to read despite conventional instruction, adequate intelligence, and sociocultural opportunity." The disorder was attributed to "functional cognitive disabilities which are frequently of constitutional origin" (Critchley, 1970). Samuel Kirk, a special educator, introduced the term Learning Disability (Kirk, 1978). He believed that Learning Disabilities are the result of processing problems that affect language and academic performance. He thought that the cause of such disabilities can be either a brain dysfunction or emotional/ behavioral disturbance (Hammill, 1990).

Parallel advances and inventions, which took place in the last decades, have helped clarify our understanding of SLD. These include improved neuropsychological methods that provided greater capability to measure cognitive ability and identify cognitive disabilities; new imaging methods that enhanced our knowledge of developmental brain anatomy and provided the ability to image the brain anatomy of cognitive processes; and the development of molecular genetic methods that enabled us to recognize the genetic origin of SLD. As a result, we have now information on the types of cognitive processes and possibly brain areas and networks affected in SLD, although there is not yet a "biological" marker diagnostic of these conditions, and no definitive cure.

SPECIFIC LEARNING DISABILITIES ARE COMMON: PREVALENCE

Specific Learning Disabilities are very common, possibly the most common medical condition of childhood. Hence, the recognition and understanding of these conditions is an important medical issue. As previously mentioned the prevalence of SLD has also become an important epidemiological and economic issue. The Education for All Handicapped Children Act (Public Law 94-142) requires states to provide free and appropriate public education to children with special needs. Approximately one-half of all children with special needs receiving special education services in the United States, or about 5% of the total public school population, are those identified as having learning disabilities. This means that a significant amount of funds is spent on special services for people with learning disabilities. What do we know on the prevalence of this condition? The best known and probably best measured form of SLD is reading disability or dyslexia. Measurements of other types of SLD (for example dyscalculia or writing abnormalities) are more difficult, and estimates of their prevalence are fewer and less accurate. Therefore, prevalence numbers for dyslexia may be more accurate than prevalence rates of other types of SLD, or of all SLDs.

The Interagency Committee on Learning Disabilities (1987) estimated the prevalence of LD as 5% to 10% of the school age population. The range of other estimates of the prevalence of learning and reading disability in the school age population varies and significantly higher prevalence has been reported. Dyslexia is the most common type of SLD. Most learning disabled children have reading problems. A conservative estimate of the prevalence of developmental dyslexia is 3% to 6%. A longitudinal study of Connecticut schoolchildren followed from kindergarten through third grade reported a prevalence rate of reading disability ranging from 6% to 9% (Shaywitz et al., 1990). The prevalence of specific arithmetic difficulties in a population of school children in England was found to be 1.3%. In the same study a larger group, 3.2%, was found to have arithmetic as well as reading difficulties (Lewis, 1994).

The prevalence of SLD has increased in the last 20 years. This may be the result of more awareness of the condition, and the presence of a clearer definition of SLD leading to better identification by clinicians and schools. Still, there is a lack of uniformity in the diagnostic process and measurement of SLD. Reported rates of SLD may be higher or lower according to the definition and the diagnostic criteria used by the various educational systems. Prevalence rates may also depend on socioeconomic status and the prosperity of the community and the school system (McDermott, 1994). A more affluent school system may give its students better access to testing and will identify a higher number of children with SLD. Also, SLD classification may be used by educational systems to provide services to children who have other problems, including autism, thus incorrectly increasing the prevalence of SLD. In a study conducted in Scotland, 14.3% of 634 children with a diagnosis of learning disabilities fulfilled the diagnostic criteria for autism (Deb & Prassad, 1994). Similarly, schools may classify children with mild mental retardation as having SLD, increasing the prevalence of SLD and decreasing the rates of mild mental retardation (MacMillan et al., 1996). Estimates of SLD in developing countries are almost impossible because of difficulties in excluding many children who have learning problems resulting from the lack of adequate schooling and socioeconomic limitations (Stough & Aguirre-Roy, 1997).

The basic pathophysiology of dyslexia is universal, despite variations in the phonological structure of diverse languages. Brain changes observed in biological investigations of dyslexia are consistent across different cultures (Paulesu et al., 2001). The core cognitive abnormality in dyslexia—deficit in phonological processing persists over time (Bruck 1992; Cirino, Israeli, et al., 2005).

The developmental course of reading disabilities speaks to the validity of these conditions: More than 70% of children identified as reading disabled in grade 3 were also reading disabled in high school (Shaywitz, Morris, & Shaywitz, 2008).

Early gender studies of reading disabilities reported a preponderance of males, with a male/female ratio of approximately 2:1, whereas later studies found an approximately equal number of reading disabled males and females (Shaywitz, Shaywitz, Fletcher, & Escobar, 1990) Another study found an equal number of male and female children with arithmetic difficulties but a preponderance of males over females in those with specific reading difficulties (Lewis et al., 1994). Schools perhaps identify more boys than girls as having SLD because boys may have a higher occurrence of disruptive behavioral comorbid with their academic difficulties, resulting in earlier referral for testing.

In summary, it is clear that SLD is a prevalent problem, eliciting greater awareness in recent years because of better recognition, and possibly because its prevalence is increasing. Large epidemiological studies with uniform criteria for the diagnosis and measurement of SLD in children are lacking. This brings us to issues of measurement, which are complex, not the least because of lack of a clear biological abnormality that can be measured.

ISSUES OF MEASUREMENT

Learning ability, like most biological phenomena, is not uniform. There are normal differences between people and, during childhood, an individual rate of development. There are faster learners and slower learners, and some students learn to read later than others. The line between "normal" and "abnormal" is frequently vague, and depends also on expectations.

There have been arguments that SLD are artificially created by schools, which judge students too harshly and do not allow for individual variability, and if children could learn at an individual pace the problem of SLD would not exist. As will be shown in the following chapters—there are specific abnormalities that separate slow or late readers from reading disabled (dyslexic) readers, and are not age or maturation dependent.

Regardless, there is a legal obligation in our society to educate children, and a legal obligation to provide special education to those who have learning problems. These factors bring about the need to measure learning ability and define disability. Ideally, there should be biological measures of SLD. In the absence of a biological measure, SLD is measured by standardized tests of academic performance, usually in reading, spelling, and mathematics (Francis et al., 1994). These tests are used to decide who receives special education services according to Public Law 94-142 (1975), the Education for all Handicapped Children Act, and the subsequent Individuals with Disabilities Education Act (1992). These tests compare the individual with the rest of the students in the state or country. Of course, it is easier to standardize the level of knowledge we require of a child than to standardize the level of educational services provided for children. We aspire to but cannot provide each child with the same level of teaching, or the same level of social and parental environment support. Therefore there may be an inherent bias in requiring all students to have similar academic achievements. Still, as long as test results are interpreted with special attention to the individual, this is the best available method to determine the presence of an SLD at the present time. Achievement tests are usually scored in one of two ways. The first is a relative measure of aptitude-achievement "discrepancy." An SLD is diagnosed if a substantial discrepancy exists between the academic achievement (as determined by achievement test) and the intellectual potential (as demonstrated by intelligence, I.Q., testing), in one or more areas of learning (including reading, mathematics, and written expression) (Fletcher et al., 1994; Lyons, 1995). A 22-or 30-point discrepancy (reflecting 1.5 or 2 standard deviation discrepancy, respectively) between lower achievement and higher intellectual ability is generally used to define a specific learning disability. Another method is an "absolute measure," using standard achievement tests to demonstrate that the individual's achievement is significantly (1.5–2 standard deviations) below age or grade levels. This measure uses low achievement as an independent measure and does not relate it to intelligence (Shapiro & Gallico, 1986).

Both types of measurement have disadvantages. Recent research suggests that people with reading disabilities are not simply the lowest 10% to 15% on the scale of normal readers, but have specific cognitive abnormalities, including deficits in phonological awareness. Reading disabled children, both with and without intelligence-achievement discrepancy may have similar deficits in phonological awareness, and similar genetic and neurophysiological characteristics. Therefore, the "discrepancy" measurement may not be valid, and may prevent children who have relatively low intelligence from getting special education help (Lyons, 1996). On the other hand, the use of the "absolute measure" of 1.5 to 2 standard deviations below grade level as a cutoff for a specific learning disability may delay diagnosis of SLD until third or fourth grade.

Ideally, we should be able to diagnose SLD long before school begins. As will be discussed elsewhere in this book, most children with specific learning disabilities have some cognitive differences present from birth (Badian et al., 1990; Bashir & Scavuzzo, 1992). Using measures of early detection along with biological measures, we may be able to identify young children at risk for specific learning disabilities and save them from the damaging experience of years of failure and reduced self-esteem. This may have to await the discovery of valid reliable biological measures and better cognitive tests for infants and toddlers. Toward this end, a better knowledge of brain mechanisms of information processing and learning is needed. In the last decades, knowledge of the neurobiology of normal and abnormal learning and behavior has expanded enormously as a result of parallel advances in neuropsychology, neuroimaging, and molecular biology, and can be applied to improved better and earlier diagnosis.

CHAPTER 2

Neuropsychological Abnormalities Underlying Specific Learning Disabilities

INTRODUCTION

Specific learning disabilities (SLD) are a group of conditions usually distinguished by academic difficulties. Such difficulties can involve reading, (including basic reading skills and reading comprehension), writing, and arithmetic (including mathematical calculation and mathematical reasoning). Other names assigned to these types of learning disabilities are dyslexia, dysgraphia, and dyscalculia, respectively. Most learning disabled children have a combination of these academic difficulties (Shapiro & Gallico, 1986) and the most common combination is a reading disability or dyslexia with other academic disabilities, for instance spelling or mathematical disability (Badian, 1983). The term "SLD" is, in many ways, a minimalistic term because it refers to, and is measured by, academic underachievement. In reality individuals with SLD frequently have other difficulties that affect their life. They may have difficulties with motor coordination, motor execution, and study organization. They may have behavioral problems, social deficits, low self-esteem, and oppositional attitudes. They are frequently referred to as being, in general, "immature." The manifestations of SLD vary with the subject's age, general ability and motivation, the presence or absence of behavioral comorbidities, and other factors. Therefore, SLD is a developmental syndrome affecting a variety of functions controlled by the brain, including learning, behavior, attention, social skills, and motor functions. Consequently, the diagnostic and therapeutic processes of SLD need to look beyond the academic difficulties, into the other components of this syndrome, and into the individual circumstances of each child.

During the last decades, parents, educators, and physicians became increasingly aware of neurologically based learning and behavioral syndromes that begin in childhood and affect school performance, among other things. This awareness benefited Attention Deficit Hyperactivity Disorder (ADHD), another neurobehavioral condition, more than SLD, possibly because of frequent media exposure of the former and its effective treatment with stimulant medications. Knowledge of SLD, on the other hand, is still lacking, outside a relatively narrow circle of academics, psychologists, and school personnel. One reason for this is the fact that SLD is harder to perceive and understand, and there have always been alternate explanations as to why a child with normal intelligence does not do well academically, including "laziness," poor schooling, or lack of motivation.

Specific Learning Disabilities are found in all societies, and persist throughout the life span. Therefore, it is not appropriate to refer to them as developmental delay or immaturity. Signs of SLD are actually present and can sometimes be detected at a very young age. The most important predictive signs are abnormal or slow development of speech and language in infancy and early childhood, reflecting abnormal language processing and impairment of phonological functions (Scarborough, 1990). It is also evident that SLD continues in some form into adulthood. In the case of reading disability, the affected individuals will learn to read slower than others and may remain slow readers. Even those individuals who have compensated for the reading problems and who can achieve a normal score on both word and nonword reading tests (which are typically abnormal in learning disabled children) may continue to have some reading and/or spelling difficulties. It is, therefore, a mistake to expect that SLD will be cured at the end of elementary or even high school. It is a lifelong condition. The affected individuals will usually acquire knowledge and make academic progress, although slower than others, in spite of their disability, by finding "detours" (compensatory methods) to bypass their specific learning disabilities. Individual prognosis depends on a complex combination of factors, including the overall intelligence and cognitive ability, which determine the ability for academic compensation strategies, the presence or absence of other neurobehavioral deficits including ADHD, and social and cultural factors.

An important need for the diagnosis and treatment of SLD is to define and characterize the learning and cognitive deficits and distinguish a subject with SLD from a regular but slow learner. We hope that in the future the diagnosis and treatment will be facilitated by the advent of specific biological tests that will identify brain abnormalities in SLD. There has been a large volume of research on specific biological markers, but no specific biological tests at the present time. For now, most SLD subjects can be characterized by cognitive abnormalities, which are confined to certain domains (e.g., language processing), leaving other cognitive domains intact. These can be demonstrated by neuropsychological testing.

HOW DOES SPECIFIC LEARNING DISABILITY PRESENT? SYMPTOMS AND SIGNS

Symptoms of SLD may present at different points of time during childhood and adolescence. Children with decoding problems who cannot learn to identify letters and cannot sound out words using phonics have difficulties by Kindergarten or the first grade, mostly because they cannot learn how to read. When reading disability involves primarily difficulties with reading comprehension, it may be detected in later grades. Some students will encounter significant difficulties in the third or fourth grade, whereas others will present in middle school or even in high school. Sometimes the presenting symptom will not be an academic failure but rather a behavioral problem. We encounter children who start being "class clowns" or who become disruptive as early as the first or second grade, and, when tested, are found to have a learning problem (causing low self-esteem and behavioral problems). A behavioral presentation of individuals with SLD is more common in adolescence, when the students may start skipping classes, refuse to go to school, or manifest symptoms of conduct disorder. Adolescents with SLD, who previously did not manifest overt academic failure, may present at that time with what seems to be a sudden academic failure with significant behavioral problems. Their parents may not be aware of any previous academic problem. Although an underlying neurological abnormality or the onset of a major affective disorder like depression should be ruled out in these cases, an adolescent with this form of presentation has quite frequently had SLD that was previously barely compensated and became more apparent because of an increased academic load and complexity in high school. A detailed history taken at that time may reveal that the student has had academic difficulties all along but those were overlooked because he or she "just passed" and were promoted. At some point, possibly in middle or even high school, they cannot keep up with the mounting academic difficulties, and an acute crisis develops on top of a longstanding frustration. By that time these students have already suffered severe blows to their self-esteem, and the prospects of remediation are less favorable.

It is desirable to detect SLD at an early age so that appropriate educational interventions and behavioral therapy can be provided, learning ability can be optimized, secondary emotional problems can be prevented, and therapy can be more beneficial.

Formal academic learning does not usually start before the age of 5 years, the age of traditional school entry. Consequently, a diagnosis of SLD cannot be made prior to that age. We know, though, that SLD is the result of genetic-biological brain abnormalities that are present at birth. We should, therefore, be able to detect some symptoms of SLD prior to the beginning of formal schooling, before reading or spelling failure occur in the second or third grade, and possibly start remediation earlier. Indeed, as noted previously, SLD children usually do have some signs of learning difficulties prior to beginning of formal schooling. There is a frequent history of delay of speech and language development and difficulties are sometimes noted in the learning of fine or complex motor activities. Abnormality of speech and language development may be in the form of dysfluency, dysnomia, and rhyming difficulties. In kindergarten, a problem with letter identification skills can be detected. Parents are frequently informed by pediatricians or pediatric neurologists that their child has some developmental abnormalities, sometimes referred to, in a nonspecific manner, as "developmental delays," but the necessary connection between these abnormalities and later reading or other academic difficulties is not always made.

A formal preschool identification of SLD remains difficult (Shapiro & Gallico, 1993). School readiness tests have not been good predictors of future disabilities, and attempts to identify a single observation or test that can predict SLD in preschoolers have, in general, not been successful. Factors that were found to be predictive of SLD include speech delay, poor parenting skills, attentional problems and enuresis, adverse social circumstances, and prematurity (<35 weeks) (Corrigan, Steward, & Scott et al., 1996). The best predictor of a reading disability is the presence of a developmental speech and language disorder. Although many children with an early language disorder no longer manifest gross language difficulties at school age, subtle dysfunctions in areas of word retrieval or other language parameters including pragmatics may be present, and can be manifested as a difficulty in following multistep directions, or during performance in unstructured settings in which maximal efficiency in language competence is necessary (Blumsack, Lewandowski, & Waterman, 1997). There is a strong relationship between the language ability of 5-year-old children and their reading ability at age 7 years, and the persistence of a language processing abnormality is a strong predictor of a reading disability (Beitchman & Young, 1997). This association is frequently unrecognized by parents and teachers. Preschoolers who are identified with a developmental language disorder are typically "declassified" when speech and language improve after the age of 3 to 4 years, and are not "flagged" as being at risk for SLD. The association of a reading disability with their history of a language disorder may not be recognized even later, in the first or second grade, when they fail to learn to read. Thereby, the opportunity for early detection of reading disability through close following of preschool children with language disorders is missed. Early, preschool manifestations of other types of SLD, including mathematical SLD or reading comprehension disabilities, are not known. These types of SLD may not be detectable until later in elementary school.

THE PROCESS OF ACADEMIC LEARNING

There is not, at the present time, a theory or a model that will explain all types of SLD. Some of the pathophysiological models proposed for dyslexia do not have a sound scientific basis. Consequently, there are dyslexic children who receive treatments intended to improve the coordination of their eye movements, although there is no proof or a solid hypothesis that explains how uncoordinated eye movements cause dyslexia. Others are treated with medications intended to stabilize a presumably abnormal vestibular system, although it is hard to find any role for this system in academic learning.

Learning is a process that consists of a sequence of cognitive steps, some of which are not yet identified. It is likely that SLD occurs when one or more of these cognitive processes are impaired. A simplified model of learning disabilities, which follows the model of brain organization and information processing, postulates that the learning process includes stages of receiving information (input), integration of information, memory processes, and "production" of the learned material (output) (Silver, 1989). A deficit or an abnormality that occurs during any one of these steps can cause SLD. The initial cognitive stage of learning (input) consists of the processing of incoming information. This stage requires intact perceptual channels, which, for academic learning, are primarily the visual and auditory channels. An inability to perceive auditory or visual information will impair learning at this early stage. Abnormalities of visual perception may interfere with the perception of the size or position of objects, affecting the ability to differentiate between letters, or may cause difficulties distinguishing an object from the background. An auditory perceptual difficulty can be manifested by an inability to distinguish subtle differences between words, such as ball or bell, or by having trouble distinguishing auditory stimuli from the background. People with an auditory perceptual difficulty can have a deficit or reduced speed of sound processing.

The next cognitive stage in the learning process is the integration of the information obtained during "input." Here the information is organized and its pieces are put in the correct sequence. This stage also includes deriving general meaning from a particular word or symbol. A good example of a problem at this stage of input processing is deficient phonological processing, which is a major etiological factor in dyslexia. Language processing abnormality, higher order visual processing abnormality, or an abnormality of information integration center in the parietal and frontal lobes can cause naming problems, difficulty in learning to read, or an inability to generalize from an example.

Memory processes play an important role during information processing including storing new information and integrating it with previously learned information. Intact short- and long-term memory are required. A significant problem with long-term memory makes the learning of new information useless. A short-term memory deficit is less debilitating but can still cause a learning disability. The child may learn a series of facts, but is unable to answer general questions that require using these facts.

The next cognitive process following input processing and information integration, is the "output" process. Here, the first step consists of an "execution scheme." A dysfunction at this stage may interfere with verbal expression, writing, drawing, or any other form of expression. Most "output" channels used in academic learning, whether in the form of oral expression, writing, or drawing, involve motor activity. Therefore "output" involves initiating and coordinating the appropriate muscle group needed for motor "production." Abnormalities of "motor production" will cause gross motor difficulties (where the "large" muscles are effected) including difficulties with walking, running or playing sports, or fine motor coordination difficulties (where the "small" muscles are affected) including difficulties with writing, drawing, catching or throwing a ball, tying shoe laces, or buttoning shirts. Examples of SLD involving abnormalities of the "production" stage of learning including some types of writing disabilities (dysgraphia), as well as maladroitness and motor clumsiness seen in some children and adolescents. These "output" difficulties, like motor clumsiness, frequently accompany other "input" and integration abnormalities, which are typically more important as causes of academic learning difficulties. Some people debate whether this last stage of "output" should be included in the cognitive chain of learning. The identification of the cognitive processes causing SLD needs to include the examination of all stages of learning.

NEUROPSYCHOLOGICAL LOCALIZATION

Neuropsychological testing attempts to identify the cognitive pathophysiology and the specific learning processes that are impaired in the individual with SLD. In the neurological clinical practice, attempts have always been made to anatomically localize cognitive functions. Thus, some cognitive impairments causing SLD were ascribed to left hemisphere dysfunction, and some to right hemisphere dysfunction (Weintraub & Mesulam, 1983). The current view is that many cognitive functions have network representations in the brain. These networks may have components in one hemisphere or in both hemispheres, which are connected by axons and dendrites. Therefore neuropsychological abnormalities are discussed more in terms of cognitive systems or modules rather than by specific anatomic localizations. For instance, a neuropsychological model suggested for SLD assumes that modular brain systems specialize in processing specific kinds of information, and that these brain systems are differentially susceptible to developmental insults (Pennington, 1991). The involved brain systems direct phonological processing, spatial recognition, social cognition, executive functions, and long-term memory. These systems emerge in early life and are "differentially vulnerable" to insults.

Abnormality of a system will cause a form of SLD typical to that system. The idea behind this model is similar to "the theory of multiple intelligences," which assumes that a number of intelligences exist, including linguistic, spatial, logical mathematical, musical, body kinesthetic, and personal intelligence (Gardner, 1983). For instance, dyslexia is the form of SLD caused by an abnormality of a system responsible for phonological processing, whereas mathematic disability may be caused by an abnormality of a system responsible for spatial cognition. Similarly, ADHD is an abnormality of the system of executive functions, and autistic spectrum disorder is an abnormality of the social cognition system. These cognitive systems or modules of brain learning may be localized in different brain regions: The left perisylvian region for phonological processing; the posterior right hemisphere for spatial cognition; the prefrontal areas for executive functioning; limbic, orbital, and right hemisphere for social cognition, and amygdala and hippocampus for memory systems. The different modules of learning have also different susceptibility to "disruption by genetic and environmental factors," with executive functions and phonological processing being the systems most vulnerable to early brain insults, including genetic insults, possibly because their evolution has been more recent (Pennington, 1991). The important part of this model is the attempt to connect cognitive functions and deficiencies (including SLD) to brain networks and systems. This relationship between a specific brain anatomical abnormality and a corresponding cognitive dysfunction is not a simple one, and will have to await more empirical proof.

TYPES OF READING DISABILITIES

Dyslexia is the best researched type of SLD, where the most advanced knowledge of the underlying pathophysiology is available. Mattis et al. (1975) described three neuropsychological types of dyslexia: a common type with language processing abnormalities, a second and less common type with visual perceptual articulatory problems, and a third type with graphomotor deficits. They later added a subgroup of dyslexics whose reading difficulties are related to abnormalities of temporal sequencing. There was also a group of children whose reading problem was not accounted for by measurable neuropsychological abnormalities.

At the present time, language processing abnormalities are believed to play the major role in dyslexia (Myklebust and Johnson, 1962). In effect, the core deficit in dyslexia is thought to be phonological, an oral language deficit, and not a visual perceptual deficit. In the past, visual factors were assumed to have a role in dyslexia (Lovegrove, Slaghuis, et al., 1986; Stein, 2001). Early theories at the beginning of the 19th century suggested that the pathology of dyslexia is in the visual system, thus explaining the reversals of letters and words thought to be typical of dyslexic reading (Orton, 1925, 1937). Although there may be a subgroup of reading disabilities with mostly visual perceptual problems, and both the phonological and visual hypotheses have received contributions from functional imaging techniques (Habib, 2000), visual factors are not the critical abnormality in most dyslexics (Ingram, Mason, & Blackburn, 1970). In some cases of dyslexia, visual and language processing abnormalities may be concurrent (Slaghuis & Ryan, 1999).

Of the group of reading disabled subjects with language processing abnormality, there may be a phonological subgroup (or a word level reading disability [WLRD]), an independent reading comprehension deficit subgroup, other subgroups (possibly including one with problems of fluency) and mixed subgroups. These subgroups may or may not be stable with age (Dmonet et al., 2004). As will be discussed later in this chapter, the most important difficulty in this type of reading disability is difficulty with single word decoding. Spelling difficulties are also characteristic of WLRD and are caused by the same phonological processing difficulties that cause the word reading difficulties. This deficit can also limit reading comprehension. In such cases, comprehension problems are considered secondary to problems with decoding (Padget, Knight, & Sawyer, 1996). Padget et al. (1996) defined dyslexia as a learning based biological disorder that interferes with the acquisition of print literacy (reading, writing, spelling), characterized by poor decoding and spelling abilities, and deficits in phonological awareness or manipulations. These primary characteristics of dyslexia may co-occur with spoken language difficulties and deficits in short-term memory. It may be appropriate to use the term "dyslexia" for this subgroup, and use the more general term "reading disability" for other subgroups of reading disability caused by reading comprehension difficulties or limitation of fluency. Children with specific reading comprehension abnormalities had similar phonological skills and nonverbal intelligence to normal reading achievers (Stothard & Hulme, 1996).

As noted previously, it is possible that there are also subgroups with deficits in some aspects of visual processing. Problems with orthography (the visual symbols associated with the sound of the language) are characteristic of at least some students with reading disabilities. A distinction between surface dyslexia and phonological dyslexia is sometime made based on the theory of dual route framework of reading (Coltheart et al., 2001).

LEARNING TO READ

Introduction

The dual route model of reading assumes that two systems for reading exist: a slower sublexical system with graphemes translated to phonemes via the phonological system, and a visual orthographic system-a fast pathway directly mapping orthographic images into word form representatives. Both routes are involved in word identification and can get activated in parallel. Nonwords that do not have a stored phonological representation, and infrequent words, are read through lexical processing (the grapheme to phoneme route) slower than frequent words. This route is also utilized when children learn to read. For low frequency words, grapheme to phoneme conversion can be faster than the direct lexical route.

In surface dyslexia the problem is primarily in the lexical system level. People with this type of dyslexia will have more problems with exception words than pseudo words. People with impairment in phonological processing will have problems with reading of pseudo words more than exception words (Fletcher et al., 2007). It is not clear whether there is evidence for a surface type of dyslexia in children (Stanovich, Siegel, & Gottardo, 1997; Manis et al., 1999).

Dyslexia caused by a phonological deficit and the lack of ability to automatize— is universal regardless of the person's specific language. The particular language has an interaction with the developmental model of dyslexia, in that in phonologically more difficult languages (e.g. English) the most pronounced weakness occurs in phonological processing whereas in phonologically easier languages (e.g. German), the crucial manifestation is the lack of skills needed to achieve automatization (Grigorenko, 2001).

Phonological Awareness and Processing

Learning to read is different from reading by expert readers. An older theory suggested that subjects who begin to read use the "whole reading" method. According to this theory each word is a "symbol" by itself, which the child learns as a whole. There is no good evidence that children learn to read this way. The way children learn to read is through an analysis of the components of the word. When children who begin to read look at the written word, they perceive a visual stimulus and then retrieve its associated lexical form, using a phonological code, and then put it into articulation (in order to read aloud). This is a similar process to the one that occurs when we name an object we see (Geschwind, 1965; Wolf, 1991). During reading, orthographic codes are postulated to have direct connections with phonological codes (Plaut et al., 1996; Zorzi et al., 1998; Coltheart et al., 2001), so words have access to phonology. In contrast, during picture naming there is access to semantics (Segui & Fraisse, 1968; Warren & Morton, 1982; Glaser, 1992). The phoneme, which is defined as the smallest meaningful segment of language, is the fundamental element of the linguistic system. The English orthography is the representation of its speech sounds (the phonology) by alphabet letters, and different combinations of 44 phonemes produce every word in the English language. To read any words, the person who learns to read has to detect phonemic sequences in words, and segment spoken words into these phonemes which are the underlying phonological elements. The reader needs to know the phonemes on which the alphabetic system is based, and also needs to have phonological awareness, which is the knowledge of the sound–letter relationship (Liberman & Shankweiler, 1991; Blachman, 1997).

This will facilitate the understanding of the relation of the spoken word to the printed word (Liberman & Shankweiler, 1991). The words' orthographic representations stay in lexical memory and can be used for future new spelling–sound relationships. When the beginning readers have a good understanding of the alphabetic principles, and after phonologically recoding words a few times, they start making greater independent use of letter-sound information to identify unfamiliar words in text. Therefore, phonological awareness and processing play a critical role in the normal development of reading. Most children become aware of the phonological structure of spoken words and are able to perform tasks requiring the segmentation of words into smaller units (syllables), at an age of 4 to 6 years—before they start school. Dyslexic children cannot do so well (Bradley & Bryant, 1983). Impaired language segmentation skills lead to phonological difficulties and prevent word recognition. The best predictor of reading ability from kindergarten and first grade performance is phoneme segmentation ability.

COGNITIVE ABNORMALITIES UNDERLYING READING DISABILITY

As previously discussed, learning to read requires learning the correspondence between letters and sounds of speech (grapheme-phoneme correspondence). Dyslexics have a specific impairment in the representation, storage, and/or retrieval of speech sounds that prevents them from manipulating phonological information and acquiring the correspondence between letters and sounds of speech (grapheme-phoneme correspondence), which is the phonological prerequisite to reading (Bradley & Bryant, 1978; Vellutino, 1979; Snowling, 1981). Consequently, dyslexic children confuse between morphologically similar letters, and have difficulties learning grapheme to phoneme rules. They also have problems with writing manifested by errors in the phonetic transcription from oral to written letters and syllables, in the spatial arrangement of letters, inversions, omissions and substitutions of letters, and segmentation of words. Tasks that demand phonological processing ability, like the nonword test, were found to be a discriminator for dyslexia. A deficit in phonological awareness and processing was found to be a core deficit in reading disability (dyslexia) (Bradley & Bryant, 1983; Habib, 2000; Ramus et al., 2003).

Clinically, dyslexics perform poorly on tasks of phonological awareness (segmentation and manipulation of speech sounds) while having normal responses to nonspeech sound stimuli. They have a deficit in the phonological but not semantic processing of pictures.

There may be more than one fundamental biological abnormality that interferes with this essential process of phonological recognition and processing. For instance, a fundamental perceptual deficit on the level of phoneme representation because the sounds are poorly represented is a form of phonological impairment. A similar effect can be caused by an inability to separate between phonemes of subtle differences, like *ba* and *da*. Manis et al. (1997) found such deficit in a subgroup of dyslexic children with phonological awareness deficit who could not pick out a phoneme within a nonword read aloud by the examiner. The deficit may be dependent on the temporal properties of the auditory stimuli (Witton et al., 1998). That could not be replicated in another study (Bishop et al., 1999). Even when dyslexics can distinguish different phonemes, they may not be able to do it fast enough (Helenius, et al., 1999).

In addition to explaining its underlying cognitive pathology, these findings have implications for the early identification and remediation of dyslexia. The best method of early identification of dyslexia is testing children for phonological recognition and processing. Similarly, a method of remediation is through teaching phonological recognition. (Lundberg, Frost, & Petersen, 1988).

How consistently the letters or characters of the language (orthography) map into speech sounds (phonology), or the "transparency' of the orthography—is important in determining how easily children learn to read. For instance, learning to read in German, Italian, and Finnish is easier than in English. Nevertheless, the effect of phonological deficit on reading is universal (Ho et al., 2004).

Spelling

Reading and spelling are very closely related, because both use the same kind of codes but in different directions. When we read, we go from letters to phonological representations, and when we spell, we go from phonological representations to letters. Learning to spell is a more difficult process than learning to read. Spelling demands a greater knowledge of the orthographic structure of the word and is a longer process. There is a close relationship between reading and spelling disorders and delays—and difficulties with language development. Speech difficulties in the preschool year have an impact on reading and spelling later., with spelling being impacted more than reading. Consequently, in children with reading abnormalities there is usually a concomitant abnormality of spelling.

Reading Comprehension Impairment

Reading comprehension requires access to the meanings of words and to higher level processes in order to develop an understanding (mental representation) of the text. That process demands, in addition to the ability to decode speech, a good language comprehension. Although phonological awareness and processing abnormalities constitute the best proven cognitive deficits underlying reading disabilities, there are other language processing abnormalities that may cause reading disabilities. These include semantics (vocabulary or word meaning), syntax (grammatical structure), and discourse (connected sentences) abnormalities. Reading disability in some children is a reading comprehension impairment. This group of children can decode printed words but have comprehension difficulties. They can read accurately and fluently but have difficulty understanding what they read. Appropriate testing may reveal a marked discrepancy between normal scores on standardized tests of reading accuracy and abnormal reading comprehension. The reason for this impairment is a language processing abnormality, difficulty understanding the meaning carried by spoken language. These children have more widespread language impairments then those found in dyslexia, including impairment in vocabulary, morphology, and syntax (knowledge of the rules specifying structural relationships in sentences). Weakness in language comprehension limits reading comprehension, making constructing meaning from text more difficult. That may explain why—in addition to phonological factors—nonphonological oral language factors (e.g., expressive vocabulary, sentence or story recall) are predictive of long-term reading outcomes (Leach, Scarborough, & Rescorla, 2003).

Reading disability is frequently mixed. This explains why preventive intervention programs for at-risk students with mixed deficits focusing mostly on phonemic awareness and phonemically based decoding strategies initially show positive effects on reading achievements (typically word reading) but may fail to maintain these positive effects in later grades when reading comprehension measures are used. At that time, components common to both oral comprehension and reading comprehension (semantics, syntax, pragmatics) become more important, and the role of broad verbal ability is large in accounting for reading comprehension difficulties.

THE RELATIONSHIP OF DEVELOPMENTAL LANGUAGE DISORDERS AND DYSLEXIA

Many dyslexic children have problems in the acquisition of speech and language. These may be leading to a reading disorder. Longitudinal studies demonstrate that children who are later found to be dyslexic perform worse than siblings and other controls on measures of language development (Scarborough, 1990). Clinically, children with language-based reading disabilities show early language processing difficulties including delayed vocabulary development. Infants with positive family history for language learning impairment were found to process temporospectral changes in both nonverbal and verbal acoustic stimuli more slowly than infants with negative family history (Benaish & Tallal, 2002). These abnormalities of language development improve but frequently stay on, so that many children diagnosed as toddlers with developmental language disorders no longer manifest a gross language abnormality at school age, but may still have subtle language processing dysfunctions, leading to the reading disorder. These can be manifested in a number of ways including reduced ability to follow instructions, which may appear to teachers as lack of attention. Other manifestations include difficulties with word retrieval or pragmatics, a subtle impairment of verbal comprehension (demonstrated on the Token test), and a slower performance on a Rapid Automatic Naming Test (Denckla & Rudel, 1976). When they get to school, those children who were diagnosed with speech and language impairment in early childhood perform less well on reading tests. Children with pervasive language impairment show the poorest academic outcome, followed by those with poor scores on tests of auditory comprehension (Beitchman & Young, 1997). Although children with decoding problems (abnormality of phonological awareness) tend to have difficulties early (by the end of the first grade), children whose reading disability primarily involves comprehension (semantic difficulties) may start having academic difficulties later.

The assessment of language skills is, therefore, an important part of the neuropsychological evaluation of SLD children because of the common presence of underlying language processing abnormalities in these conditions. The assessment should include all aspects of speech and language (language comprehension, central auditory processing, and phonological awareness).

It should be clear, though, that not all dyslexics have oral language impairment. Also, some children with severe oral language impairment learn to read well.

RAPID AUTOMATED NAMING

An important manifestation of language abnormality, dysnomia, is associated with reading abnormalities (Swan & Goswami, 1997). Rapid automated naming (RAN), whereby children have to say aloud the names of pictures presented on a sheet recurrently in random order, is the most widely recognized oral language concomitant of dyslexia. Dyslexic children

were found to differ from normal readers and from children whose reading is abnormal for age but who do not meet the IQ discrepancy criteria,
on continuous naming speed (Ackerman & Dykman, 1993). Dyslexics have
also been shown to differ from normal readers in the speed with which they
name familiar visual symbols such as letters and numbers (Denckla & Rudel,
1976; Wolf & Obregon, 1992). Phonological awareness and rapid naming abilities uniquely predict reading skills over time (Wagner, Torgesen,
et al., 1997). RAN deficit can be seen independently in dyslexics (Henry,
Ganschow, & Miles, 2000), but it is not clear whether a rapid naming deficit
results from a phonological processing deficit or is independent of it (Wolf
& Bowers, 1999). There is a "double deficit" hypothesis for dyslexia—impli-
cating both, phonological skills and RAN.

SPEED OF PROCESSING OF AUDITORY
INFORMATION, DEVELOPMENTAL LANGUAGE
DISORDER, AND DYSLEXIA

Children with developmental language abnormalities often have difficulty
coping with auditory and other information when presented at a high rate.
It has been suggested that these children have a temporal processing deficit,
impairing their ability to integrate sensory information arriving at a rapid
succession (Please see a discussion in the next chapter: Theories of Specific
Learning Disabilities). These children may have a normal ability to identify
and discriminate tones when the interstimulus interval is in the range of tens
of milliseconds, but when the interstimulus interval is shorter, their discriminating ability is significantly impaired causing them to respond slower, compared with normal children. In these children, there is a significant correlation
between the degree of temporal processing and the degree of the receptive
language impairments, suggesting that the temporal processing impairment reduces their ability to integrate sensory information arriving in rapid
succession.

Children with developmental language disorders may have difficulties processing rapid information from sensory modalities other than auditory. For
instance, they perform worse than controls on tests involving tactile processing. This means that language-impaired children may perform worse than
controls on tests demanding sensory processing, if the stimuli are given in
rapid succession, regardless of the modality of stimulation.

It was suggested that a weakness of rapid processing of speech sounds
and possibly other types of stimuli is caused by an impairment of a specific
intrinsic clock controlling the rate of neuronal firing patterns or oscillations,
leading to developmental language disorder and dyslexia. It is possible that
this problem applies to other or all sensory modalities, and the fundamental

deficit in learning-disabled children is a deficit in processing rapidly changing information. Dyslexics perform worse on tasks demanding a higher rate of information processing. For instance, dyslexics read significantly more accurately in a one-word condition than in a whole-line condition. Fluency-based reading problems leading to dyslexia include problems with rapid letter, word, and sentence reading and also the ability to perform other rapid naming tasks (Katzir et al., 2006). It has been shown that the illusion of stream segregation that exists when two pure tones are presented alternately exists in dyslexics when the presentation is slower compared with normal readers (Helenius, Tarkiainen, Cornelissen, Hansen, & Salmelin, 1999). In a group of dyslexic children who have a concomitant oral language disability, a significant deficit was found in both nonsense word reading (a test of decoding skills) and nonverbal temporal processing. The degree of deficit in nonverbal temporal processing correlated with the degree of deficit in reading nonsense words. Dyslexics with normal oral language scores, on the other hand, had neither phonological decoding nor temporal processing deficits in any sensory modality. Their reading difficulties could have been the result of a deficit at a higher level of analysis (Eden, Stein, & Wood et al., 1995).

Similarly, reading-disabled (as well as other learning disabled) children do not perform well on tests of motor sequential activity, for example the ability to make rapid sequential finger and nonverbal mouth movements. Studies report that dyslexics performed worse than controls on the Bimanual Coordination Task (a task of motor coordination and interhemispheric collaboration) (Moore, Brown, & Markee et al., 1995), and on a finger localization task (Moore, Brown, & Markee et al., 1996). These children, therefore, may have a generalized defect in the central nervous system processing of rapidly changing stimuli. Reading-disabled children were also found to have a deficiency in the processing of fast visual stimuli. There may be similar specialized subsystems for temporal processing for the auditory, somatosensory, and motor systems. Impairments of one or more of these subsystems may cause SLD, including dyslexia.

There may be a general brain system of temporal processing, a specific intrinsic clock, controlling the rate of neuronal firing patterns or oscillations. These oscillations may be important in gating or "binding" sensory information in cortico-thalamo-cortical networks. The system may be located in the left hemisphere. Studies in adult aphasics suggest that damage to the left hemisphere disrupts processing of rapidly changing acoustic spectra, verbal and nonverbal. This is corroborated by a positron emission tomography study in adults showing that the left frontal area is "significantly activated only by sets of stimuli that incorporated rapid acoustic changes" (Fiez, Tallal, & Miezin, et al., 1992). If this system is "slowed," the processing of information within the tenths of milliseconds range is impaired, whereas information presented within longer durations such as scene analysis or coordination of gross motor activities will not be affected (Llinas, 1993). It is possible that because of some cellular dysfunction, related to a lack of critical experience in early development, the ability of cellular circuits to respond in the appropriate time-related manner is modified so that it cannot process information rapidly. This may occur for processes involving a particular time range. It was suggested that a weakness of rapid processing of speech sounds, and possibly other types of stimuli, is caused by an impairment of this specific intrinsic clock controlling the rate of neuronal firing patterns or oscillations, leading to developmental language disorder and dyslexia.

The relationship between temporal fluency problems and phonological problems can be explained in different ways. These two impairments may be unrelated coexisting problems (Wolf & Bowers, 1999). Alternately, fluency type problems in the detection of auditory stimuli with certain temporal properties may be a fundamental problem which underlie the phonemic processing impairment (Witton et al., 1998), although this hypothesis could not be replicated in another study (Bishop et al., 1999).

It is also possible that motor coordination abnormalities are not related to the reading or other learning abnormalities. Rather, these may be indications that other neurodevelopmental brain abnormalities are concomitantly present in people with SLD (Fletcher-Flinn, Elmes, & Strugnell, 1997).

OTHER COGNITIVE DEFICITS ASSOCIATED WITH READING DISABILITY

There are other cognitive differences between some reading-disabled and normally reading children that may play a role in the pathophysiology of dyslexia. Working memory for verbal information is related to word recognition and dyslexia (Schatschneider & Torgesen, 2004). Children with SLD often have generalized working memory deficits, possibly due to reduced "storage" in the executive system (Swanson, 1993; Witruk, 1993; Eden, et al., 1995; Swanson, Ashbaker, & Lee, 1996; Demont et al., 2004). Tests of phonological awareness involve working memory. Therefore, it is not clear whether working memory is an independent factor for dyslexia. It was suggested that the deficit in phonological processing is a deficit of direct access to and manipulation of the retrieval of phonemic language units from long-term declarative memory. This means that there are specific neural processes responsible for coding these phonemes, which are of higher order than the auditory, motor sensory, and visual counterparts of these sound units. According to this explanation, dyslexia results from difficulty to manipulate sublexical units in working memory.

An interesting study by McCallum and Bell sheds some light on the multiple cognitive factors that may be involved in reading disabilities. This study randomly sampled 105 elementary and middle school children, age 5.5 to 13.2 years who completed the Test of Dyslexia, an instrument that provides a concise measure of all factors known to be associated with reading, according to dyslexia research. This battery included: Achievement tests (including spelling, letter-word calling, reading comprehension, listening comprehension, decoding, and written composition), processing measures (including phonological awareness, memory for letters, auditory synthesis, word memory, rapid symbol naming, visual discrimination, and visual closure), and IQ screening (including vocabulary and matrix analogies). Factor analysis of these cognitive variables produced three empirically and theoretically derived factors, each of which contributed to the prediction of reading and spelling skills: auditory processing, visual processing speed, and memory. Scores from the three factors contributed uniquely and significantly to each of the four reading and reading-related skills: letter-word calling, reading comprehension, spelling, and decoding. Factor scores from the three factors combined predicted 85% of the variance associated with letter/sight word naming, 70% of the variance associated with reading comprehension, 73% of the variance associated with spelling, and 61% of the variance associated with phonetic decoding.

Reading comprehension was most strongly predicted by auditory processing, followed about equally by visual processing speed and memory. Overall, these findings support the conclusion that auditory, visual, and memory skills are all implicated in the acquisition of reading skills (McCallum & Bell, 2001).

In summary, although phonological deficits are a major pathophysiological factor in many dislexics, other cognitive neuropsychological factors may play a role in causing reading disability—either independently or as underlying factors of phonological deficits.

CHAPTER 3

Theories of Specific Learning Disabilities

INTRODUCTION

Specific learning disabilities (SLDs) are manifested by academic underachievement in spite of normal intelligence and adequate teaching, in the absence of severe communication and emotional disturbances. The fact that some people have a learning disability has been recognized since the end of the 19th century. It has also been suspected that such disabilities are related, at least partially, to some form of brain dysfunction. However, the etiology and pathophysiology of these conditions are constantly debated.

A theory for SLDs needs to explain the cognitive and brain-related deficits that cause the specific academic difficulties. For reading disability, a theory has to explain the key academic skill deficits in word decoding and encoding. There is a question whether the deficiency is with a specific kind of academic learning (i.e., math or reading), or there is a dysfunction of more basic brain mechanisms that then affect academic learning as well as other functions, including motor functions and behavior. Another questions is whether the SLDs seen in some metabolic and genetic conditions and syndromes is different from that of "idiopathic" SLDs, or there is a final common mechanism in the brain for developmental learning disorders that encompasses all these different etiologies.

Differences Between Specific Learning Disabilities and Brain Damage

Impairment of learning ability commonly occurs in children with brain abnormalities, with congenital birth defects, chromosomal or metabolic abnormalities, brain infections, or significant head trauma. But learning impairment in these cases is frequently different from that of developmental SLDs. Although there are exceptions, learning impairment in patients with brain damage is usually more pervasive. In addition, structural brain damage is frequently demonstrated by a clinical neurological examination, neuroimaging, or neuropathological studies. Developmental SLDs, on the other hand, do not cause generalized brain dysfunction or intellectual disability, and the learning abnormalities are more specific or "focal" and asymmetrical, affecting some academic areas (e.g., reading and spelling) while not affecting other areas (e.g., mathematical calculations). The overall understanding of SLDs is that these conditions occur as a result of selective and specific brain abnormalities that interfere with certain abilities of learning. Brain abnormalities causing SLDs are, unlike acquired brain damage, developmental aberrations, probably occurring during brain development. Consequently, models of developmental disorders cannot be based on acquired brain injury (including adult acquired alexia).

Recent neuropsychological studies have demonstrated that the learning disability in some genetic and metabolic conditions is similar to that seen in developmental SLDs—"asymmetrical" in nature. For instance, learning disabilities in Williams syndrome, involve mathematical more than reading abilities. So perhaps SLDs are different from the learning abnormalities found in diffuse brain damage, but similar to those caused by a genetic defect. Or, perhaps SLDs are caused by as-yet-unidentified genetic defects.

Pathophysiology: SLD versus Basic Cognitive Abnormalities

One of the debated issues related to theories of SLDs is whether the brain impairment causing SLDs is specific to an area of academic learning (i.e., an abnormality of phonetic processing which specifically affects reading), or a more basic cognitive impairment that can affect academic learning as well as other functions (i.e., auditory sound discrimination, which may affect reading along with other language functioning). Reading and mathematics involve a number of cognitive tasks. For reading, the brain has to perform orthographical, phonetic, semantic, and motor tasks. These tasks involve many cognitive modalities, including attention, visual and language processing, and planning and motor execution, all interacting with each other in the correct order and at great speed (neuronal latencies in association cortices are in the range of 100–300 milliseconds). The pathophysiology of reading disability may involve an abnormality of one of these cognitive tasks or a number of them. If SLDs result from a more basic cognitive abnormality (i.e., visual processing, auditory processing or language processing), then other functions in addition to reading should typically be abnormal.

Pathophysiology: One Cause versus Multiple Causes

The majority of early *single factor theories* claimed that a dysfunction of visuo-spatial processing was responsible for the reading deficit in developmental dyslexia (Orton, 1925). Only a minority of early publications attributed a significant role in dyslexia to language processing problems (Lieberman, et al., 1971) or to incomplete or mixed cerebral dominance.

Multifactor theories suggested that there are different types of dyslexia, with the primary deficiencies occurring either in the auditory or visual cognition (Johnson & Myklebust, 1967; Ingram, Mason, & Blackburn, 1970; Mattis, French, & Rapin, 1975). Birch (1962) suggested three subcategories of dyslexia: Abnormal reading occurs because of failure to establish visual hierarchical dominance, resulting in figure-ground problems; because of a disorder in visual analysis and synthesis, for example, in part–whole relationship; or because of a deficiency in intersensory integration.

THEORIES FOR THE PATHOPHYSIOLOGY OF READING DISABILITY

There have been a number of theories of the cognitive and neurological mechanisms responsible for dyslexia (reviews in Habib, 2000; Grigorenko, 2001; Ramus et al., 2003; Demonet, 2004). Most recent theories have received some support from functional imaging. The theories proposed include the phonological theory, the rapid auditory processing theory (Tallal, 1980, 2000), the visual and magnocellular theory (Lovegrove et al., 1980; Livingstone et al., 1991; Stein & Walsh, 1997) and the cerebellar theory (Nicolson & Fawcett, 1990; Nicholson, Fawcett, & Dean, 2001). For a review and critique of the various theories, see Ramus et al. (2003).

Deficiency in Visual Perception

The visual perception theory of dyslexia suggested that reading disability is the result of problems in the processing and integration of visual information. This theory was prevalent at the beginning of the 20th century. It was thought at that time that the pathology of dyslexia is in the visual system, manifested as "word blindness," a very selective type of blindness that involves only written language. This would parallel adult acquired alexia, which can be caused by a lesion in the occipital lobe and the corpus callosum connecting the right and left hemisphere.

In 1891, Dejerine reported that damage to the left inferior parietal-occipital region (including the angular gyrus) in adults resulted in an impairment of reading and writing. He thought that this region played a role in the processing of the "optic images of letters" (Dejerine, 1891; Habib, 2000). James Hinshelwood and Pringle Morgan saw similarity between the symptoms of dyslexia in children and adolescents, and the neurological syndrome of "visual word blindness" (Morgan, 1896; Hinshelwood, 1917). Hinshelwood and Pringle, and later Orton, thought that the impairment of reading and writing in young children could be due to visual perceptual problem, perhaps involving a developmental abnormality of the parietal lobe (Hinshelwood, 1917; Habib 2000). Samuel Orton (1937) described it as a failure to represent print appropriately in the two occipital poles. A visual type abnormality could explain the reversals of letters and words thought to be typical of dyslexic reading (Orton 1937; Hermann & Norrie, 1958). Similarly, Bender and Hermann thought that the main problem leading to reading disability was a dysfunction of visual perceptual processing (Habib, 2000).

The question that could not be answered is the lack of other visual perceptual abnormalities of dyslexic subjects. It was also later understood that reading involves more than just orthographics (Vellutino, 1978, 1979).

Language Processing Abnormalities

Introduction

Another theory suggested that reading disability, dyslexia, is caused by abnormalities of language processing. A developmental abnormality of language processing could be a result of aberrations of the anatomy of brain cortical structures involved in language processing typically located in the left hemisphere (Galaburda, Menard, & Rosen, 1994). The theory suggests that when such abnormality occurs in the fetal brain or early in life, it causes a failure of the left side of the brain to dominate the right side and a corresponding lag in the functional specialization of language, which in turn interferes with learning to read.

The Development of Normal Asymmetry and Left Hemisphere Dominance for Language

Broca demonstrated that left hemisphere lesions affect language functioning, making a connection between a structural abnormality of the left hemisphere and language dysfunction. Such a connection also exists in other species. The song of finches and canaries is abolished by lesions of the left but not the right side of the brain. That initiated a look for anatomical hemispheral differences or asymmetries that could explain the dominance and specialization of the left hemisphere for motor and language functions.

A number of structural anatomical asymmetries have been described in the region of the sylvian fissure. The planum temporale, in the upper surface of the posterior portion of the temporal lobe, was found to have such an anatomical asymmetry, the left larger than the right. Geschwind and Lewitsky found an asymmetry of the portion of the upper surface of the temporal lobe behind the gyrus of Heschl. The asymmetry was seen in the majority of the brains studied. This area constitutes a part of the temporal speech region of Wernicke; therefore, the asymmetry in this area may account for the predominant localization of speech to the left hemisphere in the majority of humans. Wada et al. showed that planum temporale asymmetry was present in the fetus and newborn (Geschwind & Galaburda, 1985). Others (Chi et al., 1977) described such asymmetry at 20 and at 31 weeks' gestation. Therefore, it was proposed that cerebral dominance is based in most instances on asymmetry of structure. The process that leads to this asymmetry occurs during fetal intrauterine life.

In general, similar asymmetries and dominance of the left hemisphere may exist in nonhumans, demonstrating that biologically determined asymmetry has existed throughout vertebrate evolution and are not a recent development.

Why does asymmetrical brain development occur? Asymmetrical hemispheral brain development occurs because of a number of factors. The male brain matures later than the female and the left hemisphere matures slower and later than the right. Slower development of the left hemisphere during pregnancy occurs because of a number of influences (genetic, chemical, related to male sex such as testosterone, differences in the chemistry, receptor structure, or density, or immune properties). Animal research has demonstrated pharmacological hemispheral asymmetries in dopamine and GABA metabolism. It is possible that neuronal migration is slower in the left hemisphere because of lateral differences in the chemistry, receptor structure, or density, or possible difference in immune properties.

Why does the right hemisphere develop faster? The right hemisphere is dominant for types of visuospatial functions and for attention. These functions are important for survival from an evolutionary point of view. This may be a reason for earlier development of the right hemisphere. Consequently, the left hemisphere is at more risk for adverse influences on brain development during fetal and early postnatal life. Such adverse influences are more likely to affect the development of the left hemisphere, which is at risk over a longer period of time. The earlier development of the right hemisphere implies that it will be subjected to disrupting influences for a shorter critical period, whereas the left hemisphere, including language processing brain areas, are more susceptible and at risk for a longer time because of later development.

Unilateral lesions in utero and in the first few years of life may cause functions to shift to the opposite hemisphere. An intrauterine damage or delay in development of cortical regions in the left hemisphere can, therefore, favor growth of cortical regions on the opposite side. Influences that delay left hemisphere growth thus tend to create brains in which the normal asymmetry of these areas is diminished, or reverses, along with the pattern of dominance.

One of the mechanisms of normally present asymmetry is thought to be the result of asymmetrical programmed death of neurons in utero during the normal process of brain development. The factors that determine which neurons die are not all known, but a neuron is more likely to die if it fails in the competition to establish connections.

Most people have a dominant left hemisphere (and are, therefore right-handed). According to this theory, an early, prenatal, injury causes developmental abnormality, or delay in development, of the left hemisphere. Such abnormality can be in the form of a structural abnormality in the region of the planum temporale, posterior perisylvian, and the insular regions of the left hemisphere (Galaburda, 1994), or a failure of one side of the brain to dominate the other, which may occur as a result of a lag in the maturation of the left hemisphere and a corresponding lag in the functional specialization of language. In such cases, motor and language dominance shifts to the right hemisphere, clinically manifested by left-handedness and language processing abnormalities. The reading disability, according to this theory, is caused by abnormalities of language processing, which in turn cause a reading disability.

A theory suggested by Orton (1925, 1937) and later by Geschwind, claims that the lateralization of language to the left hemisphere is delayed in dyslexics, and consequently the language prerequisites for learning to read could not develop normally.

Indeed, there is a high prevalence of oral or written language deficits among reading disordered children as well as a higher incidence of left-handed people among dyslexics and a much higher percentage of SLDS among left-handed people than among right-handed people.

Neuropathology of Developmental Dyslexia

Anatomical studies demonstrate a brain hemispheral asymmetry. The planum temporale area of the temporal lobe is larger on the left in a predominance of cases (Geschwind & Levitsky, 1968). In dyslexics the prevalence of this asymmetry is reduced (Geschwind & Galaburda, 1985; Cohen et al., 1989; Habib, 2000), reflecting failure of normal asymmetrical cell loss to occur or another developmental pathology. Neuropathological studies reported microanatomical abnormalities in the brains of dyslectic people suggesting abnormalities of neuronal migration (Cohen et al., 1989; Habib, 2000). These include excessive numbers of neurons in the subcortical white matter, areas of micropolygyria, primitive layering, and neurons; a primitive left hemisphere cortical differentiation, primitive orientation of neurons; and clusters of primitive cells and abnormal myelination. These abnormal features are found significantly more in the left hemisphere, most notably in areas that are important for language.

Geschwind, Galaburda, and their colleagues have proposed an association between learning disabilities, immune disorders, and left-handedness (or non–right-handedness). This theory suggests that an abnormal effect of testosterone or related factors on the brain and the thymus during in utero development interferes with the development of left hemisphere dominance, and with that of the immune system, resulting in left-handedness, developmental language disorders and dyslexia, and autoimmune and atopic illnesses. There are studies that support some aspects of this theory. A higher frequency of immune diseases, migraine, and development learning disorders was described in left-handed individuals and their families (Geschwind & Galaburda, 1985). A study of Norwegian six graders, which used measured word recognition and phonological decoding found a significant association between handedness and dyslexia and a significant but weak association between handedness and immune disorders, but no association between dyslexia and immune disorders (Tonnessen, Lokken, Hoien, & Lundberg, 1993). Another study, using a questionnaire, found that children with reading problems and their families suffered more frequently from immune and autoimmune disorders, particularly those involving the gastrointestinal tract and the thyroid gland. There was no evidence, though, of a higher prevalence of left-handedness in these children (Crawford, Kaplan, & Kinsbourne, 1994). Other studies that examined a possible association between non–right-handedness and immune disorders (asthma, allergic disorders) did not find such association (Biederman et al., 1995). It is still possible that familial left-handedness constitutes a specific subgroup of dyslexics, or represents a risk factor, but this theory needs further confirmation.

Other authors introduced the possibility that allergies can impair learning ability and cause a learning disability. A child suffering nasal symptoms such as itching, sneezing, and rhinorrhea, may have nocturnal sleep loss, secondary daytime fatigue and, as a result, a temporary learning impairment. Some of the medications used to treat allergic rhinitis may cause central nervous system adverse effects and contribute to learning impairment, but there is no evidence of any long-term cognitive effect of allergies.

Impaired Interhemispheric Communication

In addition to theories of abnormal lateralization, another theory for the pathophysiology of dyslexia was an impaired interhemispheric communication. This theory is based on evidence of impaired interhemispheric transfer of sensory or motor information in dyslexia (Moore, Brown, Markee, Theberge, & Zvi, 1995, 1996; Habib, 2000).

Developmental Delay

An early hypothesis attempting to explain SLD claimed that learning these conditions are a specific kind of developmental delay (a "neuromaturational" delay) in which the acquisition of academic skills is delayed. Evidence used to support this theory includes other developmental abnormalities found in children with SLD (i.e., motor coordination) and electroencephalographic abnormalities in some children with SLD, manifested by a slow and disorganized background that may later normalize. The interpretation of this course that these children's neurodevelopmental abnormalities (including the specific learning disabilities) reflect a slow developmental maturation (Hamony et al., 1995). Similarly, some authors suggested that reading deficits are the results of maturational disorders affecting specifically the development of cognitive processes.

Current Theories

The Phonological Theory

Neuropsychological studies have provided evidence that the main mechanism leading to developmental dyslexia is a defect in phonological processing—segmenting and manipulating the phoneme constituents of speech (see chapter 2 of this book: The neuropsychology of SLD). This "phonological theory" of reading disability puts the main deficit in the domain of language processing (Ramus, 2003).

Learning to read requires learning the correspondence between letters and sounds of speech (grapheme–phoneme correspondence). Children need to segment words into phonemes and have grapheme–phoneme correspondence. Most of them are able to do so when they start school, whereas reading disabled (dyslexic) children cannot manipulate phonological information adequately possibly because they do not have an adequate representation of phonemic units (Bradley & Bryant, 1983; Habib, 2000; Demonet, 2004). Such a deficit prevents them from having the phonological foundation of reading. Dyslexics perform poorly on tasks of phonological awareness (segmentation and manipulation of speech sounds). It has been demonstrated that phonological training improves reading ability.

The critics of this theory agree that dyslexics have a phonological deficit, but think that the phonological deficit is a derivative of a more generalized brain disorder involving general sensory, motor, or learning processes. Dyslexics also have problems with sensory and motor deficits, short-term memory, and slow automated naming (Snowing, 2000), Which may suggest that there is a more fundamental abnormality underlying their reading disability.

Abnormal Sensory (Auditory) Processing

This theory suggests a more basic abnormality underlying reading disability. It does not contradict the phonological theory, but notes that phonological awareness of the syllables and rhymes in words that are impaired in dyslexia, develop before literacy, at the developmental age of speech rather than the age of reading. The phonological deficit in dyslexia must, therefore, arise at a developmentally earlier level of phonological representation than the phoneme. This theory suggests that the phonological deficit is a derivative or outcome of a more generalized auditory dysfunction affecting the processing of sounds or disturbing sounds from being kept in memory long enough to be processed. It may involve "a deficient buildup" or a more rapid fading of the memory trace, or a possible prolonged short-term "cognitive window" that could distort processing of rapid stimulus sequencing and the proper development of cortical representation needed for reading acquisition. In support of this theory, there is evidence that dyslexics do not perceive contrasts as well as normal readers (Mody et al., 1997; Adlard & Hasan, 1998), and have abnormal physiological responses to various auditory stimuli (Kujala et al., 2000; Temple, 2000). Dyslexics perform poorly on a number of auditory tasks, including frequency discrimination (McAnally & Stein, 1996; Ahissar et al., 2000) and temporal order judgment (Tallal, 1980; reviews by Farmer & Klein, 1995). Speech rhythm is one of the earliest cues used by infants to discriminate syllables and is determined principally by the acoustic structure of amplitude modulation at relatively low rates in the signal. Goswami et al. pursued the hypothesis that the potential deficits in frequency-modulation detection in dyslexic individuals might relate to deficits in the processing of acoustic structure at the level of the syllable. They found that individual differences in sensitivity to the shape of amplitude modulation accounted for 25% of the variance in reading and spelling acquisition even after controlling for individual differences in age, nonverbal IQ, and vocabulary, They suggested that the potential deficits in frequency-modulation detection in dyslexic individuals might relate to deficits in the processing of acoustic structure at the level of the syllable. (Goswami et al., 2002). These results support the hypothesis that dyslexics have deficits in the processing of acoustic structure at the level of the syllable.

The Magnocellular Theory

The magnocellular theory arose from observations that subjects with dyslexia showed poor thresholds for stimuli with low contrast, or high temporal frequencies, and poor sensitivity to visual motion (see also chapter 10; Lovegrove et al., 1980, 1987). These deficits are related to impaired visual processing in the magnocellular visual pathway. There are two visual systems, magnocellular and parvocellular. They differ in their preferred spatial frequencies, temporal properties, and contrast sensitivity (Steinman et al., 1997). The magnocellular system, or the "transient" system that modulates global form, movement, and temporal resolution, is also important for directing visual attention and visual search skills—all having a role in reading ability. These findings gave rise to a theory suggesting that dyslexia results from a defect in the magnocellular part of the visual system (Steinman et al., 1997; Hari, Renvall, & Tanskanen, 2001), (Demonet, 2004). Livingstone et al. found neurophysiological and anatomical abnormalities of the magnocellular system in dyslexia. They found abnormalities in dyslexics' response to low-contrast, high-frequency stimuli. The same dyslexic children responded normally to targets of lower frequencies and higher contrast (Livingstone, Rosen, Drislane, & Galaburda, 1991). They also reported that in the brains of SLDS subjects, examined by Galaburda, there were anatomical changes in the thalamic lateral geniculate body (LGB). The neurons in the magnocellular part of the nucleus were atrophied, but the neurons in the parvocellular part of the nucleus were normal.

The evidence for the theory has not been consistent, and it was criticized because the neurophysiological and anatomical findings have been difficult to reproduce, the difficulties in people with dyslexia extend beyond the frequency domain, and there are other findings suggesting that people with dyslexia might have difficulties in slowly evolving domains (Demonet, Taylor, & Chaix, 2004).

The Rapid Auditory Processing Theory

Similar to the magnocellular theory, it has been suggested that children with developmental language disorders have a temporal processing impairment affecting their ability to integrate auditory sensory information when such information is changing rapidly or arriving at a rapid succession (Tallal & Piercy, 1973; Tallal et al., 1993; see also chapter 2). They may have the ability to processes auditory information when the interstimulus interval is in the range of tens of milliseconds between stimuli, but may not be able to do so when the interstimulus interval is shorter. The result may be impaired discrimination or slower processing. A significant correlation was found between the degree of temporal processing and the degree of the receptive language impairments in these children (Tallal, 1980).

Subjects with dyslexia may be similarly affected with temporal processing impairment. The difficulty to discriminate brief, rapidly changing auditory stimuli may impair their phonological discrimination (Tallal, 2000).

Multisensory Temporal Processing Deficit Theory

Children with developmental language disorders have difficulties processing rapid information from sensory modalities other than auditory processing (e.g., visual and tactile processing), and may therefore have a generalized defect in the central nervous system processing of rapidly changing stimuli, that impairs and slows information processing. In addition, they do not perform well on tests of motor sequential activity (e.g., the ability to make rapid sequential finger and nonverbal mouth movements, and the ability to rapidly produce single or sequential speech syllables and words). If this system is "slowed," the processing of information in the tenths of milliseconds range is impaired, whereas information presented within longer durations such as scene analysis or coordination of gross motor activities is not affected (Llinas, 1993). Impairments of one or more of these subsystems may cause specific learning disabilities, including dyslexia. Dyslexia, according to this theory, is a multisystem deficit with a fundamental incapacity of the brain to perform tasks requiring processing of brief stimuli in rapid temporal succession, for instance changes in the tens of milliseconds range that characterize acoustics of ongoing speech (Tallal & Piercy, 1973). Visual, auditory, and tactile processing channels are impaired.

This theory could explain some of the other sensory, perceptual, and motor symptoms seen in dyslexia (Habib, 2000). As noted, dyslexics do not perform well on tests of fine motor skills, including motor sequential tasks such as rhythmic tapping, rapid sequential finger movements, and nonverbal mouth movements. Automation of motor skill, motor reaction time, speed of naming, and motor balance may also be impaired in dyslexics (Nicholson & Fawcett, 1990; Fawcett & Nicholson, 1992).

There may also be a general brain system of temporal processing, a specific intrinsic clock, controlling the rate of neuronal firing patterns or oscillations. These oscillations may be important in gating or "binding" sensory information in cortico-thalamo-cortical networks.

It was suggested that the left hemisphere may play an important role in rapid processing of brief stimuli (Fiez, Tallal, & Miezin, 1992). Adult aphasics with acquired left hemisphere damage are also impaired on rate processing tasks. The causes for the abnormal function of this system in dyslexia may be developmental.

This is corroborated by a positron emission tomography (PET) study in adults showing that the left frontal area is "significantly activated by sets of stimuli that incorporated rapid acoustic changes" (Fiez, Tallal, & Miezin, 1992). If this system is "slowed," the processing of information in the tenths of milliseconds range is impaired, whereas information presented within longer durations, such as scene analysis or coordination of gross motor activities, is not affected (Llinas, 1993). It is possible that because of some cellular dysfunction related to a lack of critical experience in early development, the ability of cellular circuits to respond in the appropriate time-related manner is modified so that it cannot process information rapidly. This may occur for processes involving a particular time range.

Language processing areas of the planum temporale are characterized by large pyramidal cells and rich myelination, and may form part of a fast component of the auditory system. Deficits in the processing of fast transitions in the auditory modality can lead to deficient language processing at loci where fast processing is required, resulting in abnormal phonological processing and, in turn, difficulties with learning to read. According to this theory—the phonological deficit -an accepted underlying deficit in dyslexia—is derived from the more generalized auditory dysfunction, manifested as impaired temporal processing of sounds (Tallal, 1980). Dyslexics may be unable to process fast incoming sensory information adequately in any sensory domain. Consequently, dyslexia is not the result of a single phonological, visual, or motor deficit, but rather impairment of temporal processing in all sensory systems (Stein & Walsh, 1997). According to this theory, dyslexia in fact may be dyschronia (Llinas, 1993).

Although there is some evidence that dyslexics have rate processing problems (Wolff, 1993; Farmer & Klein, 1995; Stein & Walsh, 1997), and some studies involving temporal order, in the auditory and visual modality, found group differences between dyslexics and normally reading individuals (Farmer & Klein, 1995), other studies contested these views. Also, slowing each element of a consonant cluster did not improve the performance of dyslexic children.

The Cerebellar Theory

It has been traditionally recognized that the cerebellum plays a role in motor coordination. In recent years it has been learned that it is also activated during learning (Nicolson et al., 1995, 1999; Eckert, 2003), and may participate in the automatization of learned tasks, including reading.

Anatomically (in the macaque monkey), the lateral prefrontal cortex, superior temporal sulcus, and postparietal association cortices project to the cerebellum via pontine nuclei (Levin, 1936; Schmahamann, 1996), whereas the cerebellum projects to the association cortex via the thalamus (Middleton & Strick, 1997; Eckert, 2003). The cerebellum receives input from various magnocellular systems in the brain and therefore can be affected by a general magnocellular deficit (Stein, 2001).

The cerebellar deficit hypothesis for dyslexia attributes the cognitive and motor problems exhibited by dyslexics to abnormal cerebellar development

(Nicholson & Fawcett, 1990; Nicholson et al., 2001). A cerebellar abnormality can be a cause or a contributing cause of a learning disability in a number of ways.

It can cause a learning disorder through a failure to acquire and automatize reading and writing skills. According to this theory, skill automatization, speed, and fluency of information are areas of independent deficit in dyslexia. It is similar to the suggestion that slow speed of information processing contributes to reading impairments independent of other factors, especially phonological deficits. Another way that cerebellar abnormality can interfere with normal reading and learning is through cerebellar abnormality causing procedural memory deficit or impairing motor control of speech articulation and other motor tasks, including handwriting.

Problems with the rate of reading words, suggesting cerebellar involvement were found in adults and children with dyslexia (Ivry & Justus, 2001). Some children with right cerebellar tumor had poor verbal and literary performance (whereas children with left hemispheral tumor had spatial deficits). Brain imaging studies have shown anatomical, metabolic, and activation differences in the cerebellum of dyslexics (Rae, 1998; Nicolson, 1999; Leonard et al., 2001), also, the deficit may be in the cerebellum because of a time estimate defect in dyslexia (Fawcett et al., 196; Rae et al., 1998; Nicholson et al., 1999).

The critics of this theory point to the fact that cerebellar signs are not always seen in dyslexia, and also to the fact that procedural learning is not restricted to the cerebellum. The architecture of the memory system subserving procedural learning includes cortical, subcortical, and cerebellar connections. Therefore, deficits of procedural learning can result from dysfunction of an extensive neural architecture and are not necessarily caused by a cerebellar abnormality (Demonet, 2004). In addition, phonological representation does not depend on speech development and will not be affected by dysarthria (Ramus, 2003).

However, there may be a subgroup of dyslexics with a magnocellular and cerebellar deficit.

SUMMARY

Early theories at the beginning of the 20th century suggested that the pathology of dyslexia is in the visual system, thus explaining the reversals of letters and words thought to be typical of dyslexic reading.

This viewpoint has changed, replaced by knowledge that language processing abnormalities play the major role in dyslexia. Visual factors, although playing a role in some dyslexics, are not critical abnormalities in most. In some patients with dyslexia, visual and language processing abnormalities may be concurrent (Slaghuis & Ryan, 1999). There are theories suggesting that dyslexia is the result of basic brain abnormalities in processing sensory information. Abnormal auditory processing or multisensory processing problem involve deficient building up or more rapid fading of the memory trace that may affect or distort rapid stimulus processing, interfere with phonological processing, and impair reading. These theories vary between some who claim that the abnormality is in one sensory (auditory or visual) channel to those who hypothesize multisensory channels. There is overlapping between "multisensory processing" difficulties to "auditory sensory" difficulties and to "temporal processing deficit."

The current proven theory is that dyslexia is caused by abnormal phonological processing. There are still questions whether phonological deficit abnormality is caused by a more generalized auditory processing abnormality, whether auditory processing abnormality is a part of a generalized sensory processing abnormality, and whether the nature of the processing abnormality has to do with rapid versus slow processing ability.

Those may all be pieces of a puzzle, in which each piece has a place, and different combinations explain different cases of dyslexia.

CHAPTER 4

Brain Correlates of Learning

INTRODUCTION

In Specific Learning Disability (SLD), brain developmental aberrations cause specific cognitive differences, and thus interfere with specific learning modalities. Therefore, I thought to introduce some general concepts of learning, which may provide guidance on the interaction of brain and learning. The following comments are by no means a thorough discussion of the biological nature of learning, but may suffice to establish the necessary connections between brain systems and learning abilities.

General biological characteristics of learning and memory may be common to all living systems. Many cellular structures and metabolic pathways underlying learning are similar in humans and in phylogenetically lower animals. Therefore, when scientists investigate mechanisms of learning on a cellular level, they can use models of simple neuronal systems from phylogenetically lower animals. Basic behavioral learning phenomena such as habituation (a decrease in response to a repeated stimulus) and sensitization (a strengthening of responses to a wide variety of stimuli following an intense or noxious stimulus) exist and can be manipulated in simple neuronal systems, including those consisting of only a few cells, or even in isolated nervous system preparations. The neuronal modifications underlying simple types of learning can be induced by nerve stimulation. Fictive swimming can be activated in the isolated brain preparation of the sea slug Tritonia by electrical pulses applied to the cut end of a nerve. Repeated application of the nerve stimulus produced changes in fictive swimming that resembled habituation. Similarly, other types of learning including sensitization can be studied in this simple organism.

Learning and learning disorders in humans are obviously more complicated. A "learning" process by an isolated nerve or by a small group of neurons may not resemble the complex concept of learning discussed in this book. Therefore, knowledge about learning and its disorders will continue to be derived from both basic neuronal systems, and primate and human behavior.

BASIC CONCEPTS OF MEMORY

Learning is closely associated with memory. The term learning implicates also the ability to retain learned material. Academic classroom learning is judged and measured by the ability to retrieve learned material; therefore, memory becomes almost synonymous to learning. We discuss here some concepts and definitions of memory. Much of the content of this discussion follows Fuster (1995).

Memory is the capacity of an organism to retain information about itself and the environment and utilize it for adaptive purposes. There are different types of memory, possibly utilizing different brain mechanisms. Declarative memory is the ability to remember events and facts about people, places, or experiences; to consciously recall these items; and then to express the recalled memory in a variety of ways. Procedural memory is expressed only through implicit measures of performance like altered dispositions, preferences, and judgments and is inaccessible to conscious recall. Semantic memory, the memory of word meaning and ideas, is, in general, more resistant to cortical damage than declarative memory, the memory of events and concrete associations. Semantic networks probably have many more lines of associative access than episodic or declarative networks, which is probably what makes the former less vulnerable than the later.

Neural Principles of Memory

How is memory organized in the brain? It could be a separable function of the brain that is dissociable from other cognitive functions. It could also be a property of each individual functional circuit, For instance, memory for visual information will be in the same brain locations that process visual stimuli (Eichenbaum, 1997). There is some evidence for both types of memory locations. There are brain areas that are specifically involved with memory, including anatomical brain structures that are important for the learning and retention of information. Functional magnetic resonance imaging studies found that in the prefrontal and parahippocampal cortices neural activity elicited by items that were well remembered was greater than the activity elicited by weakly remembered or forgotten items. The hippocampus is a part of the brain that is important for certain memory functions, as shown by conditioning experiments. Classical conditioning of the eye-blink response is intact in animals with hippocampal lesions. However, trace conditioning, a variant of the standard paradigm in which a short interval (500 to 1000 ms) is interposed between the offset of the conditioned stimulus and the onset of the unconditioned stimuli, is impaired in animals with hippocampal lesions and in amnesic patients with damage to the hippocampus. In humans, the medial temporal lobe was shown to be important for certain stages in memory production. It binds together information from different parts of the cortex and stores the "whole" event. Its role is important at a critical time of learning when it receives highly processed input from cortical association areas. Damage to temporal lobe impairs memory and learning but may spare general cognition. Subjects with bilateral damage to the medial temporal lobe or diencephalic midline can have a global memory impairment for declarative memory, the conscious recollection of recently occurring facts and events, which will be present for every sensory modality in which information was presented and emerges more clearly sometime after the time of learning. (Squire & Zola, 1996; Schacter, 1998). However, they do not have memory impairment for nondeclarative memory abilities that involve other skills, including motor skills and habits, thus demonstrating that these areas of the temporal lobe are not controlling all types of memory. A well-studied case (Scoville, 1968) is the case of H.M.—the patient who underwent a large bilateral excision of medial temporal lobe including a large part of the hippocampus and the amygdala, as a treatment of severe epilepsy. After surgery this patient became densely amnestic and was incapable of new learning. He could not learn his way around the hospital and could not recognize people even though they spent several hours with him immediately beforehand. Yet he remained able to retain new information for a short time and to learn new motor tasks, though not remembering the events and circumstances surrounding the performance of these tasks.

As stated above, there is also a theory that there is no one specific area responsible for memory in the cerebral cortex, and memory is the output of a cortical network. The memory storage site is, according to this theory, in the cortical networks that initially process the information. The latter view has been supported by recent functional brain imaging studies in humans that indicate that learning and memory involve many of the same regions of the cortex that process sensory information and control motor output (Ungerleider, 1995).

Working Memory, Executive Functions

The process of memory may be a graded process in which input to the brain is processed into short-term memory, which lasts only a short period of time. The information is then transformed into a more permanent long-term store in which the changes remain for days, weeks or longer. Retrieval consists of activation or reactivation of the specific network involved with the perception and memory of an item (Fuster, 1995). A large amount of attention has recently been paid to a cognitive system given the name "working memory."

This memory system, with "headquarters" in the frontal lobes is responsible for temporary storage and manipulation of information during performance of cognitive tasks (Hulme & Roodenruy, 1995). As previously discussed, some researchers do not agree that there is one executive area and think that, depending on the type of task involved, there are parallel systems, each with its own central processor. Studies, including positron emission tomography (PET) studies, support this view by demonstrating a separation between spatial and verbal working memory. The PET scans performed during a task involving remembering the locations of three dots produced activity mostly on the right side of the brain—including certain regions of the prefrontal cortex and regions involved in perceptual location. By contrast, recalling the identity of four letters produced mostly left hemisphere activity. The working memory area for facial features in the prefrontal cortex was found to be separate from the working memory of their location. Although there may be separate circuits for spatial and verbal working memories, there is an area of the prefrontal cortex that acts as a processor for working memory information regardless of its type. This area for "executive functions" is activated when choices have to be made based on previous information or when subjects have to keep track of choices they have made in previous trials. The idea that the prefrontal cortex may have "executive functions" is also suggested by studies of patients who have suffered frontal-lobe damage. These individuals often show severe difficulties in executive functions that require working memory, such as planning and organizing. They are also easily distracted or, conversely, can't switch their attention away from a task. Executive functions and working memory are important in the context of SLD because these functions may be impaired in attention deficit hyperactivity disorder—a very common comorbidity of SLD. This relationship will be discussed later in this book.

LEARNING MECHANISMS

Until recent decades there was very little information on the brain correlates of learning, and for most scholars of learning the brain has been a closed box. They could research the behavioral correlates of learning but not the neurological or brain correlates. Although we do not yet have a complete neurological model of learning, we do have many components of this puzzle. We know that it involves networks of neurons in different parts of the brain; we also know that it is composed of an afferent arm, information-processing arm and an efferent, effector arm; we know that the learning network is influenced by motivation, reward, and emotional factors; and we know some of the cellular neuronal mechanisms underlying the ability of neurons and networks to assemble and transmit information.

The following are some examples of learning processes in which at least part of the biological-brain correlates of learning has been studied.

Songbirds

Researchers of the neural correlates of learning have been interested in songbirds. Songbirds' ability to sing is a learned function. It involves central nervous system networks, sensory experience, and memory. Understanding how birds learn to sing can teach us how the nervous system handles the complex task of learning. The songbird learns a new song by first listening to the song of another bird and memorizing it. It produces its song by learning to pattern its respiration to produce distinct sequences of notes. It then rehearses its own songs, using auditory feedback, by matching the sound it produces to a memorized model. The interval between memorizing and reproducing can be as long as several months. A central circuit that governs song production has been identified in the bird's brain (Mooney & Spiro, 1997). This network occupies a relatively large volume of the bird's brain, particularly the forebrain, with nuclei also in the thalamus, midbrain, and hindbrain. There are a number of nuclei in the forebrain that produce sustained neuronal activity in the form of spike trains, before and throughout the song, in a stereotyped manner for each syllable and in a precise temporal pattern (Yu & Margoliash, 1996; Mooney & Spiro, 1997). In the canary's example, the bird's own song is the most effective stimulus for eliciting such responses. Deaf birds fail to reproduce a song from memory. The brain structures important for song learning are the hypoglossal nerve and the nucleus hyperstriatum ventrale, para caudale (HVC). There may be some lateralization of song control, similar to the lateralization of human language. In the canary, lesions of these structures on the left cause greater losses or more severe deterioration of syllables than similar lesions on the right side. There is also a correlation between the size of the song system nuclei and song learning (Wise, 1985).

This model provides insights into general neurological principles of learning. It tells us that learning involves a network that starts with obtaining information (in this case acoustic or auditory information), memory processes, and execution of a response. It also gives us more particular information on how neural activity relates to the acoustical structure of individual notes, and how the neural code for song is changed by auditory experience (Mooney & Spiro, 1997).

Olfactory Learning

Insight into the brain's functional biochemical correlates of learning can be derived from studies of olfactory learning in the rat. Olfactory preference conditioning is a form of learning that normally occurs in the course of both rat and human development. Newborn rats can be classically conditioned to odors during the first postnatal week. A functional response to odors can be measured in the rat's brain olfactory bulb by 2-DG (2-deoxyglucose) uptake patterns and single-unit recording of the mitral/tufted cells. Olfactory-associative training for as little as 10 minutes will enhance subsequent olfactory bulb responses to the learned odor as measured by enhanced 2-DG uptake. In addition to these functional changes, early olfactory experience modifies olfactory bulb structure and produces an increase in the number of juxtaglomerular neurons in odor-specific region of the olfactory bulb compared with young rats not exposed to the odor. It was also learned experimentally that the neurochemical correlate for early olfactory learning in newborns rats requires an intact noradrenergic input to the bulb.

Such events and changes may occur in human learning. A learning experience may elicit biochemical as well as structural changes in different areas and systems in the brain. Developmental or acquired abnormalities may impair either the biochemical or structural correlates of learning and cause a specific learning disability whereby a specific brain network but not necessarily the brain as a whole, is affected.

Long-Term Potentiation

Long-term potentiation (LTP) is an important concept in the process of information transfer and processing in the brain. It is an electrophysiological phenomenon in which synchronous and repeated activation of many synapses causes incremental increases in the strength of the synaptic transmission lasting for hours or longer (Dobrunz, 1998). It is experimentally expressed as a persistent increase in the size of the synaptic component of the evoked response, recorded from individual cells or from populations of neurons. It represents at least certain forms of memory and learning. These forms of learning and memory are selectively impaired by several experimental methods that eliminate or attenuate LTP.

Long-term potentiation (and another phenomenon called long term depression [LTD], discussed later) has been found in excitatory pathways of the hippocampus, and in several other regions in the brain. Induction of LTP in the hippocampus involves the neurotransmitter glutamate—the most common excitatory transmitter in the brain, especially abundant in the hippocampus and the cerebral cortex and important for learning and memory. Glutaminergic synapses have a number of receptors including N-methyl-D-aspartate (NMDA) and α-Amino-3-hydroxy-5-methyl-4-isoxazolepropionic acid (AMPA). When activated by released glutamate, the receptors depolarize the postsynaptic membrane by opening ion channels. The induction of LTP in the hippocampus with the enhancement of synaptic efficiency involves the activation of NMDA receptors, localized on dendritic spines, with an increase in transmitter release and change in the properties of the (calcium) ion channel which is important for synaptic transmission. Activity-induced change in the morphology or number of dendritic spines may also contribute to changes in synaptic efficiency (Bliss & Collingridge, 1993). Later stages of LTP may also require protein phosphorylation, protein synthesis from existing mRNAs, and gene transcription. Several labs have demonstrated that norepinephrine antagonists disrupt induction of LTP but do not impair expression of previously established LTP.

The reverse form of activity-dependent synaptic plasticity in the brain is LTD. It occurs when individual synapses are activated in isolation: Responses get smaller and stay that way for a long time (Goda & Stevens, 1996). The best studied form of LTD is that of the depression of excitatory synaptic transmission in the cerebellum. The expression of cerebellar LTD is mediated by postsynaptic AMPA receptors, and involves, similar to LTP, voltage-dependent calcium channels, intracellular second messengers including cGMP and protein kinases, and possibly an intercellular messenger, NO, found in the cerebellum. Cerebellar LTD may be important for motor learning, whereas the exact nature of the role of Hippocampal LTD in learning still remains to be explored (Zhuo & Hawkins, 1995).

The process of information transfer may also occur through intersynaptic cross-talk. Neurotransmitter released by one synapse may spill over and be detected by a neighboring synapse. Excitatory synapses in the cortex are very close to each other and information may pass through a spillover of the neurotransmitter glutamate. Also, NMDA receptors are affected by glutamate spillover. Consequently, synaptic transmission mediated by NMDA receptors could involve more cross-talk than other synapses (Dobrunz, 1998). Blocking of glutamate receptors will block LTP and diminish ability to learn. Drugs that block the function of NMDA receptor, for example the selective glutamate receptor blocker aminophosphonovaleric acid, block LTP and diminish the ability of rats to learn tasks that require spatial cues (Kentros et al., 1998).

The hippocampus is, in general, an important brain structure for learning, beyond the effects of the LTP/LTD complex. The hippocampus has learning functions that are not NMDA related (Kentros, Hargreaves, & Hawkins et al., 1998). Hippocampal lesions have a greater effect on learning than the one caused by blocking LTP/LTD (Goda & Stevens, 1996). For instance, hippocampal lesions have a profound effect on an animal's ability to learn in the water maze, whether or not the animal has practiced on a similar task. This abnormal effect on learning is more severe than the one caused by the effect of LTP/LTD abnormality. It is also evident that a deficiency in one of the elements needed for LTP (or other neural mechanisms of learning) may cause only a selective abnormality of learning. For example, the experimental deletion of one protein kinase believed to be important in some aspects of learning in mice can result in a focal but not global deficit of learning (Silva, Paylor, & Wehner et al., 1992).

It is still difficult to make direct connections between these mechanisms of learning and substrates like LTP and LTD, glutamate and other receptors—and Specific Learning Disabilities. Thinking of learning and memorizing, though, as processes conducted by a large population of stronger and weaker synapses in a digital (all or none) or analog (graded) manner, for different types of information, subserving different functions, in different parts of the brain, is helpful to the understanding of SLD. It is feasible that an abnormality of the LTP/LTD physiology affecting specific systems or specific brain areas may play a role in SLD.

EMOTIONAL AND MOTIVATIONAL EFFECTS ON MEMORY AND LEARNING

The process of learning and memory is not a "closed loop" free of influences. Processing of incoming information can be influenced at many points during the long pathway from, for instance, looking at a written word, to areas of memory, storage, and prefrontal executive control. "Epicognitive" processes, including emotional factors, motivation, and attention, can have significant effects on learning and memory.

Important influence on memory and learning comes from emotional factors. We all recognize that during periods of emotional turmoil, our ability to learn and retain new information is diminished. What is not clear is how and at which point of the learning process do the emotional factors intervene and have an effect. In the animal learning model of odor preference mentioned earlier, rat pups learned to distinguish odors. Bilateral lesions of the amygdala in these pups, differentially affected early olfactory memories. Although conditioned pups became behaviorally aroused in response to the odor compared with control pups, they no longer showed a relative preference for that odor. Conditioned activation may be easily learned but learning odor preference is more difficult, and damage to the amygdala may be more likely to disrupt the memory for more difficult, slowly acquired information than easily acquired information.

The amygdala complex in the temporal lobe may be the mediating structure of some of the emotional factors influencing memory and learning. This structure is not an essential structure for the process of long-term retention of memory and learning, but can modulate, through its adrenergic neurotransmitter system, the long-term memory storage in other brain regions. It may be the center activated by emotional factors and through which emotional factors interfere with learning and memory (McGaugh & Cahill, 1997).

A factor that plays a role in academic as well as other types of learning is motivation. Indeed, there are many parents who believe that the main reason for their children's school failure is lack of motivation. Although rarely the only reason for learning abnormality, motivation can be an important factor. It is hard to assess and measure. Research of the effects of motivation on learning ability frequently uses rewards to induce motivation, or conversely, uses stimuli with aversive properties to reduce motivation. The dopamine hypothesis suggests that the neurotransmitter dopamine plays a fundamental role in mediating the rewarding properties of all classes of stimuli, although other models claim that a number of biochemical systems make independent contributions to reward (Nader, Bechara, & Kooy, 1997).

Clinical experiments have discovered that recently formed memories and learning can be influenced, for a limited time after they are formed, by a number of interventions including drug injections or brain stimulation. Such postlearning treatments have the potential to either enhance or impair memory, depending on the experimental conditions (Cahill & McGaugh, 1996).

EFFECTS OF TRAINING ON LEARNING AND MEMORY

What are the brain correlates of training? We may get some answers from studies of brain changes during the learning of perceptual skills, although learning of perceptual skills may be different from the learning of historical facts, dates, or new mathematical facts. Among other differences, dopamine (rather than glutamate) is an important neurotransmitter in activation of prefrontal cortex during motor training (Shadmehr & Holcomb, 1997). There is an improvement of the performance of perceptual skills with practice, and gains are retained over a long time. Perceptual skill learning includes fast and slow stages: Fast learning may reflect the setting up of a task-specific processing sequence for solving the perceptual problem, which takes place on line while the stimulus is still present. Slow learning reflects an ongoing, mostly off line, perhaps structural, modification of the representations within the processing system, establishing new associations and dissociations of neuronal networks (i.e., transcription-dependent synaptic consolidation) (Sagi & Tanne, 1994). The improvement of the performance of perceptual skills with practice is the result of plasticity with, and changes in, those brain areas that are critical to the performance of the task, and is specific to these areas. This implies that when we train for a specific task, only a discrete part within the representational domain of this function in the brain is affected by the training and learning. Perceptual learning in vision, for instance, is very specific for simple stimulus attributes, and there may be no transfer of learning between two visual tasks (Sagi & Tanne, 1994). A few minutes of daily practice on a sequential finger opposition task induced large, incremental performance gains over a few weeks of training. These gains did not generalize to the contralateral hand or to a matched sequence of identical component movements, suggesting that it is a lateralized representation of the learned sequence of movements that evolved through practice (Karni, Meyer, & Rey-Hipolito, Jezzard, et al., 1998). A study of magnetic source imaging revealed that the cortical representation of the digits of the left hand of string players was larger than that in controls. No such differences were observed for the representations of the right-hand digits. The amount of cortical reorganization correlated with the age at which the person had begun to play (Elbert, Pantev, & Wienbruch, Rockstroh, & Taub, 1995). Similarly, training rats to reach for bits of cookies resulted in an increase in dendritic length and branching complexity in neurons of the motor-sensory forelimb cortex (Withers & Greenough, 1989).

As previously noted, perceptual learning may be a specific type of learning, guided by specific mechanisms and neurotransmitters. It is possible, though, that anatomical changes occur in the brain during other types of learning and practice, including glutamate NMDA-related learning mechanism in the hippocampus.

DEVELOPMENTAL ASPECTS OF LEARNING

When cognitive ability, learning, and behavior are measured, a clear developmental pattern is evident. Cognitive abilities and academic learning are constantly improving throughout childhood. A developmental pattern is also present when cognitive abilities are measured. An example of such a pattern is that of face recognition, a specialized type of visual perception, possibly governed by the right hemisphere. Face recognition is an important cognitive ability because human faces provide an important source of social information. Tests of perception and comprehension of facial expression given to children and adults, demonstrated a clear developmental pattern with increased perception of facial expression between the ages of 6 and 8 years, little further change until about 13 years, and then a second period of increased ability, to adult performance, at about 14 years. Similarly, there is clear evidence for a developmental pattern of speech and language abilities. Over the first 6 months of life infants distinguish a wide range of speech contrasts and have some capacity to differentiate voices and speaking rates, whereas over the next 6 months they acquire the ability to recognize some phonetic and prosodic characteristics of language. Eight-month-old infants exposed to recordings of three children's stories for 10 days during a 2-week period listened significantly longer to the lists of story words read to them 2 weeks later than to words not previously read to them. By comparison, a control group of infants who had not been exposed to the stories showed no such preference.

These suggest that 8-month-old infants begin to engage in long-term storage of words that occur frequently in speech, an important prerequisite for learning language (Jusczyk & Hohne, 1997).

The major developmental question is, of course, how does this happen. How does the brain acquire this ability for cognition and memory? Does it have this ability imprinted or is it all acquired? Leonard Bernstein, the conductor, and Albert Einstein, the physicist, made their great achievements because of talent and hard work. Their unique ability to process information, learn, remember, create, and produce, is believed to be partially "hard wired" in their brains, and partially acquired, through environmental stimuli and the brain's ability for plasticity. The basic claim of biological theories of learning and cognition is that both contributors to the development of cognitive and learning abilities, the "hard wiring" of the brain as well as the brain's ability for plasticity, depend on intact growth and development of the brain, a process which starts at conception and continues throughout childhood, and includes the stages of neurogenesis, migration, myelination, and connectivity. There are a number of examples that demonstrate that the period of brain development is critical for the development of normal cognition. Impaired ability to learn during the developmental period can be detrimental for future cognition and learning. Studies using nonhuman primate models found a close relationship between the development of frontal lobe functions including some aspects of memory and the ability to inhibit certain motor responses, and the electrophysiological development of the neocortex studied by electroencephalography. Conversely, when the brain does not develop and mature normally, the "imprinted" learning as well as the ability for new learning are frequently impaired. Alcohol exposure in utero can impair brain development, resulting in cognitive and learning impairment. Data obtained from an animal model of fetal alcohol syndrome demonstrates the neurobiological basis (including neurotransmitter abnormalities) of the learning impairments that occur as a result of prenatal alcohol exposure (Kirstein, Philpot, & Dark, 1997). Another example is the effect of deprivation of sensory experience during development. A 1932 monograph on the development of the awareness of space and "spatial consciousness" in congenitally blind people describes subjects who were congenitally blind or who became blind early in life. Congenitally blind people had significant problems with spatial awareness. They did not have a spatial image of objects. They had problems describing a circle, and could not assess the shape of objects they held in their hands. An intelligent blind girl who handled dogs understood that they have heads, tails, and ears, but she had no proper idea of how the parts were conjoined together.

Similarly, the biologically based Specific Learning Disabilities are the manifestations of brain abnormalities, probably mostly abnormalities of brain connectivity, which occur during brain development, and continue to have an effect on the ability to learn later. What those abnormalities are is the subject of discussion of the next chapters.

BIOCHEMICAL SUBSTRATES OF LEARNING

Basic molecular processes involved in learning include neurotransmitter release, secondary messengers (cAMP), modulation of CA^{++} channels, Na-P pump, and in long-term memory and learning—protein synthesis.

Neurotransmitters are biochemical substances that are transmitted through the synapses between nerve cells and neural processes, and carry out interneural information exchange. The neural information that is passed from a neuron can have an excitatory or inhibitory effect on the recipient neuron, enhancing or decreasing its activity. Many neurotransmitters, including dopamine, noradrenaline, acetylcholine, and glutamate, are involved in aspects of learning and behavior. Much of the pharmacological treatment of behavioral disorders involves manipulation and modification of neurotransmitters in the brain. For example, drugs like benzodiazepines, which alleviate anxiety, augment the action of gamma-aminobutyric acid (GABA), an important inhibitory transmitter. Antidepressants, such as Prozac, enhance the action of serotonin and indoleamine, whereas certain antipsychotics antagonize the action of dopamine. The biochemical mode of action of neurotransmitters involves the binding of receptors that are located on the surface of neurons. Some receptors are ion channel proteins that can form aqueous pores through which ions cross the membrane, whereas others, including the dopamine receptors, interact with a neighboring membrane protein that cleaves a high-energy phosphate bond from guanosine triphosphate. A single neuron can release one or more neurotransmitters (Nicoll & Malenka, 1998).

Glutamate is an abundant amino acid that is an excitatory transmitter in the central nervous system, especially in the hippocampus and the cerebral cortex. Glutaminergic synapses have one of two categories of receptors: quisqualates or kainates and NMDA. When activated by glutamate, both these receptors depolarize the postsynaptic membrane by opening ion channels. The currents generated by NMDA receptors have a long course, and are therefore suitable for temporal integration and mediating the synaptic changes that occur as a result of synchronous convergence of inputs. There is evidence that the activation of NMDA receptors is responsible for the induction of LTP in the hippocampus.

Knowledge regarding the biochemical substrate of learning can be acquired from addiction. At least two neurotransmitters are involved with addictive behavior: dopamine and glutamate. Dopamine has long been known to have a role in addiction because all addictive drugs cause a surge of dopamine in the brain's reward center—the nucleus accumbens. But addiction is actually a form of brain learning and involves, in addition to dopamine, another neurotransmitter, glutamate. It is possible that addictive drugs cause a surge in dopamine in the brain and this way "attract the brain's attention," followed by brain increase of glutamate, which is a more long-term change and constitutes the learning part of the addictive behavior. What dopamine is doing is reinforcing the drug-seeking behavior experience. The role of glutamate is in the learning of the drug effect. A glutamate-dependent enhancement of synaptic activity was found during addiction learning, and intact glutamate neurotransmission was shown to be essential. Compounds that interfere with glutamate signaling block the intense drug cravings that addicts feel during withdrawal. In addition, dextromethorphan, a medication with gluta-mate antagonistic properties, reduced the absolute reinforcing properties of cocaine. Compounds that prevent glutamate from acting by blocking gluta-mate receptors (like NMDA) as well as lesions of the prefrontal cortex (a place of many neurons that discharge glutamate) prevent sensitization to amphet-amine in rats.

Catecholamines and Information Processing

It is well known now that neurotransmitters participate in the transmission of neural information. Cognitive functions, including learning, involve activ-ity of a number of neurotransmitters, each playing a different role, and also interacting with other neurotransmitter systems. A neurotransmitter system that plays an important role in learning processes, as well as in motor func-tions, is the catecholamine neurotransmitter system. Examples of neurologi-cal and psychiatric disorders wherein catecholamines play an important role in the pathogenesis include Parkinson disease, schizophrenia, and drug abuse.

Dopaminergic and noradrenergic neurons of the primate brains originate in the substantia nigra, the ventral tegmental area and the locus ceruleus of the brain stem, respectively, and project diffusely to many subcortical and cortical areas. A most important characteristic of these systems is that their neuronal projections are numerous and diffuse, branching along the surface of all cortical lobes (Figure 4.1).

The pattern of their neurotransmitter release is also unique, with a low and stable baseline rate of firing, and slow conduction velocity compared with other neural systems, resulting in a steady, often synchronous transmitter release, which is independent of the source of stimulation. They are not able to sustain high levels of activity, but their effect on the target cell may last several seconds or even minutes, in contrast to the millisecond duration following release of amino acids such as GABA or glutamic acid. This anatomical and physiological organi-zation is suited to a diffuse, modulatory action rather than to precise, localized transmission of discrete sensory or motor signals. Dopamine modulates neuronal activity of target cells by enhancing the ability of neurons to transmit signals and reduce the distortion created by noise, thus increasing the signal-to-noise ratio. Indeed, the type of cognitive improvement observed in human subjects receiv-ing DA agonists is improved signal detection. The enhancement of the excitatory inputs relates to the background firing rate noise and to an absolute increase in

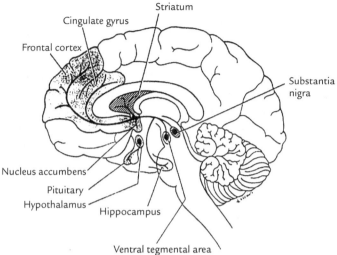

Figure 4-1:
Dopaminergic projection systems in the brain. The major dopaminergic nuclei in the brain are the substantia nigra pars compacta (*hatched*), shown projecting to the striatum (also *hatched*); the ventral tegmental area (*fine stipple*), shown projecting to the frontal and cingulate cortex, nucleus accumbens, and other limbic structures (*fine stipple*); and the arcuate nucleus of the hypothalamus (*coarse stipple*), which provides dopaminergic regulation to the pituitary.
Source: Neurobiology of mental illness (3 Ed). Edited by Dennis Charney and Eric Nestler. Publisher: Oxford University Press. Print: ISBN-13 9780199798261. Publication date: April 2011.

signal length (Cohen & Servan-Schreiber, 1993). The effects of catecholamines depend on a number of functions including the nature of the cognitive function involved. Dopamine has more significant effects on tasks that involve motivation or actions that predict a reward or an adverse outcome. A brain imaging study using PET scanning demonstrated an increased activity of dopamine during a task that involved increased motivation, compared with a task that did not involve motivation (Koepp, Gunn, & Lawrence, et al., 1998).

The cholinergic system exerts its role in memory in a number of ways including by interactions with other neurotransmitter systems. Cholinergic, noradrenergic, opiate, and GABAergic systems have been shown to interact in the amygdala, where the end result was the regulation of the release of norepinephrine (Fuster, 1995). Such interactions between the cholinergic system and several neurotransmitters and neuromodulators may be important in learning and memory (Decker & McGaugh, 1991).

There is growing evidence that insulin may affect learning and memory. Insulin may work in the brain much as it works elsewhere in the body—by helping glucose enter into brain neurons, thereby helping them maintain their energy production. It may also have other beneficial roles, such as spurring neuronal growth, although there is no specific evidence for its role in childhood learning or learning disabilities.

Nitric oxide (NO), a gaseous intercellular messenger, may have a role in cellular mechanisms of learning and memory. A role of NO in learning was found for the vestibulo-ocular reflex (VOR), a reflex that aids in the stabilization of visual images on the retina during head rotation. Cerebellar NO was found to be a mediator of the acquisition and retention of adaptive VOR gain change in the goldfish, a sensorimotor model of learning. The VOR is a reflex that aids in the stabilization of visual images on the retina during head rotation. Levels of NO increase with activation of glutamate receptors or depolarization of climbing fiber afferents. A vestibule-cerebellar injection of an NO synthase inhibitor, which specifically blocks NO production, inhibited the acquisition of VOR gain increases. Nitric oxide may also play a role in the expression of LTP, and there may be an NO-dependent form of LTP.

Genetic Effects on Learning

A factor that needs to be included in the model of normal learning is the genetic factor. How much of our ability to acquire knowledge and skill is genetically imprinted, and how much is actively learned? The importance of the genetic factor is hard to assess, but is definitely different for different types of learning. For instance, it may be stronger for the acquisition of motor skills than for learning of facts. Some motor functions are genetically imprinted in the brain and do not require active learning. Phyletic memory is the memory acquired over the course of evolution. The function of the primary sensory and motor neocortical systems involves genetically determined phyletic memory (Eichenbaum, 1997), whereas other more complex motor activity is learned.

Absolute pitch is the ability to recognize a pitch without an external reference. An interesting study on absolute pitch (AP) aimed to distinguish the genetic component of AP from a learned ability for this trait. Researchers examined absolute pitch in musicians attending music conservatories, training programs, and orchestras. Early musical training appeared to be necessary but not sufficient for the development of AP. Forty percent of musicians who had begun training at 4 years of age or younger reported AP, whereas only 3% of those who had initiated training at 9 years of age or later did so. But, in addition, AP possessors were four times more likely to report another AP possessor in their families (Baharloo, Johnston, & Service et al., 1998). This study suggests that both early musical training and genetic predisposition are needed for the development of AP.

MEMORY AND LEARNING SUPPRESSIVE GENES

Genetic factors were found to be involved with memory formation. Research groups working with organisms including Aplysia and fruit flies demonstrated that events associated with long-term memory—including protein synthesis, and growth of synapses and other changes—do not occur when certain genes (i.e., a gene called *CREB*), were blocked. *CREB* interacts with the neuron's DNA and turns on dozens of genes, which remodel synapses and effect learning and memory storage processes. Other genes may also be involved (Rugg et al., 1998).

SUMMARY

A biological model of learning and memory includes specific parts of the brain that are "dedicated" to learning. At the same time, learning of a function or attribute takes place in the same place where this function is localized, so learning is also a pervasive process that takes place at almost any place in the brain.

There is a learning plasticity in the brain. A brain area or network can anatomically or functionally change with learning, training and experience.

A network of neurons can change its pattern of connectivity. There are instructive signals that can regulate the changes.

Neurons involved in classical conditioning are found in the brainstem, cerebellum, and cortex (Knudsen, 1994). Networks that support cognitive skills, such as pattern recognition and language acquisition, can be established by the interaction of genetic determinants and unsupervised forms of learning.

Later in life plasticity mostly follows experience and training.

The brain networks involved in different types of learning may use different basic mechanisms and neurotransmitters. The basic networks of learning are also influenced, through other synaptic connections, by other factors including emotional factors, motivation, and reward.

CHAPTER 5

Neuroanatomy of Specific Reading Disabilities I

Anatomical Deviations

INTRODUCTION

Specific learning disabilities (SLDs) result from cognitive deficiencies—specific deficiencies in brain functions important for learning. Are these deficiencies the result of a structural brain abnormality, or of irregular or abnormal programming of brain networks related to learning? Discussing this question necessitates some understanding of the normal anatomy of learning. Learning to read, calculate, and write demands coordinated functioning of many brain areas. An optimal learning condition involves the ability to perceive, process, and analyze sensory information, and the ability to express learned material by the execution of a response, which can be done verbally (e.g., by answering a question), by writing, or by other means of execution. The student has to be alert, focused, motivated, and emotionally healthy. As one can imagine, there need to be a large number of brain systems, in different brain locations, participating in and supervising these actions.

Advances in neurosciences, particularly in neuroimaging, in the last decades, help identify certain areas of the brain that are important for the functions of information processing and learning. This raised the expectations that the pathophysiology of SLDs may be explained by structural or functional abnormalities of these areas and their connections.

Indeed, recent studies confirmed subtle differences in brain anatomy of SLDs. The exact significance of these differences is not yet clear.

The methods of studying the functional anatomy of cognition and learning have changed significantly in the last decades, and have evolved from observations of cognitive deficits caused by lesions—to the ability to study normal and abnormal brain functional anatomy in vivo using new brain imaging tools, including magnetic resonance imaging (MRI), functional MRI (fMRI), Diffusion Tensor Imaging (DIT), and positron emission tomography (PET) scanning. These, enhanced, more sensitive, neuroimaging methods, including quantitative methods, have been developed to investigate the existence of more subtle abnormalities. The areas of the brain that mediate knowledge about objects, words, colors, letters, and digits can now be investigated by measuring changes in regional cerebral blood flow (rCBF), oxygen utilization or tracing individual neurotransmitters, using positron emission tomography (PET) or functional MRI (fMRI). These functional anatomy methods have opened new windows into the brain, helping us understand how reading, calculating, writing, and other academic domains are acquired.

NEUROIMAGING METHODS

There have been a number of neuroimaging modalities used in the anatomical research of Specific Learning Disabilities (SLDs).

Brain Magnetic Resonance Imaging

Magnetic resonance imaging provides detailed pictures of the brain in multiple planes. It is the preferable neuroimaging method for most brain disorders because it provides the best available resolution, and can demonstrate all brain areas, including the brainstem and the posterior part of the brain—areas that are not well demonstrated on computed tomography (CT). It does not involve radiation to the brain. There have been a number of MRI applications that allow the demonstration of blood flow and cerebrospinal fluid flow, of an angiogram (magnetic resonance angiogram, MRA) or magnetic resonance venogram (MRV). Functional MRI and MRI spectroscopy (MRS) provide information about the function and chemical metabolites of the brain. Other new methods include the following:

Tractography

The brain has a complicated network of connections between different cortical and subcortical regions. Knowledge of theses tracts has been obtained by biological techniques, including histochemistry performed on postmortem specimens. Tractography is an MRI technique that demonstrates neural tracts in vivo. That is done by a technique called diffusion tensor imaging (DTI), which looks at the symmetry of brain water diffusion. Diffusion is the process by

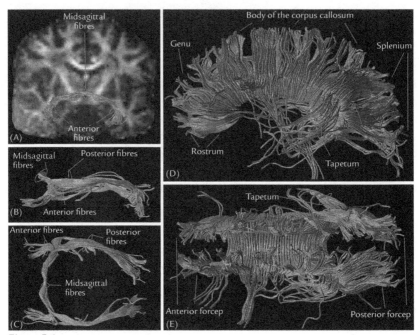

Figure 5-1:
Diffusion tensor tractography reconstruction of the anterior commissure and the corpus callosum. **(A)** Anterior **(B)** left lateral, and **(C)** superior view of the anterior commissure. **(D)** Left lateral and **(E)** superior view of the corpus callosum.
Source: Atlas of human brain connections. Marco Catani and Michel Thiebaut de Schotten. Published March 2012. ISBN 9780199541164. Chapter 9: Figure 9.1.

which molecules or other particles intermingle and migrate according to their random thermal motion. Diffusion of water in the brain, designated "isotropic" diffusion, occurs equally in all directions. If the water diffuses in a medium with barriers, the diffusion will be uneven. Bundles of fiber tracts cause the water to diffuse asymmetrically in a tensor, the major axis parallel to the direction of the fibers. This asymmetry is called anisotropy. Diffusion tensor imaging and fiber tractography can demonstrate the orientation and integrity of white matter fibers in vivo. It can delineate white matter abnormalities, including abnormal hemispheric fiber connections in cases of agenesis of the corpus callosum, and in malformations of cortical development (Lee et al., 2005) (Figure 5.1).

BRAIN ANATOMY RELATED TO SPECIFIC LEARNING DISABILITIES

The Neuron

The physiology of information processing and learning is centered on the neuron. The neurons are the building blocks of the brain networks that participate in information processing and learning. The neuron consists of a cell body and nerve processes, the axons and dendrites. In his "neuron doctrine," Ramon Cajal suggested that the neuron is the basic working unit of the brain, and that the brain works by neurons connecting, receiving, and delivering information to other neurons. Cajal's invention of the method of silver impregnation enabled him and many researchers after him to visualize the neuron and its processes, and demonstrated how the neurons interact to transmit information. He described neurons as "polarized cells that receive signals on highly branched extensions of their bodies, called dendrites, and send the information along unbranched extensions, called axons" (Cajal, 1952). Later studies demonstrated that the transmitted stimuli may be excitatory or inhibitory. A single neuron may receive inhibitory and excitatory inputs from incoming axon terminals from neighboring or distant cells through many synaptic connections on its cell body and dendrites. The transmission of information along the axons and between neurons is by a combined chemical–electrophysiological process. Transmission along the axon is by electrical potentials (action potentials), which are caused by the movement of positively charged sodium ions from the extracellular space, where sodium is normally in higher concentration, into the interior of the neuron, across the surface membrane. This causes depolarization of the neural cell membrane, and creation of action potential. The action potential propagates along the axon. When it arrives at the axon terminal, it causes the release of chemical substances, called neurotransmitters, from small vesicles in which they are packaged into the space between the two cells known as the synaptic cleft, a space 20 nanometers in width that is the contact point between neurons. Calcium ions enter the nerve terminal during the peak of the action potential and help coordinate the release of the neurotransmitter molecules. After their release, the neurotransmitters bind to postsynaptic receptors, triggering a change in membrane permeability and, as a result, another electrical potential that will travel along the processes of the connecting cell. Information is conveyed in this manner from one neuron to another. Neurons in different parts of the brain may have different neurotransmitters. More so, different parts of the same neuron may have different receptors, responding to different neurotransmitters. A large number of neurotransmitters have been identified in the brain including dopamine, gamma-aminobutyric acid, noradrenaline, and serotonin. Similarly, there are a large number of receptors in postsynaptic sites matching the neurotransmitter released from the presynaptic terminal (Fishbach, 1994). The neurons involved in information processing, learning, and memory are located primarily in the neocortex, the gray matter area on the surface of the brain. These neurons are organized in six layers. Sensory cortical areas are arranged in a modular organization. In these areas, neurons of similar function that specialize in detecting a given sensory feature are arranged in columns, 50 to 80 nanometers wide, that extend throughout the thickness of the cortex to its surface (Hubel & Wiesel, 1968). A sensory module in the visual cortex will respond, for instance, to a particular line orientation. Neurons of different cortical regions in the frontal, temporal, parietal, and occipital lobes connect by horizontally running fibers. Similarly, there are nerve fibers that form vertical connections between neurons in cortical regions and "lower" basal ganglia and brainstem areas. These extensive horizontal cortico-cortical and vertical connections provide the potential for the extensive neural interaction involved in perceptual processing, motor functioning, and other types of cognitive functions (Fuster, 1995).

Cognitive processes take place through the interaction of network of neurons. For each task some of the neurons and synapses of these networks have to be activated and be reinforced, whereas other connections have to be inactivated. All this has to be accomplished accurately, in the correct order, frequently in synchrony, and at great speed. (Neuronal latencies in association cortices are in the range of 100–300 milliseconds).

Principles of Localization of Function

One important question related to the anatomy of cognitive functions is whether these functions are permanently localized to a distinct anatomical location in the brain, or whether they are an outcome of an ad hoc association of neuronal networks firing in a certain sequence, without a "topographical" localization. There are functions that are localized in "specialized" areas and have a dedicated and segregated neural substrate, as is evident, at least in the adult brain, by the selectivity of impairments after focal brain damage, and by functional anatomical studies (Goldman-Rakic, 1988). Some functions, for instance, simple sensory motor functions, are genetically imprinted and thus develop automatically without the need for systematic learning. Other, more specialized, or phylogenetically newer functions, have to be learned, and may not be precisely localized. There is no evidence for a genetically imprinted localization of functions such as ballet dancing or chess playing in the brain. Such functions do not develop automatically without systematic learning and training. More so, even when such functions are learned, the network of neurons responsible for their knowledge may not stay permanently localized in the brain (Polk, 1998). Reading is one of the functions that has to be learned.

Recent functional anatomy studies give us some understanding of the way concepts and functions are anatomically localized in the brain. When subjects generated words describing colors and actions, generation of color words selectively activated a region in the ventral temporal lobe just anterior to the area involved in the perception of color, whereas generation of action words activated a region in the middle temporal gyrus just anterior to the area involved in the perception of motion. These data suggest that object knowledge is organized as a system in which the attributes of an object are stored close to the regions of the cortex that mediate perception of those attributes (Martin et al., 1995). Environmental factors may play a role. Functional neuroimaging demonstrates that in most normal subjects the neural substrates underlying letter recognition are segregated from those underlying digit recognition. On the other hand, subjects in a visual environment in which letters and digits occur together rather than separately show less evidence for segregated letter and digit processing. It is therefore possible that the learning of letters and numbers is associated with a specific cortical spatial organization with separate cortical location for these two functions. This suggests that the environment can lead to qualitative changes in the brain's functional organization (Polk, 1998).

Anatomy of Learning

The following is a short review of brain anatomy, particularly those parts of the brain important in information processing and learning.

The human brain, which weighs three to four pounds, contains about 100 million neurons. Its main parts are the cerebrum, cerebellum, and brainstem. The cerebrum is divided into the left and right hemispheres, connected by the corpus callosum and other axonal bridges. The cerebral hemispheres are further divided into the frontal, parietal, temporal, and occipital lobes (Figure 5.2).

A simple starting question would be, What are the brain areas involved in academic classroom learning? Although every region of the brain may be involved in some kind of learning, a likely model of academic learning in the brain includes a "sensory" and a "motor" part, and involves intake of sensory information (e.g., visual, auditory including language, somatosensory information), primary and secondary analysis of each sensory modality, integration of sensory modalities, memory pathways, planning of response and, last, the execution of a response. Anatomically, the brain areas involved include the auditory and visual primary and secondary processing areas, language processing areas, memory pathways, the tertiary processing areas in the parietal and frontal lobes, the limbic lobe, and the cerebellum.

Study of the anatomy of learning can be structured according to the information procession model. The "sensory" modules are visual, somatosensory, and auditory. Learning involves the perception of sensory information, and processing and analysis of such information. The "motor" part is demonstrated through the execution of a response, solving a problem, or answering a question (Figures 5.3, 5.4, and 5.5).

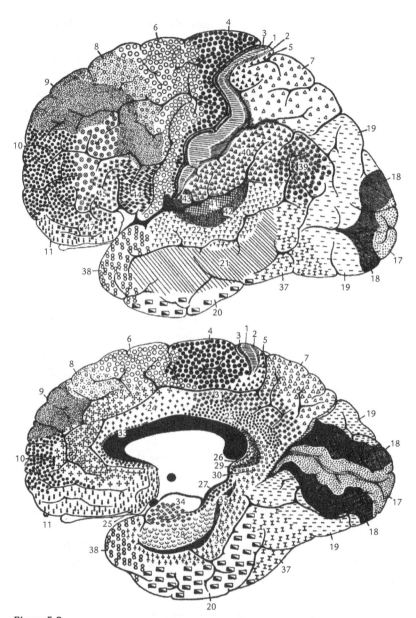

Figure 5-2:
Brodmann's regionalization map of the human cerebral cortex as projected schematically onto the lateral (*top*, left hemisphere) and medial (*bottom*, right hemisphere) aspects. Each cortical area is indicated by a different pattern of symbols and a different number. (From K. Brodmann, 1909)

Source: Brain architecture, 2nd ed. Understanding the basic plan. Larry W. Swanson. New York: Oxford University Press. ISBN-13: 9780195378580. Publication date August, 2011. Chapter 10. Figure 10.4 (Brodmann's regionalization map of the human cerebral cortex).

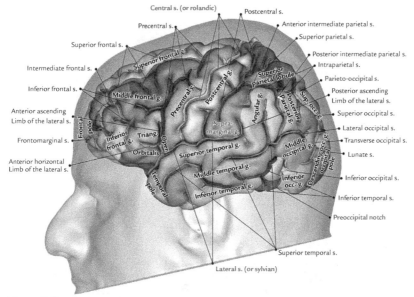

Figure 5-3:
Three-dimensional reconstruction of the brain showing the principal gyri(u) and sulci(us) of the dorsolateral surface of the left hemisphere. Interlobar sulci are in *dark grey*. Intralobar sulci are in *black*.
Source: Marco Catani and Michel Thiebaut de Schotten. Atlas of human brain connections. Published March 2012, ISBN 9780199541164. Chapter 2, Surface neuroanatomy.

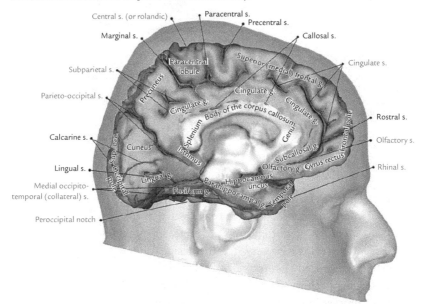

Figure 5-4:
Three-dimensional reconstruction of the brain showing the principal gyri(u) and sulci(us) of the medial surface of the left hemisphere. Interlobar sulci are in *dark grey*. Intralobar sulci are in *black*.
Source: Marco Catani and Michel Thiebaut de Schotten. Atlas of human brain connections. Published March 2012, ISBN 9780199541164. Chapter 2, Surface neuroanatomy.

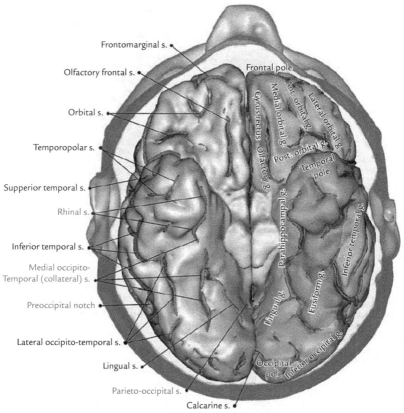

Frontomarginal s.
Olfactory frontal s.
Orbital s.
Temporopolar s.
Supperior temporal s.
Rhinal s.
Inferior temporal s.
Medial occipito-
Temporal (collateral) s.
Preoccipital notch
Lateral occipito-temporal s.
Lingual s.
Parieto-occipital s.
Calcarine s.

Frontal pole
Ant. orbital g.
Gyrus rectus
Medial orbital g.
Lateral orbital g.
Olfactory s.
Post. orbital g.
Temporal pole
Parahippocampal g.
Inferior temporal g.
Lingual g.
Fusiform g.
Occipital pole
Inferior occipital s.

Figure 5-5:
Three-dimensional reconstruction of the brain showing the principal gyri(u) and sulci(us)
of the ventral surface of the left and right hemisphere. Interlobar sulci are in *dark grey*.
Intralobar sulci are in *black*.

Source: Marco Catani and Michel Thiebaut de Schotten. Atlas of human brain connections. Published March
2012, ISBN 9780199541164. Chapter 2, Surface neuroanatomy.

Sensory Perception

The posterior part of the cerebrum is involved with input, the perception and
storing of information received from the external world. There are several layers of Sensory processing, from simple to increasingly complex, The brain sensory perception regions are assigned the designation of primary, secondary
and tertiary, organized hierarchically according to the complexity of information processing performed in these areas. Neurons in a primary processing
center can process information from only one sensory modality. The neurons
in the secondary processing areas are involved in a more complex level of
analysis, but similar to those in the primary processing areas, still specialize
in processing information of one modality only. The tertiary processing areas
can process information from more than one sensory modality.

The primary visual cortex (Brodmann area 17) and the visual association cortices (Brodmann areas 18 and 19) are part of the occipital lobe, and process simple and complex visual information, respectively. Neurons in these areas exclusively process visual information, and each neuron responds only to certain characteristics of the visual information. Studies of monkey striate cortex revealed vertical as well as horizontal organization. Stimulus dimensions such as position of objects on the retina, line orientation, and perhaps directionality of movement are mapped in the vertical, whereas the horizontal system has layers organized by hierarchical processing orders (Hubel & Wiesel, 1968; Fishbach, 1994). Brain abnormalities in these areas can cause a range of deficits of visual information processing, from cerebral blindness, a complete loss of the ability to cognitively process visual information, with no response to visual stimuli, to less severe forms of visual agnosia, including visual misperceptions, like distortion of shape or size of objects. Abnormalities of these areas may interfere with the recognition of letters, numbers, and symbols used in reading.

More complex visual processing (e.g., processing of motion and visuospatial information) continues beyond the striate cortex, in tertiary visual centers, including the inferior temporal cortex area and the posterior parietal cortex. There are two major cortico-cortical pathways connecting the visual cortex to other parts of the cerebral cortex, a ventral connection to the inferior temporal cortex, which is important for object recognition, and a dorsal pathway into the posterior parietal cortex, which is important for spatial perception (DeSimone & Duncan, 1995). As a stimulus proceeds along this pathway, the complexity of visual processing and the processing ability of the individual neurons increase. Although in the primary processing areas there is a close topographic representation of the retina, in the tertiary processing areas the cells are activated more by the relevant behavioral features of the stimulus, involving more than one modality, and get convergent inputs from other sensory modalities and information. What this means is that neurons in advanced processing areas may respond to a combination of two features of a stimulus, although not responding to any single feature of the stimulus by itself. For instance, there are cells in the monkey's visual pathway in the inferior temporal lobe that specifically respond to faces. These cells do not respond to one particular shape (lines, circles etc.) but perceive and recognize the face as a whole. Lesions in these areas can result in prosopagnosia, the loss of ability to recognize faces. The visual image perceived in these advanced processing areas and in our consciousness is not exactly the pure image registered on the retina. There is a lot of interference, or selection of information, by conscious processes, and our mental state can enhance or reduce certain parts of the image. Similar hierarchies of sensory processing are found in the temporal lobe for auditory analysis and in the parietal lobe for somatosensory perception (Luria, 1966).

Areas in the parietal lobe, primarily in the post-central gyrus, process somatosensory information, including information on position and vibration sensation; the localization, quality, and intensity of touch and pain sensation; and the complex "cortical" sensory modalities of graphesthesia, the ability to perceive the configuration of letters and numbers written on the skin, and stereognosis, the ability to assess the shapes of objects put into our hands. Acquired lesions of the parietal lobes may cause inattention or extinction of feeling in the opposite side of the body. Patients may lose their body orientation and not recognize body parts on the affected side. There may be space disturbances, astereognosis, agraphesthesia, and apraxia (an inability to perform a motor function, although no disturbance of motor or sensory functions exists). There is little known about the use of somatosensory information for reading or calculation, although we use somatosensory information to help us hold a pen or pencil or turn pages.

Areas in the temporal lobe process auditory information, from sound recognition and analysis, to language.

The Executive Brain

No less important than the brain sensory information processing loop is the motor or executive loop—which facilitate preparing and execution of a response. The motor system is an elaborate system that includes areas of the cerebral cortex, spinal cord, brainstem, cerebellum, and basal ganglia.

The frontal lobe motor center controls the body muscles including motor planning, and the initiation and execution of voluntary action. The motor execution system is hierarchical (Fuster, 1995), starting with conceiving an action, planning it, and then advancing to the execution of this action.

Accordingly, there are different regions in the brain motor area that control these different stages of the motor process, from the planning to the execution stage. Motor action starts in the prefrontal cortex where the motor plan is conceived, followed by the premotor area, where it is planned, to the frontal motor cortex. Electrical recordings from the motor cortex at the time of movement demonstrates that prefrontal cells fire first, followed by premotor cells and then by cells in the motor cortex.

A precise motor map exists where different regions of the motor cortex control specific muscle groups, primarily over distal and fine movements. This explains why a disproportionly large part of the cortical motor area is involved with the innervation of the hand and fingers, which perform fine movements. The lower part of the motor cortex designated Brodmann area 44, coordinates the muscles involved in speech.

In addition to cortical areas in the frontal lobe, there are other brain areas that are involved in planning and execution of muscle control, including subcortical areas in the basal ganglia and the cerebellum.

The Angular Cortex and Prefrontal Area

In the information processing and execution scheme of the brain there has to be an "executive" system that coordinates it all and makes the appropriate decisions. This system has to have connection to the parts of the brain involved in processing sensory information, and the part of the brain involved in the execution of the response, and has to be hierarchically more complex and have the ability to integrate different modalities of information. Such tertiary processing areas are present in the parietal and frontal lobes. Neurons in these areas are not modality specific and may respond to stimuli of different modalities. These brain areas also have elaborate connections with other cortical and subcortical structures. In the parietal lobe, the angular gyrus is important for symbolic language, allowing recognition and visualization of symbols, a function involving processing of visual and lingual information. To this end the neurons in the angular gyrus need to have the ability to decipher information from at least two association areas, visual and auditory/language. Brain abnormalities in this region may cause inability to develop symbolic language and read. In the adult brain, a lesion in this area may cause alexia, the loss of reading ability.

The other cerebral area involved in multimodal information processing is the prefrontal area. In the scheme of information processing, the prefrontal areas have two tasks. The first is a similar capacity of integration of information from sensory association areas, including visual, auditory, and somatosensory information. In this capacity the prefrontal cortex acts as a tertiary information processing center. It does not require external stimuli from the outside world because its function depends on its connections with primary and secondary sensory cortical brain areas as well as the subcortical basal ganglia and brainstem areas. Histologically, the frontal areas contain neurons typical of the tertiary processing areas, which are not modality specific. The other task of this brain area is the execution of plans and programs and the regulation of behavior.

Patients with lesions of the prefrontal areas may not suffer any isolated sensory, perceptual, speech, or motor deficit, but may lose the ability to respond and analyze brain stimuli arriving from other brain areas. They may also have a deficit in the ability to create plans and follow them, and to use proper strategies to fulfill a given task. Vigilance can be impaired. They cannot regulate their behavior by using previously obtained information, and their behavior may consist of impulsive responses to immediate stimuli (Luria, 1966).

The Emotional Brain

An important brain system that affects information processing and execution is the emotional brain. There are many brain structures involved with emotions, in particular within the limbic system. The limbic system consists of many structures, including the hippocampus, amygdala, anterior prefrontal substance, cingular gyrus, fornix, hippocampal gyrus, orbitofrontal gyrus, and inferior medial temporal lobe. This system serves as a highly developed olfactory system in animals. In humans it serves as a center for emotions and autonomic functions. It participates in the modulation and processing of sensory information, and may also participate in the modulation of motor response. The hippocampus is an important organ involved in mediation of memory, learning, and behavior. Its major outputs are to the cerebral cortex and the lateral septal part of the basal ganglia (Risold & Swanson, 1996). (For further discussion on the role of the hippocampus in learning, see the section on learning and memory in the previous chapter (Chapter 4)).

Brainstem

The brainstem is located at the "base" of the brain and includes the midbrain, pons, and medulla. All the cranial nerves controlling ocular muscles, facial movement, and sensation, tongue movements, and the apparatus of speech and swallowing, originate in the brainstem, and many important motor and sensory tracts traverse it. The medulla regulates the body's autonomic functions, including respiration, circulation, and digestion. The brainstem's contribution to the information processing scheme is through its role as a conveyer of afferent somatosensory information and efferent motor fibers to the muscles. Most important, the brainstem has a central role in the modulation of wakefulness, sleep, and vigilance, sometimes referred to as maintaining the "tone" and vigilance of the cortex (Moruzzi & Magoun, 1949), which is important in overall cognitive functioning. Brainstem lesions may cause disturbance of wakefulness, vigilance, and attention, and thus disturb the information processing sequence. Normal sleep is characterized by synchronization of cortical neurons. During the transitions from sleep to wakefulness this synchronization breaks up, marked in the electroencephalogram (EEG) by the replacement of high-voltage slow waves with low-voltage fast activity. This activation of the EEG during arousal may be produced by afferent stimuli traversing the brainstem, which arouse the subject to alertness. Electroencephalogram changes seemingly identical with those observed during physiological arousal reactions can be produced by direct stimulation of the reticular formation of the brainstem or lesions of this system (Moruzzi & Magoun, 1949). The integrity of the brainstem is necessary for maintenance of the sleep–wake cycle, arousal and vigilance, which are essential for normal information processing and learning.

The Cerebellum

The cerebellum plays a major role in motor functions, especially in motor coordination, motor planning, and programming and execution of movement. Cerebellar dysfunction causes extensive motor and coordination problems, including the inability to perform motor functions such as walking or writing in a coordinated manner, using a spoon, or opening a door with a key, thus interfering with daily adaptive functions. Neuropsychological studies in patients with cerebellar syndromes provide evidence of cerebellar participation in motor learning (Fischbach, 1994). More recent research demonstrates that the cerebellum may also be involved in cognitive processes not directly related to motor movement and coordination. Patients with cerebellar lesions demonstrate non-motor deficits in various areas, including problem solving, error detection and language, and possibly attention. Anatomical experiments demonstrate that neurons in the cerebellum innervate areas of the cerebral cortex involved in cognitive function. Researchers used a technique for demonstrating neuronal pathways by retrograde transneuronal transport of herpes simplex virus type 1 (HSV1). By injecting HSV1 to the prefrontal cortex, neurons in other brain areas that connect to this region are labeled. Thus it was found that neurons in the dentate nucleus of the cerebellum (and the basal ganglia) project to this prefrontal cortical area, with possible contribution to cognitive processing such as working memory, learning, and planning future behavior (Middleton & Strick, 1994, 1997). The cerebellum may also be involved in learning the timing of movements (Raymond, Lisberger, & Mank, 1996). Perceptual and motor cognitive tasks involve the analysis of temporal information with precise timing. Temporal information processing may, therefore, be a critical issue in learning and, consequently, in learning disabilities. There are multiple timing mechanisms in the brain, representing a kind of internal clock. It is believed that the cerebellum is the critical neural structure associated with this timing mechanism, although the cerebellum's timing capabilities may be limited to a range only relevant for motor control (Ivry & Keele, 1989).

Other studies found a role for the cerebellum in improving motor performance only.

NORMAL BRAIN DEVELOPMENT

Introduction

Brain structure and physiology are constantly changing during development, the period of our life when intensive learning takes place. This is probably also the period during which events resulting in SLDs presumably occur. Therefore, normal and abnormal brain development is of enormous importance in the study of SLDs. Methodological complexities are also derived from the fact that the brain changes constantly during development. It means that during the period of infancy, childhood, and adolescence, which is also a period of schooling and intense learning—brain anatomy is an ever-changing substrate, evolving with age. Therefore, what we can observe with still pictures of the brain may not explain why there is normal or abnormal learning. A functional anatomical observation at one age may not be valid for an older or a younger age and projection from data obtained in adults to the pediatric and adolescent age group is not always valid.

Stages and Sequence of Brain Development

Brain development starts in the first weeks of gestation, and continues throughout intrauterine life and into childhood and adolescence until the second decade of life. Although development of the main brain structures and neuronal migration, occur in utero, a significant proportion of brain growth and development in humans takes place after birth.

Brain development is a vast and complex subject and will not be discussed here in detail. It starts very early in gestation and follows an orderly detailed sequence. The development of the central nervous system starts with the neural plate which gives rise to the neural tube. The neural crest is another developing neural element located dorsal to the neural tube. Neurons migrating from the neural crest create the peripheral and autonomic nervous system and some endocrine and thymus elements. The main brain structures are grossly developed by the end of the first trimester of pregnancy.

In the central nervous system—the neural tube divides further into the cerebrum, cerebellum, and spinal cord. The germinal zone, where neural and glial precursors are creted, forms inside the neural tube, adjacent to the lateral ventricles.

The next developmental stage is neuronal migration, the movement of neurons from their birthplace, the germinal zone, into their appropriate cortical locations. These neurons, the central elements of the nervous system, migrate to their precise locations in different layers in the cortex. Cellular migration to

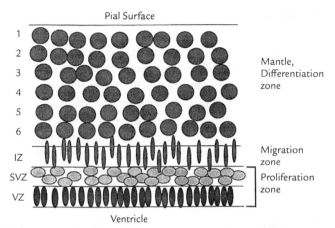

Figure 5-6:
Organization of proliferative and differentiation zones within the wall of the neural tube. This scheme shows developing cerebral neocortex. The proliferative zones (ventricular zone [VZ] and subventricular zone [SVZ]) are adjacent to the ventricle. Postmitotic cells migrate from the proliferation zones, through the intermediate zone (IZ) and stop migrating in the mantle, where differentiation is completed. The cerebral cortex is a laminar structure (six major layers); cells in the deeper layers (for example, layer 6) are generally born before cells in the superficial layers.
Source: Neurobiology of mental illness, 3rd ed. Edited by Dennis Charney and Eric Nestler. New York: Oxford University Press. Print: ISBN-13 9780199798261. Publication date: April 2011.

the cortex starts at 6 to 8 weeks of gestational age and is completed between the sixth and eighth fetal months (Figure 5.6).

At their final cortical location, the neurons grow, differentiate, and mature, and establish synaptic connections through their dendrites and axons. Neuronal differentiation begins at the 16th gestational week, before cell migration is completed and continues into postnatal life.

The next stage of brain development–myelination starts in utero but continues into the second decade, in an orderly manner, with a different pace and timetable for different brain areas. The myelin is a fatty material that engulfs the neuronal processes and allows information to flow efficiently between neurons. To a large degree, the development of motor, sensory and cognitive functions and behavior follows the developmental progress of myelination. The axons of the primary sensory and motor areas of the cerebral cortex are among the first to myelinate, allowing for the basic perception of stimuli and motor activity. The unimodal association areas (the cortical areas involved in the interpretation of stimuli related to a single sensory modality, for example, visual or auditory) myelinate next, and those of the "tertiary," polymodal association areas in the parietal-temporal and prefrontal regions (the cortical areas involved in the integration of multiple sensory and cognitive modalities), as well as the connections between various cortical areas, myelinate last. The prefrontal cortex may not become fully myelinated until puberty (Fuster, 1995).

Connectivity: The Process of Selection

Even though neurons arrive at their appropriate destinations and neuronal processes are fully myelinated, no significant sensory, motor, or cognitive activity can take place unless the brain's 100 billion neurons are connected. Synaptogenesis, an elaborate process of synapse formation and connectivity, starts once the neurons finish their migration and get to their appropriate destination. Synaptogenesis is a complex developmental process. The specific and intricate way in which the neurons are connected with one another determines the extent and quality of our perceptual and cognitive abilities (Shatz, 1992).

Connections between neurons are created, lost, and reorganized during different stages of brain development in a process that includes programmed cell death. One of the ways cell death occurs is through the scarcity of synaptic sites. A great excess of neurons is produced in fetal life. The number of synaptic sites in the cortex is smaller than the number of migrating neurons. Programmed cell death helps to match the number of approaching neurons with available synaptic sites. There are specific recognition properties that place some cells at an advantage in establishing connections. If two presynaptic cells have equal affinity for the postsynaptic site, the one arriving first has a greater chance of surviving, whereas the other neuron may die.

The phenomenon of matching presynaptic axons with neurons was studied in the visual cortex of the Rhesus monkey. The advancing tips of the axons arriving at a brain region have to select their target neuron and make the appropriate connection. One hypothesis for the process of selection is that trophic factors or signaling molecules attract advancing axons to particular neurons. There may be many axons aiming for the same neuron. The "competition" between these axons will end with only one of them connecting to the target and the permanent removal of all other axons (Gan & Lichtman, 1998). The balance between the development and elimination of synapses and axons determines the final size and form of a given pathway. Other factors that determine the final "wiring diagram" may be genetic and physiological events that occur in the brain during development, including the level of activity of the synapse. If a synapse in intrauterine life is busy with external or intrinsic stimuli traversing it, it has a better chance of survival (Catalino & Shatz, 1998). The interaction with the environment during early life, and possibly during the prenatal period, plays, therefore, a very important role in brain development. The final brain microstructures emerge through the process involving genes-circuits-experience, which takes place during brain development. In the visual system the lateral geniculate body differs in its connectivity between the immature and adult brain; specific layers do not exist initially, but are later present in the adult.

This may be, among others, an important factor in the pathophysiology of SLDs.

The physiology of the visual system consists of visual information being transmitted from the retina through the optic nerve, from the optic chiasm to the lateral geniculate body in the thalamus, from there through the optic radiation to the occipital cortex, and from there to other cortical areas, where further processing of visual information takes place. The transmission of this neural information is through neural processes and synapses. It was shown that to achieve its full functional development, the visual cortex needs to have "visual experience" during critical periods of early life. Prenatally, such experiences may be obtained through the generation of intrinsic spontane-ous synaptic activity inside the retina, whereas postnatally this experience is obtained from external visual stimuli (Shatz, 1992; Feller et al., 1996). The effect of internal prenatal experience in the retina is different from the exter-nal postnatal experience. Although the internal activity elicits coordinated action potentials in the retina, this activity disappears when the eye opens to the world. These early spontaneous neural retinal activities may be essen-tial to the function of certain genes, such as MHC-1 (major histocompatibility complex-1), which translates such activity into neural structure and to the regulation of synapses in response to activity and are therefore important for normal later neural development. When activity was blocked MHC-1 was down regulated.

In the absence of such critical experience, the structural as well as func-tional development of the visual cortex is abnormal, affecting visual percep-tion (Fuster, 1995). Lack of visual experience because of visual depravation in early life may cause structural developmental abnormalities of the visual cortex.

Studies of the behavioral and electrophysiological effects of early visual deprivation in cats and monkeys utilized blocked visual input to the retina by eye closure during a critical period of development (Wiesel & Hubel, 1965). This caused fewer action potentials to be generated in the retina of the closed eye. The result was that axons from both eyes were not organized in the cor-rect patterns, leading to abnormal development and abnormal function of the visual cortex.

Other animal studies confirmed the observation that lack of early sen-sory experience can interfere with normal behavior in later life, presumably because of the effect it has on the development of neural connectivity. When animals raised with sensory deprivation were compared with those raised in an enriched sensory environment, the latter were superior in perform-ing a number of behavioral tasks. There were also corresponding effects on the development of the cortex. Cortical neurons in the animals raised in an enriched environment had more dendritic branches and spines compared with those raised in an environment without sensory stimulation. Dendritic

branches and spines are the extensions of the neuron important in establishing connections with axons and other neurons and creating the neural
networks that determine cognition and behavior. Similar experiences exist
in humans. Children born blind because of congenital cataracts who underwent correction of their cataracts and were then able to see for the first time
had significant difficulties understanding what they saw. The reasons for that
include the fact that their visual cortex lacked the essential visual experience
needed for the normal development of the connectivity of the neural cortex.
In another reported study, functional brain MRI of subjects during sentence
processing in English and American Sign Language did not display activation
of language areas of the left hemisphere. These results suggest that the early
acquisition of a natural language is important in the expression of the strong
bias for these areas to mediate language (Neville & Bavelier, 1998).

THE NEUROANATOMY OF SPECIFIC READING DISABILITIES
Introduction

There are many examples of acquired focal brain damage causing a selective cognitive or learning abnormality without causing global dementia or a
total inability to learn. For example, in adults, acquired lesions of the angular gyrus, in the parietal lobe, can in some cases cause alexia—the loss of
the ability to read. Similarly, a left parietal lesion can cause Gerstmann syndrome—the co-occurrence of acalculia, agraphia, and right–left disorientation. Lesions of the prefrontal areas may cause specific disturbances in the
regulation and control of behavior without causing generalized brain dysfunction affecting intelligence. In the famous case of Phineas Gage described
about 150 years ago (1848), an acquired lesion of the frontal lobes caused a
dramatic change in behavior and personality (Damasio, Grabowski, Frank,
Galaburda, & Damasio, 1994). Phineas Gage was a 25-year-old foreman for a
New England railroad, who had an accident in which a tamping rod flew and
hit his face, entered the skull behind his left eye, and exited at the top of his
skull. He lost his eye, but otherwise had a good physical recovery. The most
significant effect of his injury was a change in his behavior and personality.
Before the accident he had been socially responsible and hard working. The
accident changed his character. He began using profane language, lied to his
friends, could not be trusted to honor his commitments, "could no longer
make ethical decisions," and, in general, stopped conforming to the acceptable social conventions. His memory and intelligence, though, remained
intact. Examination of his brain after his death revealed that the rod pierced
and damaged both frontal lobes causing the cognitive and behavioral symptoms. These examples demonstrate that focal brain abnormalities, such as

those following a stroke, head trauma, or resection of a brain tumor can cause specific cognitive deficiencies.

Specific learning disabilities (e.g., dyslexia or dyscalculia) are conceptually "selective" or "focal" brain abnormalities, and do not involve pervasive or generalized brain dysfunction. Therefore, it can be assumed that similar to adult cases with focal brain damage, in SLD there is a selective brain abnormality affecting specific areas or networks and causing selective cognitive deficits. These cognitive deficits cause a specific learning disability. There has been an expectation that detailed anatomical studies will reveal the location and type of such abnormalities. However, there is a significant difference between SLDs and acquired focal brain damage. The difference is the nature of brain differences underlying SLDs. These are typically not the result of brain damage but the outcome of developmental aberrations, which occur during the period of brain development. The goals of biological studies of SLDs are to identify these brain abnormalities, and assess the etiology and timing of occurrence.

A recent neuropsychological model of learning disabilities (see chapter 2) assumes that brain functions are modular, that unique brain systems specialize in processing specific kinds of information, and that these brain systems are differentially susceptible to developmental insults (Pennington, 1991). It suggests that the brain systems that are impaired in the different types of learning disabilities are phonological processing, spatial recognition, social cognition, executive functions, and long-term memory. These systems emerge in early life and are "differentially vulnerable" to insults (Fodor, 1983). For instance, dyslexia is the learning disability caused by an abnormality of the system of phonological processing, whereas mathematic disability may be caused by an abnormality of the system of spatial cognition. Similarly, attention deficit disorder is an abnormality of the system of executive functions, and autistic spectrum disorder is an abnormality of the social cognition system.

These cognitive systems or modules of learning are localized in different brain regions. Pennington suggests the location of the left perisylvian region for phonological processing; the posterior right hemisphere for spatial cognition; and amygdala and hippocampus for memory systems. (He also suggests the location of the prefrontal areas for attention deficit hyperactivity disorder, and the limbic, orbital, and right hemisphere for autism). The different modules of learning have different susceptibility to "disruption by genetic and environmental factors," with executive functions and phonological processing being the most vulnerable systems to mental and genetic insults because their evolution has been more recent (Pennington, 1991).

We also have to consider the possibility that anatomical abnormalities detected in cases of SLDs are already brain modifications or adaptations to an abnormality that occurred earlier, possibly in utero.

Although the concepts underlying this model may be valid, the relationship of a specific learning disability to a corresponding cognitive system, and to a specific brain anatomical localization is not a simple one. The aim of the following chapters is to report anatomical abnormalities detected in SLDs, using a variety of imaging techniques, and discuss whether empirical proof exists for brain localizations of SLDs.

Structural Anatomical Abnormalities

Hemispheral Asymmetries

A major focus of imaging studies in SLDs was, initially, the measurement of hemispheral asymmetry of various brain areas including the areas around the sylvian fissure, areas in the temporal cortex, the occipital cortex (Hier et al., 1978), and the caudate nuclei. One reason for the focus on hemispheral asymmetry was the issue of cerebral dominance and the capacity of each side of the brain to acquire a particular skill. The left hemisphere is usually dominant for language and manual skills, whereas the right hemisphere is more involved in certain spatial and musical abilities (Geschwind & Galaburda, 1985). A unilateral lesion in the early periods of brain development may cause loss or shift of function. An early attempt to find a morphological correlate of dyslexia was made by Geschwind and Levitzky (1968) and Galaburda et al. (1978). The most common type of abnormality found was the lack of the normal hemispheral asymmetry of the planum temporale and corpus callosum.

PLANUM TEMPORALE

The planum temporale is the superior posterior surface of the temporal lobe. In the left hemisphere, it is a part of the language area and may be involved in auditory comprehension. In the majority of people the plenum temporale is larger on the left. In an unselected autopsy population, its surface area was larger on the left in 65%, on the right in 10% and symmetrical in 25% (Geschwind & Levitsky, 1968). This observed asymmetry has been documented as early as 33 weeks of gestation, suggesting a biological prenatal mechanism. Similarly, early imaging studies (CT and MRI) demonstrated an asymmetry favoring the left planum temporale, auditory cortex, and speech region in two-thirds of normal adult brains. Postmortem studies of brains of dyslexic people revealed predominance of symmetrical plenum temporale. The symmetry was due to larger than normal areas on the right side, rather than smaller areas on the left. Imaging studies of dyslexic people have replicated the autopsy findings and commonly demonstrate reversal of the usual planum asymmetry. Hynd et al. in one of the first quantitative MRI studies of dyslex-ics, found that 90% had symmetrical plana, whereas only 30% of normal sub-jects or those with attention deficit hyperactivity disorder demonstrated this pattern (Hynd et al., 2003). Similarly, an early brain MRI study of young men with persistent, severe developmental dyslexia demonstrated that the volume of the temporal lobes was symmetrical in most cases. Other neuroradiologi-cal studies have confirmed these findings. Correlations were found between planum temporale asymmetry patterns, measures of language processing, and measures of reading (Hugdahl et al., 2003). For instance, a significant correla-tion between a reading achievement measure, the Woodcock-Johnson Passage Comprehension scores, and asymmetry of the posterior superior surface of the temporal lobe, was found in dyslexic subjects. Those with higher scores had more leftward asymmetry, and conversely, those with lower reading scores had less leftward asymmetry, suggesting that, among dyslexics, the direction of this asymmetry may serve as a risk factor and/or a marker for the severity of reading comprehension problems (Kushch et al., 1993).

There may be a link between these findings and the higher prevalence of left-handedness among dyslexics. Normal left hemisphere dominance is usu-ally associated with right-handedness. Indeed, most people are right-handed, corresponding to a dominant left hemisphere. In dyslexic people there may be a developmental abnormality of the left hemisphere with loss of domi-nance, developmental language processing abnormality, reading abnormal-ity, a shift of motor dominance from the left to the right hemisphere, and left-handedness.

It was suggested that the normal asymmetry of the planum temporale results from an asymmetrical developmental neuronal loss, with a greater "pruning" down of the right side during late fetal life and infancy. Hemispheral symmetry reflects failure of this asymmetrical cell loss to occur.

As is the case with all neuroanatomical research in dyslexia, there have been conflicting reports. A significant number of studies demonstrate that individuals with dyslexia do not exhibit symmetry or reversed asymmetry of the planum temporale (Leonard et al., 1993; Best & Demb, 1999; Robichon et al., 2000a). In some, the symmetry of brain structures in these subjects was due to small left plana, rather than to increased size of the right (Rumsey, Nace, Donohue, Wise, Maisong, & Andreason, 1997; Eckert, 2003).

Factors including sex, age, handedness, and definition of dyslexia, and the methods used to acquire images and define and measure brain anatomical regions of interest, including the planum temporale, may play an important role in the results of these studies. For instance, morphometric MRI, which compared the convolutional surface area of the planum temporale, temporal lobe volume and superior surface area, in a homogeneous sample of dyslexic children and unimpaired children, found substantial sex and age differences for all measured regions, with all the measurements in boys being significantly larger. An analysis controlling for age and overall brain size revealed no significant differences between dyslexics and unimpaired children on a variety of measures, in particular in surface area and symmetry of the planum temporale. This suggests that the structural differences found between dyslexics and normal readers may be age and sex dependent (Filipek, 1996).

ASYMMETRIES IN OTHER CORTICAL AREAS

There have been reports of deviations from the usual pattern of asymmetry in other brain areas of reading disabled people. These include reports on reduction of the normal asymmetry of other temporoparietal regions posterior to the planum temporale (Eckert, 2003); inferior frontal area (Jernigan, Hesselink, Sowekk, & Tallal, 1991); and areas 44 and 45.

As is the case with studies of the corpus callosum and planum temporale, there are other studies reporting no differences between dyslexics and normal readers (Hynd et al., 1990).

Corpus Callosum Abnormalities

Many brain tasks require communications between the left and the right hemisphere, which is carried out by axons traversing the corpus callosum—the major communication pathway between the hemispheres. Congenital abnormalities of the corpus callosum are recognized including an absence (agenesis) or partial agenesis. Damage to the corpus callosum can also be caused early in life by asphyxia or infection. Abnormalities of the corpus callosum (CC) are associated with various degrees of neurological abnormalities, including seizures and cognitive deficits. In mice, the size of the CC relates to morphological asymmetry of the cerebral cortex: Those animals with deficits in or an absence of a CC do not exhibit anatomical cortical asymmetry, a finding that may be associated with cognitive deficits.

Reading may involve inter-hemisphere transfer of information. The posterior part of the corpus callosum, the splenium, contains axons linking the planum temporale and the angular gyrus, which are important areas for language processing and reading. It is, therefore, conceivable that an abnormality of the corpus callosum may interfere with normal reading.

Neuroimaging studies on C.C. morphology and size in dyslexics reported conflicting findings. Some reported size differences between dyslexics and normally reading individuals, including a smaller anterior section (the genu), or a larger posterior section, the splenium, in dyslexic children (Hynd et al., 1995, Duara et al., 1991), although a subsequent study of dyslexic adolescents failed to confirm the latter finding. Other studies reported abnormally shaped isthmus (Rubichon & Habib, 1998; Von Plessen et al., 2002). An MRI study measuring the mid-sagittal surface area of the corpus callosum in children with learning disabilities, found callosa that were highly variable in size. Children with familial dysphasia or dyslexia had a thicker corpus callosum compared with learning disabled children who had perinatal adverse events. Corpus callosum size did not correlate with the severity of the learning difficulties. Other studies could not demonstrate any significant size differences between groups of dyslexics and controls (Larsen, Hoien, & Lundberg, 1990; Schultz et al., 1994).

Methodological factors may be responsible for some of the differences between studies, and interfere with conclusions: The range of subjects' age was not uniform, and controls were not matched for sex, handedness, socio-economic status, intellectual ability, or educational experience. The size, as well as the shape of various brain structures is different for males and females, for children and adults. Factors that influence such differences include genetic as well as environmental factors. A large MRI study observed significant sex differences in the shape of the corpus callosum, with the splenium being more bulbous shaped in females and more tubular shaped in males (Allen, Richey, Chai, & Gorsky, 1991).

There were no significant differences in the surface area of the CC or its subdivisions. These sex differences in bulbosity did not reach significance in children (2–16 years). The area of the corpora callosa increased significantly with age in children and decreased significantly with age in adults. The study authors speculated that male/female differences may be related to the effects of gonadal hormones during a critical period of development that influence the survival of neurons in sexually dimorphic nuclei (Allen et al., 1991).

Methodological problems of this nature, and the lack of uniformity in the selection of patients for the studies and in the imaging methods, affect many biological studies of learning disabilities (Filipek, 1996).

CHAPTER 6

Neuroanatomy of Specific Reading Disabilities II

Morphometry-Volumetric Studies

INTRODUCTION

More detailed morphological imaging studies of dyslexia were done using volumetric methods. Voxel-based morphometry (VBM) is a technique characterizing regional cerebral volume and tissue concentration differences in magnetic resonance imaging. Volumetric analysis can be done in two ways: with pre-chosen specific voxels or whole brain voxel-based analysis. Whole brain voxel-based analysis investigates the whole brain rather than looking at specific brain structures, and has the advantage of not limiting the analysis to predefined neuroanatomical regions.

Leonard and colleagues (2001) examined the morphology of language-related brain areas in a group of dyslexic college students who were characterized by a discrepancy between their poor phonological decoding ability and better reading comprehension. Compared with controls, dyslexic subjects were more likely to exhibit a duplication of the left Heschl gyrus, extreme leftward asymmetry of the planum temporale, small right cerebellar anterior lobes, and leftward cerebral asymmetry (Leonard et al., 2001). The probability of a dyslexia diagnosis increased with the additional presence of each of these anatomical measures). There were no frontal lobe measurements in this study. This effect may have been due to decreased gray matter rather than white matter.

A whole brain voxel-based analysis study (Brown et al., 2001) was performed with 16 young adult men with dyslexia and 14 matched control subjects, and showed evidence of decreased gray matter in many brain areas of the dyslexic subjects, including the left inferior, middle, superior, and mesial temporal region, mostly in the left posterior superior temporal gyrus (STG), and bilaterally in the temporal-parietal-occipital juncture, and in the frontal lobe (mostly left orbital gyrus and frontal pole, and bilaterally in the inferior frontal gyri bilaterally), in subcortical areas, including the head of the caudate and thalamus bilaterally. A reduction in gray matter in dyslexic patients was also found in the semilunar lobules of the cerebellum.

The findings of this study were consistent with other studies that described abnormal patters of activation of the middle and inferior regions of the left temporal lobe in dyslexics' brains (Rumsey, 1997; Georgiewa et al., 2002), but this study reveals more widespread differences, both in the cerebrum and the cerebellum, as well as changes in the basal ganglia of dyslexic subjects.

Are the changes in the brains of dyslexics widespread and do they involve the basal ganglia and cerebellum? Recent studies implicated the cerebellum in perceptual and cognitive processes, including semantic and phonological processing (Fulbright et al., 1999). Also, there are interactions between the caudate and prefrontal cortex suggesting that basal ganglia structures may be involved in cognitive processing (Parent & Hazrati, 1995).

A later study (Eckert et al., 2003) had MRI examination of a number of brain regions in 19 dyslexic children, grades 4 to 6, from a family genetics study, who were impaired in phonological coding, orthographical coding, and rapid automatic naming-three markers associated with the language phenotype for dyslexia (Berninger et al., 2001), and comparing them to controls (19 males, 13 females, with no reading abnormalities). Anatomic measurements of their posterior temporal lobe, inferior frontal gyrus, cerebellum, and whole brain were collected. The dyslexic children exhibited significantly smaller brain volume, right anterior lobes of the cerebellum, and pars triangularis bilaterally. Measures of the right cerebellar anterior lobe and the left and right pars triangularis correctly classified 72% of the dyslexic subjects (94% of whom had a rapid automatic naming deficit) and 88% of the controls (after controlling for brain volume). The anatomical variables that differentiated dyslexic from control subjects were consistently significantly correlated with real word reading, pseudoword reading, and spelling, the three language skills on which the dyslexic children were reliably different from the controls. Of the four reading-related language processes (phoneme and orthographical coding, rapid automated naming [RAN], and rapid automated spelling [RAS]) only RAN was consistently significantly correlated with the anatomical measures that distinguished dyslexic from control participants.

This study demonstrates that measures of the right cerebellar anterior lobe and inferior frontal gyrus distinguished dyslexic children from controls with a high probability, and that anomalies in a cerebellar-frontal circuit are associated with rapid automatic naming (Eckert et al., 2003). Measures of the temporal lobe did not differentiate dyslexic from control participants.

A magnetic resonance imaging study using the same method of voxel-based morphometry to examine gray matter volume differences was performed by a group of Italian researchers with 10 familial adolescents and adult dyslexics belonging to four different families (Brambati et al., 2004). The proband from each family had persistent, severe developmental dyslexia. There was, in addition, at least one first-degree relative with either clinically evident or compensated dyslexia (a positive history of reading problems and difficulties and discomfort in reading and associated impairments in meta-phonological skills and in short-term memory). The control group was composed of 11 non–reading-impaired subjects (6 females, 5 males; age range 14 to 55 years, mean 27.4 years). This mixed adult–children study of patients with familial dyslexia reported regional reductions of gray matter volume in the dyslexic subjects in comparison with controls, in the planum temporale, and cerebellar nuclei bilaterally, in the left superior and inferior temporal gyrus, and in the right middle temporal gyrus. There was a regional pattern of gray matter increase and decrease. In the left middle temporal cortex there was reduced gray matter surrounded by a region, more posteriorly and inferiorly, with higher density. In other studies, the left temporal areas, primarily middle and inferior temporal gyri, have been found to have reduced activation), to tasks requiring phonological retrieval (Price et al., 1996; Poldrack et al., 1999; Jobard et al., 2003). The authors suggested that these areas of localized gray matter volume reductions were "critical functional components of the posterior reading network." In novel readers, grapheme-to-phoneme conversion mechanisms play a central role in the decoding of written language, and parietal-occipital brain areas are important. In expert readers, the recognition of the abstract orthographical representation of familial words is important for the rapid access to the meaning and phonological representations; therefore, inferior-temporal regions, which are related to whole-word recognition, are active. Also, the cerebellum has been suggested to play a key role in reading, both at the peripheral (eye movements) and central level of written language processing.

Silani et al. (2005) tested sporadic adults with well-compensated dyslexia in a sample derived from three different countries (the United Kingdom, France, and Italy), with three different orthographies, using VBM. Gray and white matter densities were compared with reading performance. A significant reduction of gray matter density was detected in the left middle temporal gyrus (BA 21). A significant increase of gray matter density was detected in a region of the left middle temporal gyrus posterior to the area of gray matter reduction (BA 37) with a negative correlation with reading. No gray matter density change was found in the cerebellar location identified by Nicholson et al. (1999). There was a reduction of white matter density for the dyslexia subjects in the frontal and parietal portion of the arcuate fasciculus in the depth of left Broca's area (underneath BA 44, P = .02) in the left post central gyrus, and a trend of reduction of WM in the arcuate fasciculus in the depth of the supramarginal gyrus.

The same subjects had a previous positron emission tomography (PET) activation study during reading tasks that demonstrated altered activation within the reading system in the left temporal and temporal-occipital area (Paulscu et al., 2001). Using both VBM and PET done during the performance of specific tasks in dyslexia, in the same patients, helps to assess whether the altered activation seen in tests like the PET scan is related to detectable morphological abnormalities of gray and white matter densities.

This study showed that the same brain areas (in the same subjects) that were found to be dysfunctional functionally are also anatomically different.

There are differences and decreased volume in the inferior frontal gyri between dyslexic and control adults (Brown et al., 2001; Eckert et al., 2003). Left and right PTR are smaller in dyslexic than in control children. Gauger and colleagues (1997) also reported smaller PTR measurements in children with specific language impairment. These findings support the idea that early frontal lobe dysfunction may play a role in the development of dyslexia.

Frontal lobe dysfunction is the centerpiece of the motor-articulatory feedback hypothesis for dyslexia (Heilman et al., 1996). This hypothesis maintains that an inability to associate the position of articulators with speech sounds is due to a lack of awareness regarding the position of articulators during speech. While unaffected subjects had normal activation of the inferior frontal gyrus during grapheme-to-phoneme conversion (Newman & Twieg, 2001; Fiebach et al., 2002), this region is abnormally activated in dyslexic subjects (Shaywitz et al., 1998; Georgiewa et al., 2002). Also, patients with left anterior perisylvian lesions are not capable of making grapheme-to-phoneme conversions (Adair et al., 1999).

Another important finding is the comparison between studies of dyslexic children and dyslexic college students (Leonard et al., 2001; Eckert et al., 2003). The two groups had anatomical differences: The dyslexic children had smaller brain volumes than controls and an absence of duplicated left Heschl's gyrus or extreme leftward asymmetry of the PT and planum parietale. On a functional level, the dyslexic college students had superior passage comprehension and rapid naming performance compared with the dyslexic children in this study. A possible explanation for these differences is that the passage comprehension and rapid naming difficulties disappeared with age as the dyslexic children learn to compensate for their reading problems. The improving reading functions of college-age dyslexics were accompanied by anatomical brain changes. Alternatively, In this case, failure to replicate could be an artifact of the type of study (Leonard et al., 2001). The one anatomical measure that was comparable in the child and adult dyslexics was that of the right cerebellar anterior lobe. The age difference in that area was possibly due to decreased gray matter (Leonard et al., 2001). Similarly, Rae and colleagues (2002) reported that dyslexic adults failed to exhibit rightward whole cerebellum gray matter asymmetry, in part as a result of reduced volume of right cerebellar gray matter.

In summary, studies differ in many aspects related to the choice of the population of dyslexic subjects chosen for the study, but demonstrate some common findings. There is reduced brain grey matter in subjects with dyslexia in a number of brain areas including the left temporal lobe, left inferior frontal area and cerebellar areas. There is a suggestion of white matter reduction although not repeatedly reported in these studies, and of basal ganglia involvement. There is a suggestion of brain volumetric differences in adolescents and young adults, compared with children with dyslexia, concomitant with improvement of reading parameters.

CHAPTER 7

Neuroanatomy of Specific Reading Disabilities III

Diffusion Tensor Imaging

INTRODUCTION

Diffusion tensor imaging (DTI) is a neuroimaging method that demonstrates the degree and direction of water diffusion within individual voxels of the magnetic resonance image, providing clues to the structure of the tissues. Diffusion is isotropic (equal in all directions) in cerebrospinal fluid. It is anisotropic (greater in one direction than the other directions) in the white matter which is comprised of the myelinated axons organized into fiber bundles, because cell structure impedes the rate of diffusion perpendicular to the directional orientation of the axon fibers, while leaving the rate of diffusion parallel to the axon relatively unhindered, thus making the diffusion anisotropic. In cerebral gray matter, internal cellular structures and cell membranes slow the rate of diffusion in comparison with the rate in cerebrospinal fluid, but diffusion remains isotropic (equal in all directions). This quantitative information about the degree and direction of water diffusion within the magnetic resonance image, allows, by inference, the visualization and characterization of the white matter tracts in vivo. and provides information about the integrity of white matter and brain connectivity (Feldman et al., 2010). A high level of myelination causes more restriction of water diffusion perpendicular to the orientation of the axons. Therefore, a high index of anisotropy is considered an indication of a normal or mature white matter microstructure.

Diffusion tensor imaging is analyzed using the following measurements: mean diffusivity (net degree of displacement of the water molecules measured in micrometers per ms), degree of anisotropy (or fractional anisotropy, FA), and the main direction of diffusibility (orientation in space of the tissue structure). These DTI Measures can be applied throughout the brain or to regions of interest, and can be compared with normal control measures. The direction of diffusibility can also be demonstrated by color coding each voxel based on the principal diffusion direction. The resulting maps provide an indicator of whether the white matter tracts are properly oriented.

A three-dimensional visualization of white matter tracts is done through diffusion tensor tractography by sequentially piecing together the estimates of fiber orientation from the directionality of individual voxels. Tractography identifies the tracts and fibers that connect specific cortical or subcortical structures. Diffusion tensor-magnetic resonance imaging tractography (DT-MRI) is the only technique that allows the identification of large pathways and assessment of microstructural integrity of white matter in the living human brain. It can be used to compare equivalent fiber connections across individual and to study the development of white matter maturation and the development of tracts and commissures. Studies have shown correspondence between tractography-derived anatomy of white matter pathways and classical postmortem descriptions. Still, DT-MRI tractography offers only indirect indices of tissue properties, and the relationship between tractography measurements and underlying biological factors is not complete.

DTI methods have been used to link features of white matter maturation to cognitive function. Findings suggest that increases in fiber organization and axonal density support or reflect increased global cognitive abilities. Increased restriction in diffusion in frontal-striatal regions predicted faster reaction times on go/no go tasks, a paradigm that requires response inhibition, in children and adults age 7 to 31 years, even after controlling for age and accuracy (Liston, Watts, et al., 2006).

There may be gender differences in DTI (for instance white matter volume increases faster in males); therefore, male-female differences need to be considered.

APPLICATION OF DIFFUSION TENSOR IMAGING TO THE STUDY OF HEMISPHERAL ASYMMETRY

Previous studies have shown direct correspondence between tractography-derived anatomy of white matter pathways and postmortem descriptions. In humans, left–right differences have been linked to the development of language. Geschwind and Levitsky found an asymmetry of the size of the planum temporale, the region of the posterior superior temporal gyrus that is classically associated with language lateralization, in 65% of the population. However, Dorsaint-Pierre et al. (2006) found that the leftward lateralization of the planum temporale does not correlate with language lateralization as assessed by sodium Amytal. Several studies have reported a higher prevalence of leftward asymmetry of perisylvian white matter volumes. Lateralization of the direct segment of the arcuate fasciculus is high (>80%), higher than that reported for the planum temporale (65%). Therefore, asymmetry of the direct segment of the arcuate fasciculus may represent a key anatomical substrate for language lateralization. Recent DT-MRI investigations have revealed three important parts of the language network: a direct pathway connecting Wernicke's territory in the left temporal lobe with Broca's territory in the left frontal lobe through the arcuate fasciculus; an indirect pathway consisting of two segments, an anterior segment linking Broca's territory with the inferior parietal lobe (Geschwind's territory); and a posterior segment linking Geschwind's territory with Wernicke's territory.

A recent study (Catani et al., 2007) used DT-MRI tractography to examine the lateralization of these pathways and possible behavioral advantages related to the degree of lateralization. The study found interhemispheric differences in the white matter anatomy of perisylvian language networks with a very different connection pattern in the left hemisphere compared with the right, with only the left hemisphere connections containing a direct segment. Individuals with more symmetrical patterns of connections and bilateral representation of language networks performed better learning words by semantic association. The authors concluded that "Paradoxically, bilateral representation, not extreme lateralization, might ultimately be advantageous for specific cognitive functions (Catani et al., 2007)." These findings raise more questions regarding the theory of abnormal hemispheral asymmetry as a basis for reading abnormality.

APPLICATION OF DIFFUSION TENSOR IMAGING TO READING

Reading is a highly complex cognitive skill requiring the coordination of multiple distributed brain regions.

Neuroimaging procedures using DT-MRI demonstrated that white matter diffusion anisotropy in the left hemisphere was significantly correlated with reading scores for reading impaired and control readers. Klingberg et al. compared whole brain fractional anisotropy (FA) values between adults with good versus poor reading ability. Poor readers had lower FA values in a region of the temporal-parietal lobe bilaterally compared with good readers. The FA values in this region correlated with reading skills (Klingberg et al., 1999, 2000). Deutsch et al. replicated the results in children age 7 to 13 years with a range of reading abilities. They found that FA in the left parietal-temporal white matter only, correlated with word identification scores (Deutsch et al., 2005).

Diffusion tensor imaging has recently been used to demonstrate a disorganization of neural fascicles located beneath the supramarginal gyrus in dyslexics compared with controls, suggesting that abnormalities in neural structures in dyslexic individuals might not only involve gray matter, but also subcortical connectivity. The best tractography correlation with reading using word identification was in the superior corona radiate in the posterior limb of the internal capsule (Beauliew et al., 2005). Those white matter abnormalities suggest that reading disability may not involve grey matter or grey matter only, and may be a disconnection syndrome (Geschwind, 1965; Catani & Ffytche, 2005).

A case study of an adolescent with radiation-induced tissue necrosis described selective damage to the arcuate fasciculus (a part of the superior longitudinal fasciculus) associated with profound dyslexia (Rauschecker, Deutch, Ben-Shachar, et al., 2009), although another adolescent with a missing arcuate fasciculus after premature delivery had normal reading ability.

Microstructural measures of white matter on DTI in children who were poor readers showed functional improvements in reading after intense remediation (Feldman et al., 2010).

It is unclear whether measures from different centers and different scanners are comparable. In addition, white matter development and myelination are thought to be activity dependent, increasing as pathways are used more frequently or more intensively. Therefore, reduced DTI measures may be a result or a cause of inactivity (Feldman et al., 2010)

FUNCTIONAL IMAGING OF DEVELOPMENTAL LEARNING DISABILITIES

Introduction (Functional brain imaging)

Cerebral blood flow (rCBF) is an indirect measure of neuronal activity. Regional cerebral blood flow is representative of neuronal activity in that region. When rCBF is studied while subjects perform cognitive tasks, including tasks involving language processing or reading, increased rCBF in brain areas that are active during the performance of these tasks is demonstrated.

Functional imaging includes positron emission tomography (PET) and functional magnetic resonance imaging (fMRI). These methods record changes related to rCBF in different areas. Those, as previously stated, are reflective of cerebral activity. Experiments are usually based on the comparison of the signal level between different conditions. In PET, a gamma emitting isotope is injected into the systemic blood supply and its concentration is measured. In fMRI, the principal mode of action is by detection of small fluctuation in the magnetic resonance signal resulting from changes in blood oxygen level associated with brain activation. The "coupling" of functional brain activation, change in blood flow to the region, and change in blood oxygen level, form the basis of the signal obtained with PET and fMRI (Raichle, 1998), although the exact physiological relation between blood flow in gray matter vessels and local variations of neural metabolism is not completely understood (Magistretti & Pellerin, 2000).

The most studied signal in fMRI is known as blood oxygenation level dependent (BOLD). It is based on the measure of changes in magnetic susceptibility of hemoglobin (Ogawa & Lee, 1990). An increase in synaptic metabolism is thought to be followed by a transient drop in oxyhemoglobin concentration, and consequently in the BOLD signal. A major increase in oxyhemoglobin concentration then occurs as a consequence of vessel dilatation, with a peak observed approximately 5 to 6 seconds after stimulus onset time.

Both PET and fMRI have poor temporal resolution relative to typical neural firing rates of neurons (fMRI better than PET). The typical time needed to acquire a single functional brain slice is in the region of 50 ms. However, the repetition time used to acquire more than one functional slice is typically on the order of 2 to 4 seconds, and the time needed to sample the entire hemodynamic response is in the range of 12 seconds. The temporal resolution of the BOLD effect is much higher than that of the PET response.

Performing PET studies with children is difficult because these studies are invasive, involving injection of radioactive material that emits a small dose of radiation. Therefore, PET studies of dyslexics were frequently done in adults with a history of developmental dyslexia. In recent years fMRI has become much more common as the tool for functional brain studies in SLD. The advantages of fMRI over PET include a higher spatial and temporal resolution, and the fact that there is no need for an injection of a radionuclide isotope, so there is no radiation exposure. The latter is especially important for studies designed for children and adolescents.

The results of these studies vary, not the least because they differ in methodology and paradigms.

Functional Neuroanatomy of Language

The search for developmental aberrations of brain anatomy in dyslexia has been influenced by evidence that reading disabilities result from underlying language abnormalities, and it has therefore focused on the neural systems serving language, located in the left hemisphere (Schultz, 1994; Demonet, Thierry, & Cardebat, 2005). As demonstrated in previous chapters, initial studies using brain computed tomography (CT) and MRI scans demonstrated abnormalities that include alterations in the pattern of brain asymmetry of language areas, as well as cortical malformations found in the brains of people with specific learning disabilities.

More specifically, as mentioned previously, the current hypothsis of the origin of specific reading disability is that of a developmental dysfunction of the brain network underlying phonological representations, or connecting phonological and orthographical representations (Paulescu, 1996, 2001; Shaywitz, 1998; Brunswick, McCrory, Price, Frith, & Frith, 1999; McCrory, 2000; Pugh et al., 2000; Temple, 2001; Shaywitz, 2002). Phonological processing (including speech sound awareness and sound–symbol association) play a critical role in successful reading acquisition. Phonological awareness (PA), the ability to identify and mentally manipulate the constituent speech sounds, has been found to predict much of the variance in reading skills. Instruction in speech sound awareness and sound–symbol association are helpful in preventing reading failure. Therefore, research efforts have focused on elucidating the functional neuroanatomy of phonological processing (Eden & Moats, 2002).

This network is primarily in the left hemisphere including the left peri-sylvian brain areas. Brain processing of phonological retrieval in tasks of letter, color, and picture naming occurs in a common neural system initially in the left posterior inferior temporal lobe, and later in the left frontal area (Demonet, Thierry, & Cardebat, 2005). The earlier processing in the left posterior inferior temporal area has a more general function (Price & Devlin, 2003) and is less specific. This area is activated during reading, but it is also activated by a range of tasks that do not engage visual word-form processing, such as naming colors and pictures (Moore & Price, 1999; Chao et al., 2002). Dyslexics who are engaged in phonological tasks such as reading may have abnormal activation in this area (McCrory et al., 2004), but also in other areas, including parts of the lateral frontal cortex (BAs 44, 45, and 47). A language dorsal phonological stream involved in reading starts in the left inferior temporal occipital junction and progresses through the caudal part of the left superior temporal region and the inferior supramarginal gyrus to the left inferior frontal gyrus.

The posterior part of the left superior temporal gyrus can be involved in the extraction, assembly, and storage of sublexical components from auditory input. Similarly, sublexical units of visual information flowing from the visual input are organized by the inferior left temporal occipital junction and inferior parietal lobule. The supramarginal gyrus is an "abstract" area in which higher-order representations derived from sensory inputs or long-term memory are manipulated over short periods of time. This pathway can continue toward the left posterior inferior frontal gyrus (BA 44), which is involved in output programming (LoCasto et al., 2004; Demonet et al., 2005).

There are a number of brain areas involved in syntax processing, including the inferior frontal cortex and/or adjacent areas. Activation in the medial parietal posterior cingulate cortex was found for discourse-level processing, possibly active in linking the current understanding of a story with prior knowledge (LoCasto et al., 2004).

Activation of inferior frontal gyrus near the border of BA44 and BA6 has been associated with "semantic processes" in which listeners must separate speech sounds contained within syllables. When perception of words and pseudo-words were compared, Newman and Tweig (2001) found a network of areas active across the stimuli, including the inferior frontal, superior temporal, and inferior parietal regions.

In normal adults, rCBF in the left temporal region, measured during a task of *word recognition*, was positively correlated with task accuracy (Flowers, Wood, & Naylor, 1991). Deficient performance on these language tasks, specially reduced word recognition skills, was associated with reduced activation in the left temporal and left inferior parietal regions.

Surprisingly, some studies demonstrated increased regional brain activation in poor readers during the performance of language processing tasks. As compared with good readers, poor childhood readers had evidence of higher metabolic activity in the medial temporal and temporal-parietal region, during word recognition and auditory CPT tasks (Hagman & Wood, 1992). A possible explanation of this seemingly unusual result is additional effort exerted by the poor readers. Another explanation is that the increased activation is in slightly different cortical areas, which are involved in the more basic, primary auditory processing.

The Functional Neuroanatomy of Specific Learning Disabilities

Positron Emission Tomography Studies

As discussed earlier in this chapter, the reading pathway consists of a left side network with two posterior pathways for visual and orthographical information and one anterior center. The posterior pathways are: (a) the ventral pathway centered in the posterior fusiform gyrus, representing an automatically accessed visual word form area; and (b) the dorsal pathway, including mainly the angular and supramarginal gyri, representing a slow, phonologically based, assembly process.

The anterior component, in the left inferior frontal gyrus, connected to the two posterior pathways, is implicated in the output of phonological and articulatory aspects (Demont, Taylor, & Chaix, 2004).

Positron emission tomography studies in dyslexic adults during reading demonstrated brain activation patterns that are different from normal readers. In one earlier study of normalized regional metabolic activity during oral reading in dyslexics there were two brain regions that demonstrated a pattern that was different from normal: the prefrontal cortex and the lingual (inferior) region of the occipital lobe. Although nondyslexic subjects had asymmetrical metabolic activity in these areas, the dyslexic readers had a more symmetrical metabolic activity in both areas as well as higher activity in the lingual areas (Gross-Glenn et al., 1991; Habib, 2000).

Rumsey et al. (1992) studied 14 adult dyslexics using PET scanning, with: 15-O labeled water injections, who performed a rhyming task during which they had to press a button when two words within a pair rhymed (phonological awareness). The dyslexic subjects failed to activate the left temporal-parietal region—activated by non dyslexic subjects. In addition, a trend to activate the left inferior and right anterior frontal regions was not seen in dyslexics The dyslexic subjects showed activation in right middle temporal region, not seen in controls.

Paulesu et al. (1993) used a whole brain 15-O PET with a group of five dyslexics. Subjects had to remember six letters that were successively flashed on a screen and decide the letter that rhymed with the target letter. In normal individuals this condition activates a large perisylvian area, including Broca and Wernicke areas, and the parietal operculum (specific to the memory part). In the memory task the dyslexics showed blood flow increases only in the posterior part (inferior parietal cortex) of the large perisylvian area activated by controls. In the rhyming task, dyslexics activated only its anterior part. In both parts there was no activation of the insular cortex. The authors interpret the results as a disconnection phenomenon between anterior and posterior zones of the language areas, in the dyslexic subjects. These findings have not been replicated.

An unpublished work by Demonet et al. found that the only region of greater activation by controls over dyslexics during reading tasks was the left inferior temporal region, at the junction between lateral and mesial aspects of the temporal lobe. This area is possibly an interface between areas associated with processing visual features of written words, temporal-occipital regions involved in complex visual processing, and more dorsal language areas in the middle and superior temporal gyri, mediating the visual entry into the linguistic system ("combining orthographical, lexical and phonological information about words"; Demonet, 2004).

The same area has been found to be activated with Japanese kanji characters, suggesting that its role is probably more orthographical than phonological (Uchida et al., 1999).

In general, despite their inherent differences in language systems, dyslexics in French-, Italian-, and English-speaking countries all show less activity than controls at the occipital-temporal junction of the left hemisphere during word processing (Paulesu et al., 2001).

Other studies attempted to isolate the various cognitive processes involved in reading and elucidate the different cortical areas that are active during each part of the process. The different cognitive processes that occur during read-ing include orthographical, phonological, and syntactic analyses. A PET study (using oxygen 15) reported that during rest, dyslexics showed reduced blood flow in one left parietal region near the angular/supramarginal gyrus, which is thought to be critical to the reading process; however, during syntactic pro-cessing, dyslexics and controls showed similar, significant activation of left middle to anterior temporal and inferior frontal cortex (Rumsey et al., 1992). This suggests that it is not the syntactic processing that differentiates dyslex-ics from normal readers.

Rumsey et al. (1997) designed a study aimed at contrasting orthographi-cal and phonological processes. Using oxygen 15, they measured changes in rCBF in response to tasks involving orthographical, phonological pronun-ciation (reading aloud) and lexical decision making—all reading tasks that normally activate different brain areas. In the first paradigm the partici-pants had to read pseudowords aloud (phonological processing), and irregu-lar words (orthographical processing). In the second paradigm they had to read two words or pseudowords and answer either a phonological question (Which one sounds like a real word?) or an orthographical question (Which one is spelled correctly?). The results showed that dyslexic men had reduced or unusual activation in the mid- to posterior temporal cortex bilaterally and in the inferior parietal cortex, predominantly on the left, during both pro-nunciation and decision making; however, in contrast, they demonstrated normal activation of left inferior frontal cortex during both phonologi-cal and orthographical decision making. There was reduced activation and unusual deactivations in the left posterior temporal/inferior parietal areas, in the first paradigm. There was no difference between the locations of brain activation with the word and non-word versions of the task. Activation of only one area, the left angular gyrus, was correlated with reading skills (positive correlation in controls and negative correlation in dyslexics). They thought that the left angular gyrus was the site of functional abnormality in dyslexia.

These results are compatible with a hypothesis of bilateral involvement of posterior temporal and parietal cortices in dyslexia (Rumsey, 1997).

Brunswick et al. (1999) used 15-O PET to study explicit and implicit read-ing in dyslexic adults. Dyslexics activated two regions to a lesser degree than controls: the left basal temporal lobe (area 37) and the left frontal operculum. In the explicit reading condition, they overactivated a left premotor area situ-ated 20 mm lateral to the area of reduced activation.

A somewhat unusual observation was reported by Garret et al. (1997), who used PET in a letter recognition test. The left Brodmann's area 37 and the left angular gyrus showed metabolic activity that was inversely correlated with task performance. They speculated that such increased activation indicates insufficient processing and may be related to failure to inhibit competing activity, or represents recruitment of resources exceeding those necessary for a given task.

These PET studies, although different in methodology and paradigms, suggest that the neural activity accompanying language-related functions and parts of the reading process, particularly phonological functions, is different in dyslexics. Differences are reported mostly in activation of the posterior, mid-temporal, and parietal regions.

Dyslexic individuals show subtle impairments in naming pictures of objects in addition to their difficulties with reading. The following study investigated whether word reading and picture naming deficits in developmental dyslexia can be reduced to a common neurological impairment. Eight dyslexic subjects, impaired on measures of reading, spelling, and naming speed, were matched for age and general ability with 10 control subjects. Participants were scanned using PET during two experimental conditions: reading words and naming pictures in the form of corresponding line drawings. In addition, two high-level baseline conditions were used to control for visual and articulatory processes. Relative to the control group, the dyslexic participants showed reduced activation in a left occipitotemporal area during both word reading and picture naming. This was the case even in the context of intact behavioral performance during scanning. Abnormal activation in this region, as reported previously for reading, is therefore not specific to orthographical decoding but may reflect a more general impairment in integrating phonology and visual information. The authors concluded that the study suggested a common neurological basis for deficits in word reading and picture naming in developmental dyslexia.

McCrory et al. (2004) performed a PET study ON 8 dyslexic and 10 matched control adult subjects. The subjects of this study were all adults who had attended a university and were remediated in childhood, representing remedied and compensated dyslexia. Positron emission tomography scans were performed while the subjects read words and named pictures in the form of corresponding line drawings. Reading and spelling literacy skills were assessed using the Wide Range Achievement Test-Revised. Naming ability was evaluated using two tasks of rapid automatic naming (after Denckla & Rudel, 1976). There were meaningless control stimuli for both reading and naming tasks. The experimental paradigm comprised four conditions: word reading, picture naming, false fonts, and nonsense shapes.

Regional cerebral blood flow was measured using 15-O-labeled water. Behavioral measures were quantified and compared between groups using factorial analyses of variance. The two groups performed with comparable levels of accuracy. Likewise, reading and naming latencies did not differ significantly between the control and dyslexic groups. In the control group, regional blood flow was increased in the left occipital-temporal region with picture naming relative to nonsense shapes. The dyslexic group showed a much smaller effect in this region. With reading relative to false fonts, the control group activated the left occipital-temporal area but no activation was detected in this region for the dyslexic group even when lowering the statistical threshold to $P < .1$. Therefore, relative to the control group, the dyslexic participants showed reduced activation in a left occipital-temporal area during both word reading and picture naming. This was the case even in the context of intact behavioral performance during scanning. No frontal activation was detected for either reading or naming.

Horwitz et al. (1998) used PET and a method for examining the covariance, or functional connectivity, between brain regions, during the performance of individual tasks, and looking for correlated neural activity [indexed by regional cerebral blood flow (rCBF)] between network elements. They examined the functional connectivity of the angular gyrus during single word reading by measuring rCBF, using [^{15}O]-water and PET in 14 normal male readers (age 25 ± 5 years) and 17 men with persistent developmental dyslexia (age 27 ± 8 years). Two scans obtained during pseudoword reading and two scans during exception word reading, were analyzed. Correlations between standardized rCBF for each reference voxel in the left and right angular gyri—and standardized rCBF in all other voxels in the brain, were determined separately for the two tasks (pseudoword and exception word reading), and for the two groups (normal and dyslexic men).

Large positive correlations were found during the pseudoword reading task between the left angular gyrus and extrastriate visual areas in occipital and temporal cortex in the left hemisphere. These regions include an area at the junction of BA 19 and 37 that frequently includes the motion processing area V5/MT, and areas in the lingual and fusiform gyri (BA 18 and 20, respectively) that have been shown to be activated during visual stimulation with letter and word-like stimuli. There were also strong correlations between standardized rCBF in the left angular gyrus and rCBF in the posterior portion of the left superior temporal gyrus (BA 22), part of Wernicke's area. Finally, there was a significant positive correlation with blood flow in or just anterior/superior to Broca's area in the left inferior frontal gyrus (BA 45).

In contrast with these findings, when the reference voxel was placed in the right hemisphere, positive correlations with right hemisphere homologues of the preceding regions were either not significant—or in the case of the foci in the middle temporal gyrus (BA 21) and Wernicke's area (BA 22)—were smaller in extent. No significant positive correlations were found with rCBF in fusiform or lingual gyri, the BA 19/37 junction, or the inferior frontal cortex.

During exception word reading, rCBF in the left angular gyrus showed a pattern of significant positive correlations with rCBF in left lingual and fusiform gyri similar to that seen during pseudoword reading, although the significance was just missed for the foci in Wernicke's area and the inferior frontal cortex.

In the subjects with dyslexia, rCBF in the left angular gyrus showed no significant positive correlations with rCBF in many of the preceding regions during pseudoword reading, including Broca's region, BA 19/37, or regions in fusiform or lingual gyrus.

Thus, the study demonstrated that in normal men regional cerebral blood flow in the left angular gyrus during single word reading shows strong within-task, across-subjects correlations (meaning functional connectivity) with regional cerebral blood flow in extrastriate occipital and temporal lobe regions. In contrast, the left angular gyrus is functionally disconnected from these regions in men with persistent developmental dyslexia meaning an ana- tomical disconnection of the left angular gyrus from other brain regions that are part of the "normal" brain reading network including from visual areas, Wernicke's area, and the inferior frontal cortex.

Altered rCBF in the left parietal cortex has been reported in dyslexia in several studies (Paulesu et al., 1996; Rumsey et al., 1997; Shaywitz et al., 1998). In addition, Rumsey et al. (1997) have shown in these subjects that left angular gyral rCBF during single word reading was positively correlated with level of reading skill in the controls, whereas these same correlations were negative in the dyslexic men. Thus, although better reading skill was associ- ated with higher rCBF in controls, in dyslexic men higher rCBF was associated with more impaired reading (i.e., those dyslexic men who had compensated to some degree used this region less than those who had not), further suggesting an important role for this region in developmental reading disorder.

Notice that the classic neurologic model for reading, based on studies of patients with acquired alexia, hypothesizes functional linkages between the angular gyrus in the left hemisphere and visual association areas in the occipi- tal and temporal lobes. The angular gyrus (BA 39) is also thought to have func- tional links with posterior language areas (e.g., Wernicke's area), because it is presumed to be involved in mapping visually presented inputs onto linguistic representations.

The loss of functional connectivity in dyslexia between the left angular gyrus and the occipitotemporal region containing V5/MT is interesting in that several reports have suggested a fundamental abnormality in the magnocel- lular system, of which V5/MT is a part, in developmental dyslexia (Livingstone et al., 1991; Lehmkuhle et al., 1993). A recent functional magnetic resonance imaging study (Eden et al., 1996) demonstrated a failure to activate the V5/MT region in response to a moving stimulus in a subset of our dyslexic subjects.

SUMMARY

PET studies, usually performed in dyslexic adults, mostly suggest reduction of brain activation during reading or language processing–related tasks. Compared with controls, dyslexics generally underactivate regions in the temporal lobe including the left inferior temporal region, inferior parietal cortex (Rumsey, 1997), left parietal region near angular/super marginal gyrus (Rumsey, 1994), and frontal operculum (Brunswick et al., 1999). A similar phenomenon may be manifested by loss of the usual left/right asymmetry of metabolic activity in prefrontal and inferior lingual cortex (Gross-Glen et al., 1991). Some studies demonstrate overactivation or a higher metabolic activity in dyslexics, in medial temporal and temporal-parietal regions, areas close to those of reduced activation (Brunswick, 1999), suggesting perhaps additional effort in dyslexic subjects or increased activity in more basic areas (when areas of higher level analysis are defective) (Hagman & Wood, 1992).

Blood flow studies also suggest that the changes seen in the brain of dyslexic people are in response to the phonological component of word processing, but not during syntactic processing.

The exact locations of the implicated areas of abnormality vary. The left inferior temporal area may be one of interface between areas associated with processing visual features of written words, temporal-occipital regions involved in complex visual processing, and more dorsal language areas in the middle and superior temporal gyri (Demonet, Taylor, & Chaix, 2004). It can be speculated that the area of abnormality is the area in which orthographical, lexical, and phonological information translates into words.

CHAPTER 8

Neuroanatomy of Specific Reading Disabilities IV

Functional Magnetic Resonance Imaging

INTRODUCTION

An fMRI signal is obtained when deoxygenated blood is replaced by oxygenated blood. It changes by a small amount in regions that are activated by a stimulus or a task, as a result of the combined effects of increase in the tissue blood flow, volume, and oxygenation. The methods used to record the changes (such as echo-planar imaging) are methods that can provide images at a rate fast enough to capture the time course of the hemodynamic response to neural activation (Anderson & Gore, 1997; Jezzard, Matthews, & Smith, 2001; Frackowiak et al., 2004). As noted in the previous chapter advantages of functional magnetic resonance imaging (fMRI) over positron emission tomography (PET) include a higher spatial and temporal resolution, and the fact that there is no need for an injection of a radionuclide isotope, meaning no radiation exposure.

FUNCTIONAL MAGNETIC RESONANCE IMAGING IN THE INVESTIGATION OF NORMAL READING

Similar to PET, fMRI studies identified cortical areas, mostly in the temporal lobes, which are activated during tasks of language processing. For instance, a single-phoneme monitoring task in adults activated the following regions: Heschl's gyrus and the transverse temporal sulcus, the lateral surface of the anterior/superior temporal gyrus, and the planum temporale (anterior to Heschl's gyrus). As the rate of presentation of the phonemes increased, there was a correlated increase in bilateral temporal activation (Habib, 2000).

Lexical tasks (i.e., reading and spelling) require processing of unimodal stimuli (i.e., auditory or visual), a task performed by unimodal brain centers (the fusiform cortex [Brodmann area (BA) 37] for visually presented words and the superior temporal gyrus (BA 22) for auditory presentation of words), and an interaction between stimuli of different modalities, which requires integration of inputs by heteromodal cortical centers (i.e., the supramarginal gyrus [BA 40] and the angular gyrus [BA 39]). Neural networks that process reading are in posterior brain structures and in the inferior frontal gyrus. Eight- to 12-year-old children reading sentences and stories activated the left middle superior temporal gyrus, left middle frontal gyrus, and (less) left inferior frontal gyrus (Gaillard et al., 2003). Activation was strongly lateralized. Other studies find consistent activation in the left temporal cortex, mostly in the inferior temporal occipital area. and variable degree of activation of the inferior temporal and fusiform gyrus, middle or superior temporal gyrus, anterior temporal gyrus, angular gyrus, inferior frontal gyrus, and premotor area.

A study to determine the pattern of cerebral activation with lexical tasks performed with 10 graduate student young adults revealed that better performance on intramodal tasks (determining if visual words were spelled the same or if auditory words rhymed) was correlated with more activation in unimodal regions corresponding to the modality of sensory input, namely the fusiform cortex (BA 37) for written words and the superior temporal gyros (BA 22) for heard words. Tasks requiring cross-modal conversation (determining if auditory words were spelled the same or if visual words rhymed), was correlated with more activation in posterior heteromodal regions, the site for the integration of inputs from modality specific areas, including the supramarginal gyrus (BA 40) and the angular gyrus (BA 39).

This corresponds to the presumed sequence of cerebral processing for reading: The relevant sequence of events for lexical processing is initiated by encoding of sensory inputs into word forms within specialized unimodal association areas of the fusiform gyrus for written words and the superior temporal gyrus for spoken words. These modality-specific word forms then access heteromodal components of the language network, including those of the temporal parietal cortex (Wernicke's area) and inferior frontal gyrus (e.g., Broca's area), so that they can elicit the associations that encode their meaning (Booth et al., 2003).

Another study of the dynamics of brain activation during normal reading was performed by Fiebach et al. (2002). They performed event-related fMRI of 12 German normal readers and found differences between brain activation to words and pseudowords stimuli as well as differences between activation in response to more and less frequent words. Word stimuli activated areas in the occipital gyri; the fusiform gyrus bilaterally and the posterior left middle temporal gyrus. Low-frequency words (and pseudowords) produced more activation in the left inferior frontal gyrus (IFG), pars triangularis (IFG, BA

45); in the left superior pars opercularis (IFG, BA 44); in the anterior insula bilaterally; in the superior lateral head of the caudate; and in the low anterior thalamus.

The left inferior occipitotemporal cortex is activated during word processing between 150 and 250 ms after word stimuli onset (Kuriki, Takeuchi, & Hirata, 1998). There are still questions whether activation in this area, including in the fusiform cortex, is specific to words, but this area is an early processing area for visual word forms in which the visual word form is computed. The posterior part of the left middle temporal gyrus (MTG) was activated stronger for words than for pseudowords. Other studies also demonstrated that phonological word form representations are stored in the posterior segments of the middle and superior temporal gyri (Beauregard et al., 1997; Indefrey & Levelt, 2000). Activation of MTG was associated with lexical semantic processing (Pugh, 1996). It is, therefore, likely that posterior aspects of middle and superior temporal cortex are areas in which visual word forms are processed and stored.

Left inferior frontal gyrus activation is often associated with phonological processing, phonological retrieval, or phonemic analysis. The increased activation of superior left pars opercularis (BA 44) for low-frequency words and pseudowords suggests that lexical search is mediated more strongly by phonological information in these areas.

It seems, therefore, that the reading process involves different brain regions including word recognition in an occipital temporal network, leading to access to the higher level semantic or phonological information in the posterior left MTG. When word reading is more difficult, as in the case of infrequent words or pseudowords, additional structures including the left IFG, the anterior insula, and subcortical structures become active.

Binder et al. (2005) studied event-related fMRI while subjects were identifying concrete and abstract words. Concrete and abstract words activated areas in the left lateral temporal cortex. Concrete words also activated the bilateral angular gyrus and dorsal prefrontal region. Abstract words activated areas in the left inferior frontal region. Their conclusions were that "The results show overlapping but partially distinct neural systems for processing concrete and abstract concepts, with greater involvement of bilateral association areas during concrete words processing, and processing abstract concepts almost exclusively by the left hemisphere."

Other assessments of the brain reading system again include posterior and anterior pathways. Posteriorly, there is a distinction between a faster ventral posterior pathway and a dorsal, slow, phonologically based pathway. The ventral pathway is centered in the posterior fusiform gyrus, representing an automatically accessed visual word form area. The dorsal pathway includes mainly the angular and supramarginal gyri, representing a slow, phonologically based, assembly process. An anterior component is in the left inferior frontal gyrus, connected to the two posterior pathways, implicated in the output of phonological and articulatory aspects (Demonet et al., 2004).

This discussion is mostly related to the processes of morphology and phonology. Additional processing involves access to stored lexical representation of word form and meaning.

FUNCTIONAL MAGNETIC RESONANCE IMAGING STUDIES IN DYSLEXIA

In adults with dyslexia, activation for word reading in posterior pathways is reduced compared with normally reading people, including reduced left occipitotemporal activation (found also for picture naming), that corresponds to the peak of the "word form area." Activity in the left angular gyrus, a key component of posterior pathways, was positively correlated with reading scores in normal readers, and negatively correlated with reading in adults with dyslexia. Activation of left inferior frontal and right hemisphere is more variable—less activated in some studies, and more activated than normal readers in other studies, possibly suggesting compensation (Demonet et al., 2004). Functional MRI combined with event-related potential for visual language tasks, revealed differences between dyslexia and control groups in left inferior frontal areas, at 250 to 600 ms after stimulus onset.

Using fMRI, Shaywitz and associates (1998) carried out a detailed investigation of regional metabolic activity in 29 dyslexic adults and 32 controls. They performed fMRI while the subjects were performing a series of tasks, tapping various levels of processing during reading (including perceptual mechanisms, orthographical mechanisms, phonological processing, and a semantic category judgment task). Subjects performed five cognitive tasks associated with reading that are "hierarchically structured," starting with visual spatial processing (line orientation task, e.g., do IIV and IIV match?), orthographical processing (letter case judgment task, e.g., do bbBb and bbBb match in the pattern of upper and lower case?), to simple phonological analysis (single letter rhyme: Do the letters T and V rhyme?), complex phonological analysis (nonword rhyme: Do Leat and Jete rhyme?), and semantic category judgment (are corn and rice in the same category?). Functional MRI performed during this sequence of tests measured metabolic activity in 17 brain regions of interest including inferior frontal, posterior superior temporal, angular, inferior lateral extrastriate, calcarine, anterior cingulate, supramarginal, insula, superior medial extrastriate, superior lateral extrastriate, and lingual. Each subject was used as his or her own control. The primary dependent variable was a count of the number of activated pixels in a given region of interest for a given task. The average percent signal change measure was also examined.

Dyslexics made more errors than normal readers on each test, but the differences were most evident on the tests of phonological analysis. Functional MRI demonstrated significant group-task interactions in four regions: Posterior superior temporal gyrus (Wernicke's area), angular gyrus, striate cortex, and inferior frontal gyrus (Broca's area). Unlike normal readers, dyslexics did not show an increase in activation when phonological coding demands increased. Hemispheric differences between normal readers and dyslexics were found in two regions: The angular gyrus and the posterior aspects of the inferior and middle temporal gyri. In each case, activation was greater in the left hemisphere in normal readers and greater in the right hemisphere in dyslexics. In addition, differences between the two groups were present also in anterior brain areas wherein dyslexics showed a pattern of overactivation.

The relative activation for a phonological processing task in normal readers was in the posterior temporal region, BA 21; supramarginal and angular gyri, BA 39 and 40; and inferior lateral temporal region, BA 37; and a reverse pattern (more activation in dyslexics) in anterior areas. The study authors proposed a general explanation of posterior hypoactivation in dyslexics during phonological processing, suggesting a disruption of this system. The hyperactivation of Broca's area reflects "increased effort required of dyslexics in carrying out phonological analysis" (Shaywitz, 1998).

In a later similar fMRI study done with a large group of children, Shaywitz et al. (2002) studied 144 right-handed children, 70 dyslexic, and 74 nonimpaired readers as they read pseudowords and real words. Similar group differences in brain activation patterns during phonological analysis were elicited, with less activation in predominantly left hemisphere sites (including the inferior frontal, superior temporal, parietal-temporal, and middle temporal–middle occipital regions) in the dyslexic group (Figure 8.1, Figure 8.2).

During the most difficult and specific phonological task (nonword rhyming), older compared with younger dyslexic readers had activation in the left and right inferior frontal gyrus. Fewer such differences between younger and older subjects were found in normal readers.

There was a significant positive correlation between reading skill and brain activation in the left occipital-temporal word form area, and a negative correlation between brain activation and reading skill in the right occipital-temporal region, with poorer readers having greater activation (Shaywitz, 2006).

It is interesting that although the pathophysiology of developmental dyslexia is different from that of acquired alexia, the anatomical metabolic disruptions found in this study are in the same brain areas involved in acquired alexia—visual areas, language areas, and the angular gyrus—the areas that link visual representations of the letters to the phonological structures they represent (Shaywitz, 1998).

An fMRI study of 14 8 to 14 years old, children with dyslexia, and 14 age-matched controls, employing visual word rhyming judgment (Cao

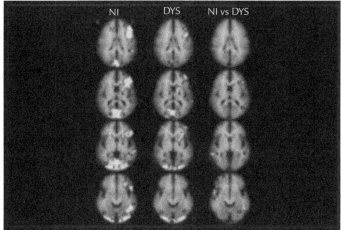

Figure 8-1:
Composite maps (column 1 and 2) demonstrating brain activation in nonimpaired (NI) and dyslexic (DYS) readers during the nonword rhyme task and composite contrast maps (column 3) directly comparing the brain activation of the two groups.
Source: Shaywitz BA, Shaywitz SE, et al. Disruption of posterior brain systems for reading in children with developmental dyslexia. Biol Psychiatry 2002;52:101–110, Figure 1.

et al., 2006), had trials of words necessitating mapping orthography to phonology and using more- and less-difficult conflicting words as well as nonconflicting words. The words in conflicting trials had similar orthography but different phonology (pint-mint), or similar phonology but different orthography (jazz-has). Trials of nonconflicting words had similar

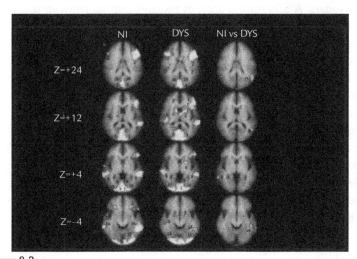

Figure 8-2:
Composite maps (columns 1 and 2) demonstrating brain activation in nonimpaired (NI) and in dyslexic (DYS) readers during the category task and composite contrast maps (column 3) directly comparing the brain activation of the two groups.
Source: Shaywitz BA, Shaywitz SE, et al. Disruption of posterior brain systems for reading in children with developmental dyslexia. Biol Psychiatry 2002;52:101–110, Figure 2.

orthography and phonology (e.g., gate-hate) or different orthography and phonology (e.g., press-list).

There was no difference in brain activation between controls and dyslexic children in the easier, nonconflicting trials. For the more difficult conflicting trials there was less activation in dyslexic children in the left inferior frontal gyrus (BA 45/44/47/9), left inferior parietal lobule (BA 40), left inferior temporal gyrus/fusiform gyrus (BA 20/37), and left middle temporal gyrus (BA 21). Children with dyslexia did not show greater activation than controls for any comparison. The authors' conclusions are that children with dyslexia have deficient orthographic representations in ventral temporal cortex as well as deficits in mapping between orthographic and phonologic representations in the inferior parietal cortex. Underactivation in the inferior frontal gyrus may be found in tasks that involve difficult phonological processing.

ACTIVATION LIKELIHOOD ESTIMATES

Activation likelihood estimates (ALE) metaanalysis of nine published VBM (voxel-based morphometry) reporting 62 foci of gray matter reduction in dyslexic readers, found six significant clusters of convergence in temporal-parietal areas bilaterally and in the left occipital-temporal cortical regions and in the cerebellum bilaterally. Additional ALE metaanalysis of imaging studies reporting functional underactivation or overactivation in dyslexics was then performed, to identify possible overlaps between structural and functional deviations in dyslexic readers. A conjunction analysis revealed overlap between the results of VBM metaanalysis and the metaanalysis of functional underactivation in the fusiform and supramarginal gyri of the left hemisphere. An overlap between VBM results and the meta analysis of functional overactivation was found in the left cerebellum. Functional overactivation co-localized with gray matter reductions in the left cerebellum (Linkersdorfer et al., 2012). Another metaanalysis study used ALE from 17 original activation studies to identify brain regions with consistent under- or overactivation. The stimuli used in these studies were reading or reading related. Maximum underactivation areas were in the inferior parietal, superior temporal, middle and inferior temporal, and fusiform regions of the left hemisphere. There was underactivation in the inferior frontal gyrus accompanied by overactivation in the primary motor cortex and the anterior insula (Richlan, Kronbichler, & Wimmer, 2009).

DIFFERENCES BETWEEN ADULTS AND CHILDREN

Are there differences between the ways the adult and the younger brain process lexical information? Using fMRI, in experiments that employ the cross modal lexical tasks (the visual rhyming task, which required conversion from orthography to phonology, and the auditory spelling task, which required the conversion from phonology to orthography), adults showed greater activation than 9- to 12-year-sold children in the angular gyrus—a region proposed to be involved in the interaction between orthographical and phonological representations. The greater activation for adults suggests they may have a more elaborate posterior heteromodal system for mapping between representational systems during lexical processing (Booth et al., 2004).

DYSLEXIA IN OTHER CULTURES AND LANGUAGES

It is assumed that the brain origins of dyslexia are universal. In English, impaired reading of alphabetical script is associated mostly with dysfunction of left temporoparietal brain regions. These regions perform two central cognitive functions that mediate reading acquisition: phonemic analysis and conversion of written symbols to phonological units of speech (grapheme to phoneme conversion).

Chinese writing is logographic rather than alphabetic. The letter-sound conversion rules for alphabetic languages do not exist in Chinese. Unlike the alphabetic reading system, which maps grapheme (visual forms) into phonemes (minimal phonological units of speech), the Chinese logographic system maps graphic forms (characters) into morpheme (meaning).

Experiments with reading-impaired Chinese children and controls using MRI revealed that the left middle frontal gyrus (LMFG) is activated during Chinese reading, and functional impairment of the LMFG is associated with reading impairment (Wal Ting Sing, 2004). This means that anatomic brain differences can be produced by differences in cultures. It is interesting that The LMFG was found to be larger in Chinese speaking Asians than in English speaking Caucasians, supporting the idea that cognitive strategies for reading development tune the cortex.

Another study of Chinese children with dyslexia examined the question of whether Chinese dyslexics have larger deficits in the semantic system (compared with phonological system)—a question that stems from the logographic nature of Chinese characters. The study used a rhyming judgment task and a semantic association judgment task. The children showed less activation for both tasks in the right visual (BA 18, 19) and left occipital-temporal cortex (BA 37), suggesting a deficit in visual-orthographical processing, and less activation (for both tasks) in the left inferior frontal gyrus (BA 44). Activations in these areas were correlated suggesting a deficit in the connection between brain regions. There were no larger differences between the normal and dyslexic groups for the semantic compared with the rhyming task, suggesting that Chinese dyslexia is similarly impaired in the access to phonology and to semantics from the visual orthography.

FUNCTIONAL MAGNETIC RESONANCE IMAGING OF SENTENCE COMPREHENSION

A study by Mayler et al. (2008) used fMRI to examine brain activation during a visual sentence comprehension task in good and poor readers in the third (N = 32) and fifth (N = 35) grades. The study also investigated whether any aberrant brain activation among poor readers changes with age. The main finding was parietal-temporal underactivation (compared with controls) among poor readers at the two grade levels.

A positive linear relationship (spanning both the poor and good readers) was found between reading ability and activation in the left posterior middle temporal and postcentral gyri and in the right inferior parietal lobule, with activation increase with reading ability.

In the left angular gyrus, activation increased with age among good readers but not among poor readers.

A central finding was that poor reading ability was associated with reduced activation relative to good readers in the parietotemporal cortex bilaterally. A positive linear relationship between reading ability and cortical activation was found in the superior aspect of the left middle temporal gyrus (Wernicke's area), the right inferior parietal lobule, and the left postcentral gyrus. In another parietotemporal region, namely, the left angular gyrus, the degree of underactivation observed among poor readers during sentence processing was greater in the older age group, suggesting that the relationship between reading ability and brain activation was additionally influenced by age.

Previous brain imaging studies of dyslexic children performing single word reading tasks show that dyslexic readers have abnormal parietotemporal activation (Shaywitz SE & Shaywitz BA 2003, 2005). This study found that the regions found to be underactivated among poor readers during sentence comprehension are largely consistent with those found to be underactivated in studies of word-level processing. The occurrence of a similar pattern of underactivation in a sentence comprehension task suggests that this area continues to be a discriminating factor in the development of reading ability beyond the level of reading single words. In the case of sentence reading, parietotemporal underactivation among poor readers could be related to problems associated with phonological working memory functions at different levels of analysis, as both the left and the right parietal-temporal regions have been linked to verbal working memory processes during reading comprehension (Keller et al., 2003).

This study also pointed to a developmental trend. The age at which poor readers are examined may influence the expression of impaired cortical function. This finding centered on the left angular gyrus, with diverging patterns of activation among good and poor readers with increasing age.

Other work has also pointed to the left angular gyrus as playing a crucial role in the development of skilled reading (Pugh et al., 2000; Booth et al., 2004).

EFFECTS OF THERAPY STUDIED WITH FUNCTIONAL MAGNETIC RESONANCE IMAGING

There have been animal studies and early human studies suggesting that training and remediation resulting in improved function are accompanied by brain anatomical changes. In animals, neuroplasticity studies showed that direct training alters the sensory maps on a single cell level (Habib, 2000). Intensive training in the auditory modality can modify the degree of asymmetry in the posterior auditory region, increasing the size of the left planum (Habib, 2000).

There are brain changes presumed to be compensatory, which are noted when older dyslexic patients are compared to younger ones. Compensatory systems (manifested in activation on fMRI) involve areas around the inferior frontal gyrus in both hemispheres and, perhaps, the right hemisphere homologue of the left occipital-temporal word form area as well.

That is better noted during difficult and specific phonological task (nonword rhyming). There was a significant positive correlation between reading skill and brain activation in the left occipital-temporal word form area, and a negative correlation between brain activation and reading skill in the right occipital-temporal region, with poorer readers having greater activation. A few studies have examined the ontogeny of these systems in typical readers and in children with dyslexia (Schlaggar et al., 2002).

Functional MRI studies show evidence of brain plasticity related to remediation. Two studies have used fMRI to examine the effects of a commercial reading program (Fast Forword), initially on adults and then in children with dyslexia. The first study examined three adults with dyslexia who received Fast Forword training during a task requiring that participants respond to a high-pitched stimulus. Following 33 training days, two of the three subjects demonstrated greater activation in the left prefrontal cortex. These two adults also showed post training improvement on both rapid auditory processing and auditory language comprehension. The one adult who did not show a change in fMRI after training failed to show behavioral improvement (Temple et al., 2000).

In a more recent study, functional MRI was performed on 20 children with dyslexia during phonological processing tasks before and after a remediation program focused on auditory processing and oral language training (Temple et al., 2003). Behaviorally, training improved oral language and reading performance. Repeat fMRI showed increased activity in multiple brain areas including increase in the left temporal-parietal cortex, and left inferior frontal gyrus, bringing brain activation in these regions closer to that seen in normal reading children. Increased activity was observed also in right hemisphere frontal and temporal regions and in the anterior cingulate gyrus (Figure 8.3, Figure 8.4).

The authors interpreted the results as a partial remediation of language processing deficits that resulted in improved reading, ameliorated disrupted function in brain regions associated with phonological processing, and produced additional compensatory activation in other brain regions. Similarly, Eden et al. described differences in brain activity of adult dyslexic subjects during a phonological manipulation task, before and after behavioral intervention. They found that behavioral changes were associated with signal increases in left hemisphere regions, usually activated by normal readers (i.e., left parietal cortex and left fusiform cortex), and in areas in the right perisylvian cortex (Eden et al., 2004).

Another fMRI study demonstrating brain plasticity in response to remediation was performed in normally reading children and dyslexic children

A   Childern with no remediation

Normal reading children
while rhyming

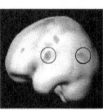

Dyslexic reading children
while rhyming
before remediation

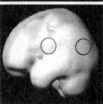

B   Dyslexic children
increases after remediation

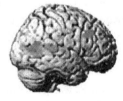
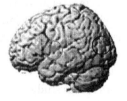

Right   Left

Figure 8-3:
Neural effects of remediation in children with developmental dyslexia.
Source: Temple E et al. Neural deficits in children with dyslexia ameliorated by behavioral remediation. Evidence from functional MRI. Proc Natl Acad Sci USA 2003;100(5):2860-2865, Figure 1, page 2863.

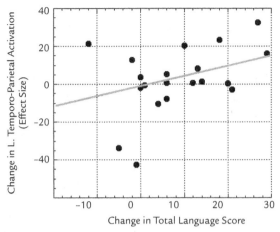

Figure 8-4:
Language improvement and increased brain function.
Source: Temple E et al. Neural deficits in children with dyslexia ameliorated by behavioral remediation. Evidence from functional MRI. Proc Natl Acad Sci USA 2003;100(5):2860-2865, Figure 2, page 2864.

during phonemic processing and morpheme processing (Aylward et al., 2003). The dyslexic children then had an evidence-based therapeutic instructional reading program (2 hours/day × 14 days = 28 hours) in linguistic awareness, alphabetic principles, fluency, and reading comprehension. The 10 dyslexic children improved significantly from the beginning to the end of the 2-week intervention. Functional MRI in the dyslexic children demonstrated initially very small areas for phoneme activation (right cerebellum; right inferior temporal gyrus; orbital, inferior, middle, frontal gyri bilaterally right more than left; superior frontal gyri bilaterally, right more than left; left superior parietal gyrus). Those increased after treatment.

Shaywitz et al. (2004) reported the response to specific phonological intervention in second- and third grade poor readers. The intervention provided 50 minutes daily of individual tutoring centered on phonological processing (relation of letters, letter sounds, and phonemes).

Functional MRI imaging was performed before intervention, immediately post intervention, and 1 year after the intervention was completed. Compared with their preintervention images, participants in the EI group were activating bilateral inferior frontal gyri, left superior temporal sulcus, the occipital-temporal region involving the posterior aspects of the middle and inferior temporal gyri, and the anterior aspect of the middle occipital gyrus, the inferior occipital gyrus, and the lingual gyrus. The authors concluded that the phonologically based reading intervention lead to the development of reading neural systems both in anterior (inferior frontal gyrus) and posterior (middle temporal gyrus) brain regions.

Richards et al. (2000) used proton magnetic resonance spectroscopy to measure brain lactate concentrations at two time points, 1 year apart, in eight boys with dyslexia and seven boys in a control group, before and after 3 weeks of a phonologically based reading intervention. Before treatment, the boys with dyslexia demonstrated increased lactate concentration (compared with controls) in the left anterior quadrant during a phonological task. After treatment, reading improved and brain lactate concentrations in the boys with dyslexia were similar to those in the boys in the control group. More recently, this same group reported fMRI changes in inferior frontal gyrus, parietal regions, and fusiform gyrus (regions which we have also found to be important in reading) following a 28-hour intervention in which phonological and morphological awareness activities were embedded in lessons also containing instruction in decoding, fluency, comprehension, and writing (Aylward et al., 2003).

SUMMARY: FUNCTIONAL ANATOMY OF DYSLEXIA

Deficits in phonological processing are expressed as problems in identifying, representing, and manipulating basic speech sounds (phonemes), which in turn lead to difficulty in mapping sounds onto letters and acquiring letter-sound correspondences. This deficit in phonological processing, especially in identifying and manipulating the sound structure of the word, leads to inadequate word recognition and to reading difficulty (Vellutino et al., 2004).

Because this basic deficit appears to be a main cause for dyslexia, much of the neuroimaging research has focused on letter- and word-reading tasks that involve phonological processing (e.g., Paulesu et al., 1996; Rumsey et al., 1997; Shaywitz et al., 1998, 2002, 2003, 2004; Brunswick et al., 1999; Georgiewa et al., 1999; Pugh, 2000; Simos et al., 2000, 2002; Corina et al., 2001; Temple et al., 2001, 2003; Aylward et al., 2003; Eden et al., 1996, 2004).

Functional MRI studies during reading have shown reduced activity in left hemisphere posterior brain systems during reading related tasks (Rumsey et al., 1992; Salmelin et al., 1996; Horwitz, Rumsey, & Donohue, 1998; Brunswick et al., 1999; Helenius et al., 1999; Temple et al., 2000; Paulesu et al., 2001; Seki et al., 2001; Shaywitz BA et al., 2002; Shaywitz SE et al., 2003) as well as during nonreading visual processing tasks (Eden et al., 1996; Demb, Boynton, & Heeger, 1998; McCandiless and Noble, 2003, Shaywitz & Shaywitz, 2005).

The two areas of reduced activation are in the parietotemporal region of the left hemisphere (including the posterior aspects of the superior and middle temporal gyri, the supramarginal gyrus, and the angular gyrus) and in the occipital-temporal region of the left hemisphere, including the left fusiform gyrus (Rumsey et al., 1997b; Shaywitz 1998; Brunswick et al., 1999; Paulesu et al., 2001, Shaywitz et al., 2002, 2003; Shaywitz & Shaywitz, 2005—review). The left fusiform gyrus is important for processing the orthographical structure of well-learned visual word forms (Cohen et al., 2000; Tarkianen et al.,

2003). The left occipital-temporal system is more involved with the development of fluent (automatic) reading when word recognition skills become more automatic and direct visual access to the mental lexicon is the predominant reading strategy (Logan 1988; Pugh et al., 2000; Shaywitz et al., 2002, 2006). This is a rapid whole word system (Salmelin et al., 1996, McCandliss, Cohen, & Dehaene, 2003). Brain activation in this region increases as reading skill increases (Shaywitz et al., 2002).

Another brain area involved with reading is the left prefrontal area, which in some studies is activated in dyslexia (Shaywitz et al., 1998; Brunswick et al., 1999; Pugh et al., 2000; Shaywitz et al., 2002) possibly suggesting compensatory engagement. Other studies do not show a difference from control (Paulescu, 2001; Shaywitz 2003) This could be the manifestation of a compensatory mechanism by adults with dyslexia. In children, most studies show either less activation in this area compared with regular readers, or no difference (Georgiewa, 1999).

Radiological imaging provides, therefore, evidence for the current main theoretical framework for dyslexia, which argues that a central problem in patients with dyslexia is a deficit in phonological processing—demonstrating abnormalities in brain areas involved in phonological processing (Pugh et al., 1997).

The brain substrate for reading is a set of areas functioning as a large-scale cortical network. Reading abnormalities may be the result of abnormalities in one or more of the components of this network, or abnormalities of the connections between the components of the network.

Experiments with reading impaired Chinese children and controls using MRI revealed that the LMFG is activated during Chinese reading, and functional impairment of the LMFG is associated with reading impairment (Wal Ting Sing, 2004).

There have been studies suggesting that training and remediation resulting in improved function are accompanied by brain anatomical changes, with increased activity in multiple brain areas including increase in the left temporal-parietal cortex, and left inferior frontal gyrus, bringing brain activation in these regions closer to that seen in normal reading children.

CHAPTER 9

Neuroanatomy of Specific Reading Disabilities V

CEREBELLAR ABNORMALITIES IN DYSLEXIA

Introduction

Traditionally the cerebellum has been thought to be important in motor-related functions, including motor planning and implementing movement (Lisberger, 1988; Horne & Butler, 1995). It was thought that its role is largely limited to these functions. Its involvement in cognitive functions like language has been ascribed to control and coordination of the motor output of speech. Recent evidence points to the cerebellum having a potentially broader role in perceptual and cognitive processes, including cognitive tasks that relate to word identification in reading.

Cerebellar Anatomical Connections with Cortical Areas

There are known anatomical connections between the cerebral cortex and the cerebellum (Middleton & Strick 1994; Schmahmann, 1996), including connections to the frontal, temporal, and parietal lobes - the parts of the brain engaged during reading.

In the macaque monkeys the lateral prefrontal cortex, superior temporal sulcus, and posterior parietal association cortices project to the cerebellum via pontine nuclei (Levin, 1936, 1990). The cerebellum also projects to these association cortices through the thalamus (Middleton & Strick, 1997). Therefore, cerebellar anomalies can affect the architecture and function of the temporal or parietal regions.

Cognitive Effects of Cerebellar Lesions

Cerebellar lesions are associated with impaired language processing, and deficient attentional control and problem solving. For instance, infarct of the right cerebellum was associated with deficits in errors detection and a verb generation task. Studies of children with cerebellar tumors demonstrate a critical role for the right cerebellar hemisphere in linguistic performance (Riva & Giorgi, 2000). For example, children with right cerebellar tumors exhibited poor verbal and literacy performance, in contrast with children with left cerebellar tumors who had had spatial deficits. Akshoomoff and colleagues (1992) reported poor naming performance in a child with a right cerebellar hemisphere tumor.

Cognitive Functional Anatomical Studies

Functional neuroimaging studies of unimpaired subjects report cerebellar activation in response to a variety of cognitive tasks, including problem solving, working memory, verb generation, tactile stimulation, olfaction, and attention tasks (Kim, Ugurbil, & Strick, 1994; Raichle et al., 1994). Similarly, functional imaging studies show activation in the left inferior frontal and right cerebellar hemisphere during fluency tasks, passive listening to clicks (Ackermann et al., 2001), linguistic working memory tasks (Desmond et al., 1998), and rapid production of consonant–vowel stimuli.

A positron emission tomography study of aphasic patients with left inferior frontal damage found hypoactivation of the right cerebellar hemisphere.

The Cerebellum and Reading

There have been studies to assess the role of the cerebellum in word identification and reading.

Fulbright et al. (1999) performed fMRI in normal adults with an aim of assessing the cerebellar involvement in word reading. They used hierarchical reading tasks designed to identify cerebral areas engaged by each of the components of reading (Pugh et al., 1996). Subjects had to indicate whether pairs of words were written in the same case (orthographical processing), whether pairs of words and nonwords rhymed with each other (phonological processing) ("rice" and "mice"), and whether pairs of words belonged to the same semantic category (semantic processing) (words like "man" and "boy" and nonwords like "leat" and "jete"). A baseline test was a line orientation task—a perceptual task, the results of which were always "subtracted." The answers the subject had to give were yes/no (same/not same) answers.

When the word rhyming condition was contrasted with the case line condition, there was no significant difference. But when the nonword rhyming condition was performed there was differential activation in cerebellar areas, including areas of the posterior superior fissure, simple lobule, and superior semilunar lobule bilaterally. For the semantic processing they found cerebellar activation in the right deep nuclear region and the inferior vermis in addition to posterior areas active in phonological processing (including the simple, superior semilunar and inferior semilunar lobules).

It seems, therefore, that the cerebellum is engaged during reading and activates differentially in response to phonological and semantic tasks. Different cerebellar sites activate with different tasks. There is also more activation when the cognitive demand is higher (when performing the semantic condition there is a need to access the lexicon). The circuits of the cerebellum that are activated during the learning phase differ from those activated during the automatic phase following practice and learning (Nicolson et al., 1999).

Cerebellar Abnormalities in Dyslexia

The cerebellum may be affected in dyslexic adults and children (Ivry & Justus, 2001; Zeffiro & Eden, 2001; Bishop, 2002). These subjects may have problems in the rate of reading single words and text, which is consistent with the role of the cerebellum in precise timing. Cerebellar involvement can be present even without a noticeable effect on motor skills associated with learning to read including oral–motor for mouth movements during oral reading and graphomotor for hand movements during spelling, although.

Eckert et al. (2003) studied dyslexic children using magnetic resonance imaging (MRI) scans, with measurements of posterior temporal lobe, inferior frontal gyrus, cerebellum, and whole brain. Dyslexic children had significantly smaller right anterior lobes of the cerebellum, pars triangularis bilaterally (which correctly classified 72% of the dyslexic subjects and 88% of controls), and brain volume. The neuroanatomical measurements were significantly correlated with reading, spelling, and language measures related to dyslexia. These findings are consistent with Fawcett and Nicolson's cerebellar deficit hypothesis, which attributes the cognitive and motor problems exhibited by individuals with dyslexia to abnormal cerebellar development (Nicolson & Fawcett, 1990; Nicolson, Fawcett, & Dean, 2001).

A number of dyslexic children have a double deficit in rapid automatic naming and phonological awareness (Wolf & Bowers, 1999). A frontal-cerebellar network may be critical to the precise timing mechanism that Wolf and Bowers hypothesize to underlie the double deficit. Dyslexic subtypes could be produced by processing deficits anywhere in the frontal-cerebellar phonological system. Each region may play a distinct, but related, role in reading that is responsive to instructional intervention.

Nevertheless, the role of cerebellar deficits in dyslexia is not completely clear. Dyslexics may have impairment in motor learning and eye movements, poor balance and general clumsiness, and structural brain studies of dyslexic subjects compared with good readers find differences in cerebellar asymmetry and gray matter volume. However, many dyslexics do not have cerebellar signs or cerebellar differences on brain imaging; many patients with cerebellar disease do not have reading problems, and brain differences between dyslexics and normal readers on imaging are found in many other brain areas. Therefore, impaired cerebellar function is probably not the primary cause of dyslexia (Stoodley, 2012).

POSTMORTEM ANATOMY

Brain Parenchymal Abnormalities in Developmental Dyslexia

Pathological studies of brains of people who had developmental dyslexia (and died of unrelated conditions) are uncommon. Three types of neuroanatomical abnormalities were described: absence of the normal cerebral asymmetries; the presence of cortical developmental abnormalities, such as microdysgenesis (ectopias and cell loss); and abnormalities of the visual pathways.

The main studies are those of Galaburda and his group, who found mostly loss of asymmetry and some specific brain abnormalities (Galaburda & Kemper, 1979). In the brains of people without a history of learning disabilities, the left planum temporale is usually larger than the right (Geschwind & Galaburda, 1985), whereas in the brains of people with learning disabilities it is symmetrical (Galaburda et al., 1985; Humphreys et al., 1990).

In addition to the loss of the usual hemispheral asymmetry, there were ectopias and dysplasias), and an abnormally high frequency of microdysgenesis. These abnormalities are manifested by focal microgyria, neuronal nests, missing or duplicated gyri, fewer layers and primitive orientation of neurons, and gliosis (Galaburda & Kemper, 1979). Cortical abnormalities can be bilateral but have been found more on the left side (Geschwind & Galaburda, 1985).

These abnormalities were found in a number of regions, including the perisylvian regions (important for language functions), and in the orbital frontal and lateral frontal and opercular areas (which are important for attention and impulse control). The presence of ectopias and dysplasia suggest an abnormality of migration, the stage of brain development when neurons migrate from their place of birth in the subcortical periventricular areas to their appropriate location in the cortex (Leonard et al., 1993). The second type of brain pathology found in these brains—the glial scars—suggests potential injury to the brain and neuronal loss during a later part of brain developmental in utero (Galaburda, 1985; Humphreys et al., 1990). The injury leading to the scars may also create minor cortical malformations, the difference being only in the time of occurrence during cortical development: malformations earlier (at around the middle of pregnancy); and scars later (the second half of gestation and early postnatal period). It was proposed that autoimmune damage to vessel walls—arteritis—reduces blood flow and causes ischemic injury to the developing cortex, predominantly to areas of vascular watershed, leading to cortical injury, scars, and malformations. Whether learning deficits are a direct consequence of ectopia or the ectopias are a marker for aberrant development in general with concomitant learning deficits, is not known at present (Demonet et al., 2004).

Other anatomical abnormalities found in the brains of learning disabled people were in the thalamus, in structures associated with visual processing (Livingstone et al., 1991). Galaburda and Eidelberg reported that the medial geniculate nucleus and the lateralis posterior nucleus were distorted in shape and had clusters of primitive cells and abnormal myelination. The thalamic abnormalities were more symmetrical.

Abnormalities were also reported in the cerebellum, where larger mean cell size was found in the medial posterior regions.

Although these findings are very important in the search for etiologies for specific learning disabilities and dyslexia, their usefulness is limited by the small samples of the studies, heterogeneity, the presence of comorbidity, unknown education history, and the restriction of analyses to preselected regions.

SUMMARY OF ANATOMICAL FINDINGS

Introduction

Knowledge of the neurological bases of learning and cognition has expanded over the last decades. This has taken place largely because of advances in three fields: neuroimaging, with improved MRI spatial resolution, the use of fMRI, and other imaging methods, including volumetrics and diffusion tensor imaging; Molecular genetics; and improved neuropsychological testing. The research on developmental learning and language disabilities has benefited from this knowledge (Lyons, 1995)

What Are the Aims of Anatomical Brain Studies in Specific Learning Disabilities?

Neuroanatomical studies have become a major research tool in the study of SLDs. Like most biological studies of SLD—the majority of data is obtained from studies on dyslexia. The aim of anatomical brain studies is to find and localize cognitive domains that are involved in reading or arithmetic and may be abnormal in SLDs. For reading, this includes localization of parameters of language processing, phonological mechanisms responsible for decoding words, and cortical areas involved in reading comprehension (Eden & Zeffiro, 1998). These domains, including phonological processing, may involve multiple cortical and subcortical regions, functioning as coordinated networks.

It is clinically evident that the pathogenesis of SLDs involves a developmental aberration resulting from a genetic abnormality, some deprivation during development, or an early insult that occurred during the period of brain development. The exact pathogenesis is not yet known, however. We look to neuroimaging as one of the most important sources that will shed light on this issue.

Summary of Results

Functional Neuroanatomy of Reading

Functional imaging of reading processes demonstrates that several left hemisphere regions are involved in reading. Some of these areas have been found to also have a role in receptive and expressive language functions. The functional anatomy of reading consists mostly of the left network with two posterior pathways. One is a ventral pathway—in the ventral occipital-temporal area—traversing the left posterior inferior temporal lobe, and centered in the posterior fusiform gyrus, representing a visual word form area. These areas are involved in storing or gaining access to abstract orthographical representations. The ventral pathway is automatically accessed.

The other is a dorsal pathway, going through the left temporoparietal cortex, including mainly the angular and supramarginal gyri. It is a slow, phonologically based assembly process. Inferior parietal cortices are involved in converting print to sound, rather than in accessing stored visual word forms.

The third component in the brain reading network is an anterior component in the left inferior frontal gyrus connected to the two posterior pathways.

A pathway for reading may function in the following way: travel from occipital cortices along the inferior longitudinal fasciculus to the left fusiform gyrus. Inferior parietal regions connect to posterior temporal cortices through the arcuate fasciculus (Catani & Ffytche, 2005). There are direct fiber tracts connecting posterior temporal and inferior parietal areas with inferior frontal regions.

There are differences in the brain regions and networks that are in action during learning to read, and those that are in action during expert reading. In novel readers, grapheme-to-phoneme conversion mechanisms are more important and parietal-occipital brain areas play a larger role in the decoding of written language. In expert readers, the recognition of the abstract ortho-graphical representation of familial words is important for the rapid access to the meaning and phonological representations; therefore, inferior-temporal regions that are related to whole-word recognition are important.

Brain Imaging in Dyslexia

Structural brain MRI studies of dyslexic subjects (computed tomography [CT], MRI, and volumetric MRI) have demonstrated differences between dyslexics and regular readers in a variety of brain regions. Initial findings (mostly CT and r MRI studies) have centered around the loss of the commonly present hemispheric asymmetry. Magnetic resonance imaging morphometric stud-ies have demonstrated, in addition, mostly gray matter volume reductions in parietal occipital areas and other areas, including the cerebellum, insula, caudate, corpus callosum, and thalamus (Pennington et al., 1999; Eliez et al., 2000; Brown et al., 2001; Leonard et al., 2001; Rae et al., 2002; Robichon et al., 2000a,b).

One of the pitfalls of some morphological studies is inadequate controls. Two such necessary controls are gender and age. The size as well as the shape of various brain structures is different for males and females, children and adults. In animals, some differences are already present in the neonatal period. Factors that influence such differences include genetic as well as environmen-tal factors. A large MRI study observed significant sex differences in the shape of the corpus callosum, with the splenium being more bulbous in females and more tubular in males. Also, the area of the corpora callosa increased sig-nificantly with age in children and decreased significantly with age in adults. Male/female differences may be related to the effects of gonadal hormones during a critical period of perinatal development on the survival of neurons in sexually dimorphic nuclei. In mice, the size of the corpus callosum relates to morphological asymmetry of the cerebral cortex: Those animals with deficits in or the absence of a corpus callosum do not exhibit morphological cortical asymmetry (Allen et al., 1991). Therefore, it is important to match subjects by age and sex.

On diffusion tensor imaging (DTI) studies, poor readers had lower frac-tional anisotropy (FA) values in a region of the temporal-parietal lobe, com-pared with regular readers. The FA values in this region correlated with reading skills (Klingberg et al., 1999). Deutsch et al. replicated the results in children age 7 to 13 years with a range of reading abilities. They found that FA in the left parietal-temporal white matter correlated with word identification scores (Deutsch et al., 2005).

Important disadvantages of these studies are that many of them measure a limited range of structures and even fewer have tried to replicate findings prospectively in a new sample.

Functional Brain imaging in Dyslexia

Given the complex nature of the reading process, one may expect that possible changes in the brains of dyslexics may be widespread and multiple neuroanatomical measures will be necessary to predict a diagnosis of an SLD such as dyslexia in children.

Indeed, functional neuroimaging studies do not find a single anatomical marker that differentiates dyslexic from controls (Brown, 2001). Rather, as noted, abnormalities of reading may be reflected in many brain areas, including posterior and frontal cortical areas, mostly in the left hemisphere, cerebellum, and basal ganglia.

Recent functional neuroimaging research has been guided by the established theory that developmental reading disability (dyslexia) is caused frequently by an abnormality of phonological processing. Therefore, many functional imaging studies employ experimental paradigms that involve reading and/or phonological processing.

Such studies reveal differences between dyslexics and regular readers in brain areas involved in phonological coding, reading words (Fiez & Petersen, 1998), and retention of verbal information in working memory.

Results have repeatedly provided evidence for brain differences in two left hemisphere posterior brain systems—the parietal-temporal, and the occipital-temporal, as well as anterior systems around the inferior frontal gyrus and possibly another posterior (right occipital-temporal) system. reduced activity was found in posterior temporal inferior parietal and left occipital-temporal cortex, mostly the fusiform gyrus, for tasks requiring phonological decoding (Salmelin et al., 1996; Rumsey et al., 1997; Brunswick et al., 1999; Paulesu et al., 2001; Temple et al., 2001; Shaywitz et al., 2002; Cao et al., 2006; Hoeft et al., 2007). The left parietal-temporal area and the left frontal operculum may represent aspects of the same phonological retrieval system (Price & Friston, 1997). The differences in activation of subjects with dyslexia in comparison with regularly reading subjects have been interpreted in the context of impaired phonological processing in dyslexia (Rumsey et al., 1997; Brunswick et al., 1999; Paulesu et al., 2001; Shaywitz et al., 2002; McCrory et al., 2004).

Activation of the left angular gyrus, a key component of the posterior pathways, positively correlated with reading scores in regular l readers and is negatively correlated in adults with dyslexia, but involvement of the angular gyrus in developmental RD is not uniformly reported (Shaywitz et al., 1998; Temple et al., 2001; Simos et al., 2006). Similarly, reduced activity in the left fusiform gyrus in children with reading disability was not always found.

Activation of the left inferior frontal and the right hemisphere is more variable. Some studies reported decreased activity in the left frontal gyrus in children with RD (Shaywitz et al., 2002; Cao et al., 2006), whereas other studies reported increased activity (Hoeft et al., 2007), possibly suggesting compensation.

Shaywitz et al. (1998) reported that dyslexics show deficient phonological task-related activity in the posterior superior temporal gyrus, angular gyrus, and extrastriate cortex, but showed relative increased phonological task-related activation in the inferior frontal gyrus (Shaywitz et al., 1998). An enhanced activity in the inferior frontal gyrus may represent a compensatory response to the failure of phonological processing mechanisms in the posterior cortical areas.

Other brain regions involved in reading may include the cerebellum (Fulbright et al., 1999) and the caudate nucleus (Parent & Hazrati, 1995).

The deficits in activation in dyslexics were shown irrespective of language.

Other representation of brain abnormalities in dyslexia include the finding that activity in temporal and parietal reading areas during pseudoword reading tasks was coordinated in normal readers and uncoordinated in dyslexics (Horwitz et al., 1998).

Magnetoencephalography demonstrated that the failure to engage these posterior brain regions was in the late stages of processing of reading (250–700 ms after stimulus onset). Also, although regular readers and dyslexics activated the frontal cortex and the posterior superior temporal cortex during rhyme judgment tasks, regular readers activated both areas as well as the insula during both tasks. The insula is the area that links these two areas. This may suggest that dyslexia is a disconnection syndrome (Paulescu et al., 1996).

There is plasticity in the brain's systems for reading, and their disruption in children with dyslexia may be remediated by provision of an effective reading intervention. A restoration of close to normal activity in the left temporal region after phonological training has been demonstrated (Demonet et al., 2005).

Postmortem Anatomical Studies

Postmortem brain anatomy of dyslexic subjects demonstrated microscopic abnormalities in perisylvian regions consisting of cortical ectopias and dysplasias, suggesting developmental aberrations. Other anatomical microscopic studies reported that neurons in the magnocellular layers of the lateral geniculate nucleus and the left medial geniculate nucleus were smaller than normal. The problems interpreting these data include small samples, subject heterogeneity and comorbidity, and uncertainty regarding the diagnosis and subtype of learning disabilities in these subjects. However, neuroanatomical studies, in general, support the theory that specific reading disability represents a congenital dysfunction of left hemisphere perisylvian brain areas underlying phonological representations, or connecting phonological and orthographical representations (Galaburda et al., 1985; Paulescu et al., 1996, 2001; Shaywitz et al., 1998, 2002; Brunswick et al., 1999; McCrory et al., 2000; Pugh et al., 2000; Temple et al., 2001).

Pitfalls in Neuroimaging Research. What Do Anatomical Studies Mean?

The most significant problems in analyzing neuroimaging findings are the diversity of clinical presentations, imaging methods, techniques, and experimental paradigms (tasks). Results are also affected by the degree of resolution of the images. Such changes from one study to the other make it more difficult to compare studies and draw universal conclusions. Differences in task and control conditions can be associated with significant differences in the localization of task-related activity (Eden & Zeffiro, 1998). For these reasons, studies have been hard to replicate.

A theoretical methodological limitation of fMRI and PET imaging is the fact that we do not have direct measurement of neural activity. We cannot even have direct metabolic measurements. We rely on a vascular filter interposed between neural activity and sensors that make the relationship between the measures of neural activity and the academic functions of learning/reading imprecise, limiting the understanding of brain–reading relationships.

One of the possibilities that needs to be considered when evaluating studies of adult subjects with dyslexia is the question whether their neuronal brain activity recorded in response to tasks such as reading or phonological processing is a primary biological abnormality or a derivative of the fact that they have a specific learning disability and cannot read and write normally.

A study of the morphology of the corpus callosum of illiterate adults (with otherwise apparent normal functioning) demonstrated that an area of their corpus callosum, in which parietal fibers cross from one hemisphere to the other, was thinner than that of normally reading controls (Castro-Caldas et al., 1990, 1999). There are studies demonstrating a significant growth of the corpus callosum until late in life (Witelson, 1991; Cowell et al., 1992; Pujol et al., 1993). This means that the corpus callosum is exposed to environmental influence for a long time. Castro-Caldes et al. (1999) argue that because there should not be any a priori reason for differences in brain anatomy in illiterate subjects (the reason for illiteracy was purely a lack of social opportunity), the thinning of this area of the corpus callosum is secondary to the fact that these subjects did not read or write, and thus there was no stimulation of the posterior association areas that give rise to the fibers crossing at that part of the corpus callosum. This means that the anatomical abnormality was the result of the fact that they did not read, not the result of a developmental brain abnormality. A similar sequence can be imagined for dyslexia.

CHAPTER 10

Neurophysiological Studies
of Specific Learning Disabilities

INTRODUCTION

The previous few chapters discussed the anatomy of specific learning disabilities (SLDs). There were a number of sections, starting chronologically
with a review of structural neuroimaging, which is essentially taking still pictures of brain anatomy, and ending with a discussion of a type of anatomical studies that, in the last decade, has proved to be more promising for SLD
research—functional imaging studies. This type of imaging examines physiological changes that occur in the brain of people during sensory, motor, or
cognitive events, thus combining anatomy with physiology. There are other
types of physiological methods that investigate brain activity. These include
electroencephalography, event-related potentials (ERP) and, more recently,
magnetoencephalography.

ELECTROENCEPHALOGRAPHY

In the past, the most common clinical tool used for the study of central nervous
system physiology was the electroencephalogram (EEG). The EEG is a recording of brain electrical activity. The recording is done through electrodes that are
attached to the scalp in standard locations. Electrical activity is a major vehicle
for the conduction of information in the nervous system. Therefore, the EEG
could be used to study abnormalities of the conduction of information within
the central nervous system in people with SLDs. Electroencephalogram "background activity" is the ongoing cortical electrical activity, which consists of a
mixture of waves with various frequencies and voltages. Wave frequencies are
in the alpha (8–12 cycles per second), beta (12 and above cycles per second),

theta (4–7 cycles per second), or delta (1–4 cycles per second) range. The EEG background changes constantly during infancy and childhood. Typically as the child grows up, the EEG background activity in the awake state contains more of the faster alpha waves and fewer of the slower theta and delta waves.

The EEG of subjects who have SLDs is frequently normal. When abnormalities are present, these are usually nonspecific and consist of a disorganized EEG background with relatively slower background activity and reduced amount of the normal alpha activity for the age of the patient. In some children with SLDs initially slow and poorly organized EEG may later normalize, a finding that led to the belief that SLDs reflect slow developmental maturation (Hamony et al., 1995). There have been reports of more specific EEG abnormalities in SLD subjects, including focal abnormalities over the left hemisphere. One such specific type of focal abnormality found in children with developmental speech, language, and reading disorders consists of intermittent left parietal alpha desynchronization (ILPAD) (Rothenberger & Moll, 1994). This finding is interesting in light of the common location of language centers in the left temporal parietal regions of the brain and the clinical correlations between language processing abnormalities and reading disability.

In general, specific EEG abnormalities are not common in people with SLDs, so the EEG cannot serve as a clinical tool in the diagnosis of SLDs or as a reliable research tool.

Quantitative EEG techniques have provided better tools for research in SLDs and attention deficit hyperactivity disorder (ADHD). Instead of the clinical practice of visually estimating the relative frequency of the various brain waves, these techniques can actually assess the amount of alpha, beta, theta, and delta range waves in various brain areas, and draw topographic maps. In general, quantitative EEG studies demonstrate that children with reading disabilities have increased amount of slower frequency "theta and delta power" and less "alpha power" (Harmony et al., 1995). An EEG power spectra study of reading disabled children performed during reading revealed that a combination of more low beta power (13–18 cycles/second) and less theta power predicted better reading and spelling. There are other quantitative EEG studies that differentiated between people with and without SLDs, or between people with SLDs and those with ADHD (Chabot et al., 1996). Brain electrical activity mapping (BEAM), which provides regional quantitative EEG power spectra, was recorded from dyslexic and nondyslexic boys during resting and cognitive activity. It demonstrated electrophysiological differences between the groups in the left temporal and left posterior quadrant regions and in the frontal areas bilaterally. These results suggest that aberrant neurophysiology in dyslexia is present in a number of cortical areas, anteriorly and posteriorly, in the right as well as the left hemisphere (Duffy et al., 1980). As noted in the section on the anatomy of SLDs, fMRI studies reported similar findings (Shaywitz,

1998). The applicability of these findings to the clinical diagnosis of SLDs is still unclear. The authors of earlier EEG power spectra studies predicted that using these statistical techniques, 80% to 90% of subjects with dyslexia could be successfully diagnosed (Duffy et al., 1980). This expectation has not yet materialized, not the least because there are problems with replication of the results of these studies. Therefore, at the present time these methods are not routinely used for diagnosis in the individual patient.

EVENT-RELATED POTENTIALS

Event-related potentials (ERPs) are brain electrical responses to specific stimuli, recorded over the scalp at characteristic times after stimulus onset. Event-related potential recording involves presentation of stimuli by a generator, the recording of electroencephalographic responses by electrodes attached to the scalp, and averaging of the responses. The results are series of distinct positive and negative waves that are reproducible. Characteristics of the response can be measured. These include the latencies and amplitudes of the various peaks, conduction times between peaks, pattern configurations, and symmetry. Event-related potentials can be elicited by basic sensory stimuli (auditory, visual, or somatosensory). ERP can also be elicited when the stimulus involves more complex cognitive processing (e.g., while performing language processing, learning a memory paradigm, reading, solving a mathematical problem). When ERPs are elicited by simple sensory stimuli, the resulting waveform is determined by the parameters of the physical stimulus such as intensity, frequency, modality, and interstimulus interval. Event-related potentials responses elicited by cognitive processing, on the other hand, do not depend on the physical properties of the stimulus, but vary as a result of the amount of cognitive processing done by the brain. Cognitive ERP responses are influenced by many factors, including the state of the subject (awake, attentive, involved with one or more competing tasks), the age, sex, neurological, and psychological status of the subject, and the use of medication or other drugs. Cognitive processing usually give rise to long latency ERP waves starting about 100 to 150 ms after the stimulus.

Event-related potentials have an important role in tracking brain correlates of cognitive functions because they can point to the temporal characteristics and cortical locations of these functions. There are a number of cognitive neurophysiological events that can be studied, including MMN (mismatch negativity), P300, and N400. Event-related potentials abnormalities in the form of increased latencies or decreased amplitudes were described in clinical conditions involving learning and memory deficits, including dementia, depression, schizophrenia, head injuries, and SLD.

Mismatch negativity is a frontocentral negativity that appears when a deviant physical stimulus occurs within a group of ongoing stimuli. It is an automatic change detecting response, is pre-attentive, and appears 150 to 200 ms after the event.

Using speech stimuli (i.e., /da//ba /wa) it was found that children with SLDs could not discriminate speech sounds as well as normal children. Impaired discrimination was associated with diminished MMN (Kraus et al., 1996; Leppanen & Lyytinen, 1997). These differences between dyslexics and controls were found for language stimuli but not for pure tone discrimination (Schulte-Korne et al., 1998a,b). Another study found that when the period between stimuli was lengthened to 80 ms, the dyslexics' response became closer to that of nonaffected readers (Habib, 2000).

An example of long latency ERP response to a cognitive stimulus is the P3 wave, which is one of the most reproducible and clinically useful of all cognitive ERP components. The response is related to conscious processing and memory updating. It is elicited in response to a stimulus that demands a "decision" by the brain. P300 is elicited in "oddball" paradigms in which subjects attend to a train of stimuli and have to respond to a different, deviant, stimulus. For instance, a subject may be given a series of auditory tones. Most of the tones are similar, but a different tone, higher or lower, is given intermittently. The rare, different tone will elicit a P300 (P3) wave, which is a broad, positive wave peaking at about 300 to 500 ms after stimulus onset, with maximal amplitudes at parietal and central midline recording sites on the scalp. P3 latency is thought to reflect processing time. It increases when the memory load involved with a task gets larger (Frank, Seiden, & Napolitano, 1996). P3 amplitude is thought to reflect capacity allocation. It decreases if there is a competing task (Donchin et al., 1986). Studies have shown smaller amplitude or increased latency responses in dyslexics (Taylor & Keenan, 1990). Event-related potentials studies in children with SLDs reveal significant differences from normal readers, usually reduced P3 amplitudes and increased P3 latency (Frank, Seiden, & Napolitano, 1994). Studies using a memory paradigm found decreased P3 amplitude and increased latency for learning disabled and reading disabled children, compared with regular readers, when memory set size was increased. This suggests abnormality in information processing because both P3 amplitude and latency would be expected to increase proportionally with increasing cognitive demands (Barnea et al., 1994; Frank, Seiden, & Napolitano, 1996).

Other cognitive paradigms are used in ERP studies, including learning and memory paradigms. P400 may reflect long-term semantic memory processes. Anomalous P400 was observed in subjects with developmental language disorders (Stelmack et al., 1988; Neville et al., 1993). Event-related potentials studies done during the performance of learning tasks demonstrated enhanced late positive wave elicited by verbal material, which was later recalled or recognized- compared with that elicited by material that was later forgotten, providing an electrophysiological correlate of learning (Paller, Kutas, & Mayers, 1987).

Event-related potentials elicited when words are presented usually include a surface negative late wave, N400–450. The characteristics of this wave depend on the subject's phonetic skills. ERP, reaction time, and response accuracy measures were obtained during rhyming and semantic classification of spoken words in average and reading-impaired children. Rhyme processing produced more pronounced ERP group differences than did semantic processing at about 480 ms, with a relatively more negative distribution for the impaired readers at centroparietal sites. This testifies to the fact that the important cognitive abnormality underlying reading disabilities, at least in some learning-disabled subjects, is in phonetic processing. Within a group of reading-disabled subjects, some had a stronger and some a weaker effect on the N400–450 wave, supporting the position that specific subtypes of reading disability exist (McPherson et al., 1996). An interesting study of ERP mapping performed during silent reading of correct and incorrect sentence revealed an abnormal pattern of early (P110) as well as late (N400) ERP waves. Short latency waves such as P110 usually reflect sensory-visual processing, whereas later waves such as N400 reflect cognitive-linguistic processing. These results were, therefore, interpreted as suggesting that sensory-visual processes as well as cognitive-linguistic processes are affected in dyslexic children.

Similar to neuroimaging studies, some ERP studies suggest that the normal hemispheric asymmetry of ERPs to simple visual, auditory, and tactile stimuli is reduced in children with SLDS. For instance, dyslexics failed to show increased left hemisphere negativity to linguistic stimuli, suggesting that their left hemisphere "treats" linguistic stimuli similarly to nonlinguistic stimuli (Sutton et al., 1986). In another study, a verbal stimulus elicited a late ERP response in the left parietal area that was of higher amplitude compared with a nonverbal stimulus, in normal but not in SLD subjects (Ostrosky-Solis et al., 1987). Event-related potentials recorded during short-term memory tasks from dyslexic children and normal-reading controls demonstrated right hemisphere prominence in dyslexics, in contrast with controls who had left hemisphere prominence. The results were interpreted as suggesting that dyslexic children relate to the physical features of stimuli as opposed to skilled readers, who rely more on the linguistic features of the stimuli (Barnea et al., 1994).

An interesting question is whether the ERP elicited in response to reading letter strings changes when a child learns to read, compared with those who cannot read yet. N1 early waves obtained in response to letter string in adults was specifically localized ("specialized") in the inferior posterior temporal cortex, and was maximal in the vicinity of the fusiform cortex. N1 early waves obtained in response to letter strings in 5-year-old Kindergarten before they learn to read, was not "specialized" (Maurer et al., 2005), although there was some specialization in children with high letter knowledge, possibly suggesting that one need to learn to read in order to "specialize." The importance of this finding is not clear, but it is possibly suggestive of brain plasticity.

MAGNETOENCEPHALOGRAPHY STUDIES IN DYSLEXIA

Magnetoencephalography (MEG) records spontaneous or evoked brain electrical activity and its topography. In addition, it can time electrical brain activities in response to stimuli. Its advantage is good temporal resolution, which cannot usually be done by functional magnetic resonance imaging (fMRI). At the same time, localization is only approximate.

Magnetoencephalography studies of pseudowords reading in normal readers show early activity in lateral occipitotemporal regions bilaterally followed after a significant delay by near simultaneous peaks of activity in the fusiform, angular, and middle temporal gyri. Subsequent activity peaks are seen in the areas of the right inferior frontal gyrus and later in left inferior frontal gyrus.

Magnetoencephalography studies helped the understanding of brain abnormalities underlying dyslexia. Salmelin et al. (1996) used MEG and compared six dyslexics and eight controls on reading of Finnish words and nonwords. Normal controls activated a left inferior temporal-occipital region (area 37) 180 ms after the presentation of words. This is the processing time estimated by the authors for "early visual processing or immediate phonological processing occurring before any conscious recognition has occurred." Dyslexics failed to activate this region. The authors state: "That dyslexics do not activate this process suggests either an inability to achieve these early operations of global word form perception or inefficient immediate phonological extraction." A left inferior frontal area was activated within 400 ms in four out of six dyslexics but none of the controls. The authors interpreted this unusual activity as a compensatory activity seen in the dyslexic subjects.

A MEG study employing face stimuli (Tarkiainen et al., 2003) elicited normal left occipital-temporal activation in dyslexic participants, in the time window of category-specific activation (150–200 ms after the stimulus). This contrasts with the reduced left occipital-temporal activation that has been observed in dyslexic participants during reading and suggests that the reduced activation of the left occipital-temporal cortex to letter string stimuli in dyslexics is a specific abnormality of reading.

A whole brain MEG study by Simos et al. investigated the relative degree and timing of cortical activation associated with phonological decoding (2008) of varied difficulty. It measured regional brain activity during performance of a pseudoword reading task and a less demanding letter-sound naming task.

The three study groups were reading disabled, nonaffected, and ADHD students. Results demonstrated a significant group main effect for performance on the pseudoword reading task: Performance was significantly higher for the nonaffected and ADHD group. The reading disabled children had decreased amplitude (indicating decreased degree of activity) compared with typical readers, in the temporoparietal regions (STG, SMG, and ANG), mostly of the left hemisphere, regions that have long been postulated to be crucial components of the brain mechanism for reading and are involved in phonological processes of print. These effects were noted as early as 350 ms after the stimulus and persisted for up to approximately 650 ms, similar timing to that delineated by Georgiewa et al. (2002) in the left inferior frontal area for visual language tasks.

There was no significant group difference of the activity in the inferior frontal gyrus, no differences in the degree of activity between typically performing students and students with ADHD, and no significant group difference for the easier phonological letter-sound naming task. Differences between normal readers and children with RD were restricted to the more demanding pseudoword reading and were not found during less demanding tasks, suggesting that aberrant brain activations are largely dependent on demands for phonological decoding.

In addition, a correlation between neurophysiological activity and reading achievement was demonstrated. For normal readers—significant positive correlations were obtained between word attack scores and the degree of activity in the left SMG, STG, ANG, IFG, and fusiform gyrus. The fact that there were no loci of brain activity that were positively associated with reading performance in children with RD is consistent with previous fMRI findings, and may reflect underdeveloped functional organization of cortical networks to support reading (Hoeft et al., 2007).

Simos and his associates (2002) used MEG in eight children with dyslexia and eight controls before and after 8 weeks of a phonologically based reading intervention. Before intervention, the dyslexic readers demonstrated little or no activation of the posterior portion of the superior temporal gyrus. After intervention, reading improved and activation increased in the left superior temporal gyrus.

Other studies used MEG to examine the brain responses to deviant auditory stimuli in dyslexics (Hari & Renwall, 2001; Renvall & Hari, 2002; Renvall, Hari, & Riitta, 2003). They used a monotonous sequence of 50 ms, 1000 Hz binaural tones, given 86% of time, and deviant tones of 920 and 1080 Hz occurring with 7% probability. A whole scalp neuromagnetometer recorded magnetic mismatch fields (MMFs) to the frequency deviant stimuli in a group of eight Finish adults with developmental dyslexia and 11 healthy controls. The reading tests employed by this research group to diagnosed

reading disability were reading aloud a Finnish story: reading speed, recognition of words versus pseudowords, speed of word recognition, naming
speed, and working memory. The dyslexic subjects were significantly slower
than the control subjects in reading, and their word recognition times were
longer. Mismatch responses to infrequent sound deviations are generated
in the superior temporal auditory cortex and are likely to reflect automatic
change detection in auditory cortex. The results demonstrated that MMFs
elicited in responses to infrequent sound deviations were diminished in
the left hemisphere of the dyslexic patients. Latencies were not different.
The results of this MEG study mean that dyslexics had markedly weaker
reactivity of the left auditory cortex to infrequent changes in tone pitch
compared with normal reading adults, suggesting an auditory processing
abnormality.

These findings may provide a clue to the source of the phonological processing abnormality in dyslexics. The deficit in phonological processing in dyslexics may derive from a more generalized auditory dysfunction, manifested as
impaired temporal processing of sounds (Tallal, 1980). The neurophysiological abnormality in dyslexia may be a persistent sensory deficit in monitoring
the frequency of incoming sounds (Baldweg et al., 1999). The authors discuss a possible existence of a short-term "cognitive window." This "cognitive
window" may be prolonged in dyslexics causing distorted processing of rapid
stimulus sequencing and the proper development of cortical representation
needed for reading acquisition (Hari, 2001).

Using MEG, Loveless et al. demonstrated that dyslexics have an abnormal enhancement of the 100 ms responses to the second tone of a pair, at
intersound intervals of less than 300 ms. The enhancement decreased significantly earlier in dyslexic patients (Loveless & Koivikko, 2000). Again, these
results demonstrate weaker activation of the left auditory cortex in dyslexic
children. Based on these results it was suggested that the decreased enhancement responses may be a result of a deficient buildup or a more rapid fading
of memory track. The fact that the abnormalities were demonstrated in the
left hemisphere suggests left hemisphere weakness. This ties up with the current hypothesis for reading disability in dyslexics, which involves deficits in
phonological skills. The neurophysiological abnormality discussed above may
explain the neural mechanism of the phonological deficit, localizing the deficit
to basic auditory processing abnormalities.

Early cortical processing of faces is similar, in location and timing, to
the processing of letter strings. A recent MEG study (Tarkiainen et al.,
2003) showed that face stimuli elicited normal left occipital-temporal activation in dyslexic participants, in the time window of category specific activation (150–200 ms). This contrasts with the reduced left occipital-temporal
activation that has been observed in dyslexic participants during

reading. In other words, although face recognition elicits activity in left occipital-temporal area of normals and dyslexics, word reading elicited reduced or deviated activity in the same area in dyslexics. So the dysfunction in this region found in dyslexics is specific to the processing of letter strings—an abnormality of reading.

The reduced left occipital-temporal activation found in the dyslexic participants for word reading (and for picture naming) corresponds almost precisely to the peak of the "word form area" proposed by Cohen and colleagues (McCandliss et al., 2003). This may suggest that the reduced activation of the left occipital-temporal cortex to letter string stimuli in dyslexics is a specific abnormality that dyslexics have in reading. Because the face stimuli and task used by Tarkiainen and colleagues did not require any phonological processing, it is not known whether this abnormality in dyslexics is related to phonological processing. The left occipital-temporal activation to faces might be abnormal if faces or objects had to be named (Tarkiainen et al., 2003).

The effect of intervention was also examined with MEG. Simos and his associates (2002) used MEG in eight children with dyslexia and eight controls before and after 8 weeks of a phonologically based reading intervention. Before intervention, the dyslexic readers demonstrated little or no activation of the posterior portion of the superior temporal gyrus. After intervention, reading improved and activation increased in the left superior temporal gyrus.

Last, studies that had functional MRI combined with ERP found differences between dyslexic and control groups in left inferior frontal areas, at 250 to 600 ms, for visual language tasks (Georgiewa et al., 2002).

SUMMARY: ELECTROPHYSIOLOGICAL METHODS IN DYSLEXIA

In summary, electrophysiological methods, including ERP, reveal important differences between subjects with SLD and normal learners, mostly when brain electrical activity is recorded during the performance of cognitive processes, including learning or reading. The demonstration, in dyslexic people, of aberrant brain electrophysiology during phonological processing and other cognitive processing associated with reading goes along with the finding that abnormal phonological processing is a determining factor underlying reading disability. There have been very significant advances in electrophysiological methods and tools, mostly consisting of increased ability to map and compute the event-related potentials. It is likely that these advances will make ERP more useful for the clinical diagnosis of SLD. The use of these methods for the clinical diagnosis of SLD is limited, however, mostly because of inconsistent methodology and results. In addition, many of the cognitive ERP parameters do not have norms for the pediatric age group, and when norms are available, the inter-individual variability is usually large limiting the ability to use these parameters for clinical diagnosis. Many of those deficits can be corrected.

VISUAL MAGNOCELLULAR SYSTEM
ABNORMALITIES

Starting in the retina, the visual system divides into two major processing pathways: a ventral pathway—the magnocellular—and a dorsal pathway—the parvocellular. This division continues in the lateral geniculate nucleus (LGN), the primary visual cortex, and higher-order visual cortices. Cells in the ventral, magnocellular layers are larger than cells in the dorsal or parvocellular layer. This is most apparent in the lateral geniculate nucleus.

The two systems differ in their preferred spatial frequencies, temporal properties, and contrast sensitivity. In primates, fast low-contrast visual information is carried by the magnocellular division, and slow, high-contrast information, by the parvocellular division. As discussed, recording of visual evoked potentials (VEP) is an electrophysiological technique used to assess the brain response to visual stimuli. It involves presentation of visual stimuli by a generator and the recording of electroencephalographic responses by electrodes attached to the scalp. Using VEP, a number of studies, suggest that dyslexics have an abnormality of the visual system, and process visual information slower than normal readers. The pattern of results suggested an abnormality affecting specifically the fast processing pathway of the visual system—the magnocellular visual pathway. Livingstone et al. found abnormalities in dyslexics' response to low-contrast, high-frequency stimuli. The same dyslexic children responded normally to targets of lower frequencies and higher contrast (Livingstone, 1991). When stimuli, in the form of flickering checkerboard patterns, were fast and with low contrast, evoked responses were slower in the dyslexic children compared with nondyslexic children. At a lower contrast (0.02)—an early negative wave, normally found at about 50 ms, was delayed in dyslexics. When the alternating checkerboard contrast was higher (0.2), the VEP of normal and dyslexics were the same. In other words, in response to visual stimuli in the form of flickering checkerboard patterns, brain responses in the dyslexic children were slower than the nondyslexic children when the stimuli given were fast and low contrast. The interpretation was that dyslexics can have normal responses to slower, higher contrast, visual stimulation frequency, but have difficulties with stimuli of faster frequencies and lower contrast (Livingstone, 1991). Studies also show a slower flicker vision rate (the fastest rate at which a contrast reversal of a stimulus can be seen) in dyslexics (Martin & Lovegrove, 1987). That means that dyslexics need much slower spatial frequency to perceive the same contrast as nondyslexic children. Again, it has been suggested that these differences in contrast sensitivity and visual persistence reflect abnormality of the transient system. This may affect many dyslexic individuals, "especially those with evidence of associated phonological deficit" (Lovegrove et al., 1980; Eden et al., 1996; Cornelissen, 1998). Visual detection of motion, another function usually ascribed to the magnocellular system, has been correlated with a lexical detection task.

These dyslexic subjects have a deficiency of the magnocellular pathway, which mediates the processing of rapid visual transitions at low contrasts (and is also involved in motion perception), causing visual information to be slower in these children (Greatrex & Drasdo, 1995). Indeed, the early negative wave, which was found to be slow in dyslexics, originates in the magnocellular system. The other visual pathway, the parvocellular, which is slow and relatively contrast-insensitive (and color selective), appears to function normally in dyslexics. It was suggested that it is this deficiency of the "transient" system in dyslexics, which makes it difficult for them to handle information presented at speed (Stein & Walsh, 1997; Stein, 2003). There is also a suggestion that normal magnocellular development may promote normal hemispheric asymmetry, whereas impaired magnocellular development is associated with the loss of normal asymmetry seen in dyslexia.

Histological measurement of neurons of the magnocellular and parvocellular layers of the lateral geniculate nucleus in five dyslexic and five control brains, revealed that the usually larger magnocellular cells are smaller in the dyslexic group, complementing the physiological findings. The parvocellular layers in the same brains were normal. These findings have not been replicated.

The evidence for this theory has not been consistent (Kubova et al., 1996), and there are research reports that question a specific magnocellular system deficit in dyslexia. Attempts to replicate Livingstone's visual evoked response findings failed to distinguish the responses of dyslexics from those of normals or other controls. A decrease in contrast resulted in an increased latency of the transient VEP in all groups, and did not distinguish the responses of dyslexics from those of controls. Response variability was similar in dyslexics and normals, but was increased in subjects with ADHD (Victor et al., 1993).

Another criticism of this theory questions the localization of the suspected abnormality within the magnocellular visual pathways. Judging from the fact that the evoked potentials abnormality in dyslexics was seen in an early evoked potential wave, which originates in the retina, the LGN, and/or the V1, and it is likely that the abnormality occurs very early in the processing of the visual stimuli. None of these structures is currently thought to be involved in cognitive processing of words (Galaburda, 1994). Therefore, the possibility that there is a cause–effect relationship between these findings and reading disability continues to be debated.

In spite of this criticism, an interesting theory suggests that similar to the visual system, subdivisions processing rapid stimuli exist in the other sensory systems that are also slower in dyslexics compared with normal readers. For instance, language processing areas of the planum temporale are characterized by large pyramidal cells and rich myelination, and may form part of a "fast" component of the auditory system. Deficits in the processing of fast transitions in the auditory modality can lead to deficient language processing at loci where fast processing is required, leading in turn to abnormal phonological processing and difficulties with learning to read. According to this theory, dyslexics may be unable to process fast incoming sensory information adequately in any sensory domain. Consequently, dyslexia is not the result of a single phonological, visual, or motor deficit, but rather a result of impairment of temporal processing in all sensory systems (Stein & Walsh, 1997) (see chapter 3).

OCULOMOTOR ABNORMALITIES

There have been ongoing questions on the role of vision and eye movement abnormalities in SLDs. The magnocellular system is important for directing visual attention, control of eye movements, and visual search—three skills that have a role in reading ability. Some authors emphasize the importance of visual and oculomotor defects in dyslexia, and suggest a link between these visual processes and reading abilities, showing a correlation between motion sensitivity and orthographical performance in an unselected sample of children.

It has become evident, though, that developmental learning disabilities stem from cognitive brain difficulties, and are not the result of a visual defect. Nevertheless, a visual abnormality should be ruled out in all learning disabled children. Optic nerve disease decreases visual acuity, whereas a visual field defect or a significant abnormality of eye movement makes it difficult for a person to fixate an object on the fovea. There may also be interplay between sensory-perceptual and cognitive factors in reading, in which a visual processing defect accompanies a "peripheral" visual abnormality. The ability to fixate, saccades (rapid eye movements that allow binocular, conjugate turning of the eyes from one fixation point to another), and smooth pursuit (movement of eyes made under visual guidance), have been studied in patients with developmental reading disabilities. Although some abnormalities were found, including fixation instability at the end of saccades and poor smooth pursuit (Eden et al., 1994; Poblano et al., 1996), it has been hard to prove a causative relationship between abnormalities of eye movements and reading abnormalities. It is possible that along with language processing abnormalities and phonological deficits, which are present in many dyslexic subjects and constitute a cause for reading disabilities, oculomotor abnormalities, when present to a significant degree, may contribute to reading as well as nonreading difficulties in those subjects.

CHAPTER 11

Genetics of Specific Learning Disabilities

INTRODUCTION

Some of our learning ability is genetically determined. The genetic component in the ability to learn is different for different types of learning. It may be stronger for the acquisition of motor skills than for learning of new facts.

Genes were found to be involved with memory formation. Research groups working with organisms including Aplysia and fruit flies demonstrated that by blocking certain genes (i.e., a gene called *CREB*), events associated with long-term memory—including protein synthesis and growth of synapses—do not occur. *CREB* interacts with the neuron's DNA and turns on dozens of genes, which remodel synapses and affect learning and memory storage processes. Other genes may also be involved (Rugg, 1998).

GENETICS OF SPECIFIC LEARNING DISABILITIES

This section summarizes available data of genetic transmission in Specific learning disabilities (SLD), especially reading disability. Genetic factors are probably the single most important factor in the etiology of SLD. Demonstrating that there is genetic transmission of SLD and establishing the pattern of transmission is important for the understanding of the biology of this common condition and for management, including early detection (Pennington et al., 1991).

Although some learning disabled people have only reading difficulties, many have, separately or in addition to reading disability, difficulties with other academic subjects, including mathematics. Genetic factors of SLD may, therefore, affect one area of deficit, for example reading, or can affect covariance of reading, mathematics, and possibly other academic deficits (Light & DeFries, 1998). Most of the genetic studies in learning disabilities involve specific reading deficits. The reasons for this are mostly historical, because reading disability, with or without other types of learning disabilities, is the most common type of SLD, and because there are better norms for reading than for other academic subjects. A chronic problem affecting advances in SLD research is that studies have used different methodologies, as well as different SLD definitions, and are, sometimes hard to compare.

Early Genetic Observations

The presence of familial aggregation of learning disabilities has been evident from some of the earliest reports on SLD, suggesting that SLD are heritable. In many families, reading difficulties are found in a number of first-degree relatives, including parents and siblings. Early familial studies suggested that reading disability is familial and that inheritance is autosomal dominant (Hallgren, 1950; Finucci et al., 1976) with genetic heterogeneity. The Colorado Family Reading Study, a family study of children with dyslexia, their parents, and siblings, with matched controls, which included longitudinal testing of reading and cognitive abilities, found that reading performance of relatives of children with this disorder was substantially lower than in controls (DeFries et al., 1978). Estimates of the risk to first-degree relatives are 35% to 45%. Along with a history of developmental language abnormality, the presence of a first-degree relative with a learning disability is a major component in the prediction of reading abnormality in a proband (Reynolds, Hewitt, & Erikson, 1996).

Twin studies, traditionally used to distinguish between genetic and environmental effects, demonstrated a high concordance rate of monozygotic twins for dyslexia and a much lower one for dizygotic twins, thus providing evidence for a genetic etiology of dyslexia. In twin studies, the concordance rate for monozygotic twins (68% and 100%) was significantly higher than the concordance rate for dizygotic twins (20% and 38%) (Bakwin, 1973; DeFries & Alercon, 1996; DeFries, Alercon, & Oison, 1997).

There may be a difference in the heritability of reading disabilities between higher and lower IQ subjects. Pennington et al. (1992) found a small difference between the heritability estimate of children with reading disabilities and lower IQ (<100; 0.43) and the heritability estimate of the group with higher IQ (>100; 0.72). The proportion of inherited factors in dyslexia is 40% to 80%, with the highest estimate for the phenotype word reading and spelling (Olson, 2002; Plomin & Kovas, 2005).

Although LD is frequently found along with Attention Deficit Hyperactivity Disorder (ADHD), these two conditions are transmitted in families independently (Faraone et al., 1993).

HOW IS SPECIFIC READING DISABILITIES GENETICALLY TRANSMITTED?

The question of how a genetic abnormality is transmitted in dyslexia has been actively investigated recently, using modern molecular genetic methods and tools. Initially, it was observed that males are affected more than females (Shapiro & Gallico, 1993), and consequently a sex influence on inheritance was suggested. It is evident now that the male to female ratio of reading disability in population samples is about 1.5:1.0, smaller than previously suggested. In addition, there has not been significant evidence for an X-linked disorder, or of parental sex effects on transmission. Other different modes of transmission have been proposed, including autosomal dominant, recessive, and polygenic transmission.

Segregation analyses of family studies (Pennington et al., 1991) and multiple regression analyses of twin data (DeFries & Fulker, 1985) confirmed that dyslexia is a genetically heterogeneous and complex trait that does not show classical mendelian inheritance. It is believed that the normal variation in reading skill is genetically transmitted in an autosomal dominant manner, but the deficits may be genetically heterogeneous. Several genetic loci seem to have an effect on reading. Molecular genetic linkage studies in families with dyslexia have identified chromosome regions in which the presence of dyslexia susceptibility genes is suspected. Links between dyslexia and markers on chromosomes 15, 6, and 2 have been confirmed by several independent studies. A locus on chromosome 15 was identified (Smith et al., 1983) and confirmed (Grigorenco et al., 1997; Grigorenco, 2001) although the locations differ. Similarly, linkage to dyslexia was found and replicated on chromosome 6 (6p21.3) (Grigorenco et al., 1997; Fisher et al., 1999; Gayan et al., 1999) and on chromosome 2 (Fagerheim et al., 1999; Petryshen et al., 2001, 2002). A complete quantitative trait loci analysis based on genome-wide scans for dyslexia in two large independent sets of families found, similarly, linkage for chromosome 6, 2, 3, and 18 (Fisher et al., 2002). Altogether, linkage analyses in families with dyslexia have reported nine chromosomal regions in which the presence of susceptibility genes is suspected. These are dyslexia susceptibility 1 (DYX1) to dyslexia susceptibility 9 (DYX9), on chromosomes 1, 2, 3, 6, 15, and 18. DYX1 is in chromosome region 15q21; DYX2 is in chromosome region 6p21-p22; DYX3 in chromosome 2p15-p16; DYX4 in chromosome 6q11-q12; DYX5 in chromosome 3p12-q13 region; DYX6 in chromosome 18p11 region; DYX7 in chromosome 11p15 region; DYX8 in chromosome 1p34-1p36 region, and DYX9 in chromosome Xq26-q27 (Schumacher et al., 2007).

GENES INVOLVED IN READING DISABILITY

Following the knowledge that reading disability is familial and heritable, genetic reading disability research began to focus on identifying the responsible genes. Genes that affect a quantitatively measured trait such as reading are termed quantitative trait loci (QTL). It is assumed that because reading is a complex construct—reading disability may have a multifactorial etiology in which any single QTL is neither necessary nor sufficient to cause the disorder (McGrath, Smith, & Pennington, 2006).

There is indirect evidence of the existence of a number of dyslexia candidate genes, identified by polymorphism in these areas that are statistically associated with increased risk of dyslexia.

The most significant ones are *DCDC2* and *K1AA0319*, both identified within DYX2 on chromosome 6p22. *DCDC2* (doublecortin domain containing protein 2) and *KIAA0319* were identified in a sample drawn from 114 US-American nuclear families of predominantly Europian origin. *DCDC2*, associated with reading disability, contains a doublecortin homology domain, modulates neuronal development in the brain, is possibly involved in cortical neuron migration, and is expressed in fetal and adult CNS (Meng et al., 2005; Plomin and Kovas, 2005).

A study by Antoni et al. (2006) searched for linkage disequilibrium in 137 triads with dyslexia in this region. The dyslexic patients in this cohort were selected based on a discrepancy between spelling ability and IQ. They found associations between the condition and markers within a locus containing the *DCDC2* gene area. This association was confirmed by further studies of 239 German triads with dyslexia, in particular in those with a severe phenotype of dyslexia. *ROBO1* (roundabout Drosophila homolog1) was discovered through mapping of a translocation in a Finish family (Hannula-Jouppi et al., 2005; Meng, Smith, et al., 2005).

Another candidate gene, *DYX1C1* was cloned in a two generation Finish family with a translocation, in a region on chromosome 15. It is expressed in the brain and is, supposedly, involved in the functional cell state (Taipale et al., 2003) although its exact function is not known. Similar to *DCDC2*, *DYX1C1* and *KIAA0319* are also involved in cell migration, and knockdown of any of these genes is associated with disrupted cell migration and presence of ectopic cells in the ventricular zone and layer 1. Almost all these candidate genes are implicated in global brain development process such as neural migration and axonal guidance. It is hard to explain how a genetic deficit, which may cause widespread migration abnormality, results in a very "specific" deficit causing reading disability. The abnormality may be a deficit in the ability to integrate the information needed for learning to read (Mitchell, 2011).

A condition known as periventricular nodular heterotropia is characterized by clusters of immature neurons in the white matter near the surface of the lateral ventricles. It is caused by mutation in the x-linked gene *Filamin-A* and a defect in cell migration is associated specifically with reading deficit (Dubeau et al., 1995).

Ectopias were also found in postmortem studies of subjects with dyslexia (without periventricular nodular heterotropia). These findings suggest that abnormality in neuronal migration may be a factor in reading disability (Gabel et al., 2010).

Although studies suggest that there may be a major locus transmission in a large proportion of dyslexic families, it is possible that the genetic model for dyslexia is a polygenic or multifactorial model. There may be a number of quantitative trait loci that underlie the transmission of both the normal variations in reading skill and dyslexia.

There are a number of possible reasons why some of the genetic findings have been hard to replicate. It is possible that some of the linkages exist in subgroups of families, though not in all. There may also be genetic factors like genetic heterogeneity, and incomplete penetrance. An important complicating factor is that the absence of consensus on the definition of dyslexia can account for variability of inclusion criteria across studies and for contradictory results (Demonet et al., 2004).

WHAT IS GENETICALLY TRANSMITTED IN READING DISABILITY?

It is not specifically known what the genetically transmitted components of specific reading disabilities are and how these are transmitted. Possibilities are that what is transmitted are phenotypes of dyslexia, including word reading, spelling, and writing. It is more likely, though, that genetic transmission will involve simpler and more basic cognitive processes rather than the very complex task of reading or of calculating. Therefore, it is more likely that what is genetically transmitted is not the deficiency in reading or spelling but one or more of the many cognitive abilities that underlie learning to read. These include, for instance, phonological awareness, orthographical and phonological coding, and short-term memory. An important cognitive factor for reading is phonological coding—the knowledge of the sound structure of the language. It is possible that the factor that is inherited in dyslexia is the abnormality of phonological coding or phoneme awareness.

It was demonstrated that the contribution of phonological coding to the heritability of the reading deficit, tested by single word reading in a twin study, was high, whereas orthographical coding did not contribute to this heritability (Reynolds, Hewitt, & Erikson, et al., 1996). One recent study reported a linkage analysis of dyslexic families that had at least four affected individuals. Family members were genotyped with markers in a number of chromosomal regions. The study analyzed five factors involved with reading ability: (1) phonological awareness, (2) phonological decoding, (3) rapid automatized naming, (4) single word reading, and (5) discrepancy between intelligence and reading performance. Phonological awareness and single word reading, each contributes to different processes related to reading skills. Rapid automated naming and single word reading are commonly abnormal in dyslexic people, and a discrepancy between intelligence and reading performance still serves as a criterion for dyslexia. The study demonstrated linkage between phonological awareness and single word reading and two different chromosomal regions on chromosome 6 and chromosome 15 respectively (Grigorenko et al., 1997). The chromosome 6 locus had a role in phonological awareness, and to a lesser extent in single word reading, whereas the locus on chromosome 15 affected single word reading only.

Other genetic studies with phenotyping support these findings, with a positive linkage between dyslexia and measures of phonological processing with genetic markers on chromosomes 1, 2, 3, 6, 15, and 18 (Cardon et al., 1994; Grigorenko et al., 1997, 2000, 2001; Schulte-Korne et al., 1998; Fagerheim et al., 1999; Fisher et al., 1999, 2002; Gayan et al., 1999; Nothen et al., 1999; Nopola-Hemmi et al., 2000, 2001; Petryshen et al., 2001). This means that a combination of genes within these regions may have a developmental effect on reading systems, leading to a reading disability (Eckert MA et al., 2003).

Genetic evidence also exists to show that both word recognition and listening comprehension are subject to genetic influence, which accounts for individual differences in reading comprehension (Keenan et al., 2006). As is the case with many other biological observations in LD, more and larger studies are necessary in order to assess the validity and importance of these findings. In the future, we might be able to link subtypes of dyslexia with particular loci.

CONCLUSIONS

The etiology of developmental dyslexia is, to a large degree, genetic (Pennington et al., 1991, 1999; Schulte-Korne, 1996; Smith et al., 1998; Fogerheim et al., 1999; Fisher et al., 1999; Gayan, 1999). The Genetic transmission is probably complex and nonexclusive. Genetic findings for dyslexia support this perspective. Phenotyping in genetic studies has resulted

in positive linkage between dyslexia and measures of phonological processing with genetic markers on chromosomes 1, 2, 3, 6, 15, and 18 (Cardon
et al., 1994; Grigorenko et al., 1997, 2000, 2001; Schulte-Korne et al., 1998;
Fagerheim et al., 1999; Fisher et al., 1999, 2002; Gayan et al., 1999; Nothen
et al., 1999; Nopola-Hemmi et al., 2000, 2001; Petryshen et al., 2001). One
gene or a combination of genes within these marker regions could have
developmental effects on a variety of neural systems involved with reading,
leading to a common behavioral outcome but heterogeneous neurobiological findings (Aylward et al., 2003).

Different genes may be implicated in different aspects of the reading disorder (e.g., genes on chromosome 15 related to performance on a single word
reading task or genes on chromosome 6 related to phonological awareness
task; Grigorenco, 1997).

GENETIC ASSOCIATION BETWEEN DYSLEXIA
AND AUTOIMMUNE DISORDERS

A potentially important finding in the genetic study of reading disabilities is a
possible association between reading disabilities and autoimmune disorders.
Studies pointed to a correlation between autoimmune disorders, particularly
those involving the gastrointestinal and the thyroid glands and reading problems (Crawford et al., 1994). As noted above, a linkage to loci on chromosome
6 was found in some families with reading disabilities. One of these loci is
near the HLA region, which codes for genes affecting the immune system. This
gave support to the theory of a complex link between non–right-handedness,
immune disease, sex hormone, and verbal learning disorder (the theory of
Geshwind-Behar-Galaburda). There are some factors that support the theory
Including the common presence of oral or written language deficits among
reading disordered children, suggesting a special vulnerability of the left
hemisphere cortical systems, and the locus for dyslexia gene in chromosome 6
(Cardon et al., 1994) which is part of the HLA complex, known to participate
in the immune system control. Still, this theory stays speculative.

GENETIC ASSOCIATION BETWEEN DYSLEXIA
AND MOTOR CONTROL

Dyslexics frequently have deficits in motor control of bimanual coordination. Wolff and others found that half of affected relatives of probands with
developmental dyslexia had motor coordination deficits and they came from
families in which probands also showed impaired motor coordination (Wolff
et al., 1995). In addition, they found that affected family members with motor

coordination deficits made significantly more dysphonetic spelling errors (measure of impaired phonological deficits) than dyslexic family members without motor deficits (Wolff, Melngailis, & Kotwica, 1996). They also found that these difficulties were more common and more severe among affected offspring in families in which both parents were affected than among affected offspring in families in which only one parent was affected. They suggested that the genetic model of dyslexia should include two co-dominant major genes (Wolff et al., 1995).

LEARNING DISABILITIES ASSOCIATED WITH SYNDROMES OF CHROMOSOMAL ANOMALIES

The subject matter of this book is the specific developmental learning disabilities, wherein the cardinal, and frequently the only, manifestations are learning difficulties. Specific learning disabilities can also be a component of a broader genetic condition in which other cardinal manifestations are present. Looking at these genetic conditions is important because it may shed more light on the genetics of learning disabilities.

Kleinfelter Syndrome

Dyslexia is found in syndromes of abnormal sex chromosome number, specifically 47 XXY (Kleinfelter syndrome). This is a chromosomal anomaly characterized by an additional X chromosome. Neurodevelopmental problems noted in early childhood include hypotonia, language delay, and fine motor coordination difficulties. Later in adolescence, the affected boys are tall, with long, thin torso and delayed sexual development. Their testicles are small and they may have gynecomastia (increased breast growth). Behaviorally, 47 XXY boys are initially introverted, quiet, passive, insecure, and have peer relationship problems. They are called lazy and unmotivated. In adolescence they may start having significant disruptive behavioral problems with impulse control abnormalities, at least partially related to continuous frustrating academic difficulties not recognized by school and parents.

Neuropsychological tests reveal specific patterns of cognitive impairment. The affected children may have normal intelligence but abnormal language abilities, with reduced verbal fluency and word retrieval, and difficulties with auditory processing and short-term auditory memory (Bender, Linden, & Robinson, et al., 1993). These abnormalities lead to a learning disability that is language based, affecting reading and writing while math skills are unimpaired.

Turner Syndrome

Turner syndrome is caused by loss of X chromosome material, and affects 1 in 2,500 females. It is characterized by short stature, sexual infantilism, and infertility. Specific learning disability is mostly in arithmetic, possibly due to reduced visual-spatial and memory abilities. Behavior problems include poor social competence (Rover, 1993), and the social isolation adds to school related problems.

Neurocutaneous Syndromes

Neurofibromatosis

Subjects with neurofibromatosis type 1 (NF1), an important genetic condition with autosomal dominant inheritance frequently have a learning disability as well as ADHD. The protein responsible for the neuropathology of NF1 is neurofibromin.

It is classified with a group of conditions known as neurocutaneous diseases or phacomatoses. With an estimated incidence of 1 in 3500, it is the most common single gene disorder affecting the human nervous system. The protein responsible for the neuropathology of NF1 is neurofibromin. Learning disabilities are very common in NF1, occurring in more than 50% of affected people (North, Joy, Yuille et al., 1994). It is now one of the clinical criteria for the diagnosis of the condition. Patients with NF1 frequently have brain abnormalities seen on MRI scan as areas of increased T2 signal intensity and referred to as "unidentified bright objects," or "UBO." The effects of these UBOs, present in more than half of the children with NF, on the brain and on cognitive functions, is not clear, and studies yield contrasting results. Some studies demonstrate that their presence was correlated with impaired visuomotor integration and with impaired academic achievements. In one study, which compared NF1 children to their unaffected siblings, significantly lower full-scale IQ and deficits in judgment of line orientation (a visuospatial test), reading disability, and motor deficit were found in the NF1 children and correlated with the number of hyperintensities on magnetic resonance imaging (Hofman, Harris, & Bryan, Denckla, 1994). Another study, found that children without T2 signal hyperintensity on MRI (UBO-) did not significantly differ from the general population in any measure of ability or academic performance (North, Joy, & Yuille, et al., 1994). A third study found that hyperintensities in the thalamus had an impact on neuropsychological functioning while hyperintensities in the cerebral hemispheres, basal ganglia, brainstem, or cerebellum did not have an impact. (Moore, 1996). It has been suggested that NF1 subjects have a specific type of SLD characterized by selective visuospatial and motor deficits, with a discrepancy between a better verbal and lower performance IQ. But recent studies have demonstrated that children with NF1 do not have a specific profile of learning disabilities (North et al., 1995; Chapman, Waber, & Bassett, et al., 1996), that visuospatial cognitive deficiencies are present in only a minority of NF1 children (Brewer, Moore, & Hiscock et al., 1997), and that language-based learning problems are at least as common. Children with NF1 who have SLD, especially girls, also have more problems of hyperactivity, impulsivity, and executive functions compared with children with developmental, nonspecific learning disabilities. Together, SLD and neurologically based behavioral problems may have a significant deleterious effect on academic and social functions of NF1 patients.

Tuberous Sclerosis

Another neurocutaneous condition is the tuberous sclerosis complex with an incidence of approximately 1:6000 to 1:10000. Like neurofibromatosis, it is a genetic condition, of autosomal dominant inheritance. Two gene loci have been proposed and there is a considerable phenotypic variation. Up to 80% of cases, though, are new mutations. Tuberous sclerosis has been characterized by a clinical triad of mental retardation, a typical cutaneous manifestation (adenoma sebaceum—sebaceous cysts over the nose bridge), and seizures of various types, including infantile spasms starting in infancy. Other manifestations of this syndrome include brain and other organ tumors. It is mentioned in this chapter because some patients with the condition do not have mental retardation but may have more selective cognitive deficits and learning problems (Clarke, Cook, & Osborne, 1996; Webb, Fryer, & Osborne, 1996). Among those are pervasive developmental disorder and hyperactivity.

Tourette Syndrome

Another genetic disorder where learning and behavioral difficulties are common is Tourette syndrome (TS). It is a familial neurobehavioral disorder characterized by involuntary motor and vocal tics, accompanied by obsessive-compulsive symptomatology, and ADHD. Other behavioral abnormalities as well as learning difficulties frequently occur (Singer, Scheurholz, & Denckla, 1995). It is suggested that the neuropathology is in the cerebral deep-seated basal ganglia, and involves an imbalance of the dopaminergic neurotransmitter system. Magnetic resonance imaging scans demonstrated abnormalities in some cases of TS, such as mild ventricular dilatation or prominent sylvian fissures, whereas SPECT and PET studies demonstrated abnormalities in the basal ganglia and in cerebral frontal cortical regions.

Although TS subjects have a variety of school difficulties, it is not clear whether they indeed have a specific learning disability or specific cognitive deficits. Although as a group TS subjects usually perform normally on neuro-psychological tests, some patients have demonstrated impairments in some of these tests, especially those with a later onset of tics and those with com-plex tics. Impaired neuropsychological scores are found on written arithmetic and visual-motor tests, expressive language, measures of problem solving, complex abstract reasoning, visual attention span, dexterity, and graphesthe-sia with comparatively better reading and word spelling. It is possible that although TS patients do not have a specific learning disability, some may have a relatively characteristic pattern of neuropsychological performance abnormalities with difficulties on "output" measures, similar to a pattern found in ADHD (Pauls, Leckman, & Cohen, 1993). It is also possible that the school-related difficulties of TS children are due to a combination of problems including tic severity, the use of tic-suppressing medication, a consequence of having a stigmatizing disorder, and the coexisting behavioral conditions including ADHD and obsessive-compulsive behaviors.

These examples of genetic disorders, which include significant learning disabilities and brain abnormalities, may help us understand the relationship between gene disorders and the various learning disabilities.

CHAPTER 12

Dyscalculia

INTRODUCTION

Knowledge of mathematics is important for the individual and for society. For the affected individual, low numeracy causes daily difficulties, and, similar to low literacy, is a handicap for life chances. It constitutes an impediment to employability, reduces lifetime earnings, and is a risk factor for depression. For society, improvement in mathematics and science performance has been associated with an increase in gross domestic product (Butterworth et al., 2011).

Mathematics is a complex subject involving language, space, and quantity. Even simple numerical abilities such as arithmetic or counting, involve transcoding between spoken number words and Arabic numerals, relating these to semantic representations of set size ("numerosity"), reasoning about relative set sizes (if 1 is added to 2, the result should be 3), and understanding the relations between set size and counting order.

The skills affected in mathematical disorders can be linguistic skills, perceptual skills, and attentional skills. In addition, as will be discussed later in this chapter, there may be specific deficits in mathematical skills, including following sequences of mathematical steps, counting objects, or learning multiplication tables. Therefore, there may be a conceptual distinction between "primary dyscalculia," in which the deficit is a specific inherent abnormality, and cases in which the dyscalculia is "secondary" to other cognitive impairments including attention deficits or visual perceptual spatial deficit (Rosenberger, 1989).

HISTORICAL BACKGROUND

Phrenological maps from the 19th century included "calculation" and "size" as two of the brain faculties—the first as an aptitude for the comprehension of numbers and the second as an aptitude for judgement of proportion and space

(Temple, 2006). It seems, therefore, that it was understood that at least some mathematical ability was determined in the brain from birth (Temple, 1990).

Early references to dyscalculia were by Henschen (1920), Berger (1926) and Gerstmann (1940). Luria (1946) noted the fact that dyscalculia is common in cases of diffuse higher cortical function impairment. Developmental dyscalculia was noted later by Kinsbourne and Warrington (1963). Cohn (1968) was the first to employ the name "developmental dyscalculia." They and others understood that dyscalculia stems from abnormalities of cognitive processes and is the result of a biological dysfunction, and that this entity is reserved to cases in which the deficit is specific and the rest of cognition is grossly preserved.

Some of the early knowledge of the neural basis of arithmetic skills came from the patients described by Henschen in the 1920s and the observations by Gerstmann on the effects of damage to the angular gyrus in the parietal lobe on calculations. Henschen (1920) wrote that "the calculation ability is a highly composite cerebral function that results from the collaboration of various posterior areas of the left hemisphere." Gerstmann and others found that left parietal damage causes deficits in calculation, and damage to the left angular gyrus disturbs the neural representation of fingers, causes right-left confusion, and agraphia (a tetrad known as Gerstmann syndrome).

These and other observations demonstrated that acquired brain disease or brain damage (i.e., stroke or brain tumor) can lead to a disturbance in the ability to perform calculation tasks, known as acalculia or acquired dyscalculia. A structural lesion to parietal areas in infants, leading to severe arithmetic deficits, is seen in children born prematurely. Decrease in parietal grey matter density in these premature babies is associated with lower math performance at the age of 15 years (Isaacs, Edmonds, Lucas, & Gadian, 2001).

It has been more difficult to determine that a developmental defect in the acquisition of numerical ability, known as developmental dyscalculia (DD), exists and is the result of brain dysfunction for this ability. But, as is the case with reading disabilities, cumulative genetic, neurobiological, and epidemiological data indicate that DD stems from abnormalities of cognitive processes and is the expressions of a biological brain dysfunction (Kucian et al., 2006).

DEVELOPMENT OF ARITHMETIC SKILLS

The development of arithmetic skills and knowledge consists of early numerical skills that are inherent and exist without learning, and more complex skills that are acquired and learned. Animals and young infants possess biologically determined, domain-specific number concept and numerosity including relational concepts such as more, less, and the ability to arrange objects according to size, as well as simple counting skills. Behavioral studies in animals reveal number perception, discrimination, and elementary calculation abilities in chimpanzees, showing that a sense of numerosity exists even in animals (Kawai & Matsuzawa, 2000). Basic numerical skills are probably innate and develop in infants without formal schooling. Infants, in the first week of life, seem to discriminate visual arrays on the basis of numerosity. Throughout the preschool years children develop early numeracy skills that are precursors to the acquisition of formal mathematical skills. Number concept refers to relationships such as more, less, and the ability to arrange objects according to size. Development can be seen in terms of an increasingly sophisticated understanding of numerosity and its implications, and in increasing skill in manipulating numerosities. The impairment in the capacity to learn arithmetic—dyscalculia—is, in many cases, a deficit in the child's concept of numerosity (Butterworth, 2005).

Toddlers can add and subtract numbers up to three. At 3 to 4 years they can count up to four items, and by 5 years, up to 15. Four year-old-children can use fingers to aid adding. Five year-old-children can add small numbers and are able to count out sums. Eight-year-olds can recognize arithmetic symbols and perform elementary exercises in addition and subtraction. Multiplication and division is acquired at 9 to 12 years.

DEVELOPMENTAL DYSCALCULIA DEFINITIONS

Developmental dyscalculia is a specific learning disability affecting mathematical skills and numerical competence, found in children with normal intelligence who do not have acquired neurological injuries (American Psychiatric Association, 1987). These difficulties disrupt the academic achievement or daily living of these children, and they underachieve on a standardized test relative to the level expected given age, education, and intelligence (e.g., DSM-IV, American Psychiatric Association, 1994).

The disorder has been designated a number of different names including Mathematical Disorder in the DSM-IV (American Psychiatric Association, 1994), and Specific Disorder of Arithmetic Skills in the ICD-10. The diagnostic criteria delineated in the DSM-IV under "Diagnostic criteria for 315.1 Mathematics Disorder" state that "Mathematical ability, as measured by individually administered standardized tests, is substantially below that expected given the person's chronological age, measured intelligence, and age-appropriate education." The disturbance also has to "significantly interfere with academic achievement or activities of daily living that require mathematical ability."

Different criteria measuring mathematical disabilities exist. Shalev and Gross-Tsur (2001) use the criterion of two grades below chronological age.

Butterworth's *Dyscalculia Screener* requires scores on two tests to be in the lowest two stanines (11th percentile) or a criterion of 3 standard deviations (SDs) below the mean of the control group (Landerl, Bevan, & Butterworth, 2004). Some researchers include children who fall under 25% to 35% in various achievement tests (Hanich et al., 2001; Jordan et al., 2002). Standardized tests for mathematics are diverse and include different components, so that the definitions of dyscalculia will differ between studies.

It is evident that, for now, DD is a clinical syndrome. We use low achievements on mathematical achievement tests as the criterion for this condition without identifying underlying cognitive or biological phenotypes.

SYMPTOMS AND SIGNS

Relatively basic numerical abilities, such as arithmetic or counting, involve semantic representations of set size ("numerosity"), understanding the relations between set size and counting order, reasoning about relative set sizes (if 1 is added to 2, the result should be 3); and transcoding between spoken number words and Arabic numerals (Landrel, 2004).

Children with dyscalculia have different combinations of difficulty in mathematics, including difficulty learning mathematical concepts, remembering and retrieving arithmetic facts (Shalev & Gross-Tsur, 2001), automatic processing of numerical information, executing calculation procedures, and developing problem-solving strategies. They have long solution times and high error rates (Geary, 1993; Landrel, 2004). They fail tests in mathematics, and may suffer the social and emotional consequences of academic failure.

Although symptoms can be seen in the first grade, such are much more evident at 9 to 10 years. Children with DD may not be able to retrieve previously learned information; learn the procedures needed for completion of problems of addition, subtraction, multiplication, or division; match written Arabic numerals to quantities; understand concepts of more and less; and determine which pair of numerals is larger or smaller. They may not be able to handle money (Shalev & Gross-Tsur, 2001).

As is true for other types of learning disabilities, children with dyscalculia, unless they have the comorbidity of another learning disability, can be very successful in areas that do not involve heavy use of numbers.

PREVALENCE AND NATURAL HISTORY

The prevalence of DD across countries is relatively uniform, with estimates of 3% to 6% or 5% to 7% in the normal population, which is similar to that of developmental dyslexia and ADHD (Kucian et al., 2006). Other studies found prevalence rates of 3.6% to 6.5% (see work by Kosc 1974; Badian, 1983; Lewis, Hitch, & Walker 1994; Gross-Tsur, Manor, & Shalev, 1996). It is likely that about 6% of school age children suffer from this disorder.

A study by Koumoula et al. (2004), which aimed to achieve a Greek validation of the Neuropsychological Test Battery for Number Processing and Calculation in Children, used a community sample of different schools, grades 2 to 5, and a clinical sample, grades 2 to 5. In their sample 15% performed on their battery below –1 SD, 6.3% performed below –1.5 SD, 4.5% less than 2.0 SD, and 1.3% below –3 SD. This example demonstrates how findings of mathematical disability depend on the achievement tests done and on the cut-off definition of disability (along with other factors like the family's socioeconomic status, and the presence of comorbidity).

A difficulty in assessing prevalence stems from the fact that DD is frequently found together with other developmental disorders including dyslexia and ADHD (Gross-Tsur et al., 1996), and also in children with epilepsy and in Turner syndrome.

Girls and boys seem to be affected by DD equally. There is not a significant body of knowledge of the ultimate outcome of dyscalculia but it seems to be an enduring specific learning difficulty, persisting into late adolescence and adulthood (Shalev et al., 2005). Almost half of a cohort of 140 dyscalculic children, tested at age 10 to 11 years, were still dyscalculic when retested 3 years later, at age 13 to 14 years. Factors associated with persistence of DD were severity of the arithmetic disorder and arithmetic problems in siblings. Socioeconomic status, gender, the presence of another learning disability, and educational intervention were not associated with persistence of DD (Shalev et al., 1998). In other studies, the family's socioeconomic status and the region appear to play a substantial role in children's mathematical performance.

GENETICS AND COMORBIDITY

Developmental dyscalculia, like other learning disabilities, has a significant familial aggregation, and high heritability. A study of monozygotic and dizygotic twins found that 30% of the genetic variance was specific to mathematics. Still, because the biological pathophysiology of DD and mathematical learning disability (MLD) is not known, we do not know how much of this disorder is genetic and how much is environmental.

It is frequently present in association with other learning impediments including a reading disability. Similarly, dyscalculia is also frequently found in combination with attentional problems. More than 25% of children with developmental dyscalculia have ADHD as well (Gross-Tzur et al., 1996). Of a cohort of children with developmental dyscalculia, 26% had ADHD and 17% also had dyslexia (Shalev & Gross-Tsur, 2001). Other estimates of the comorbidity of dyslexia with dyscalculia are higher (Lewis, Hitch, & Walker, 1994). A causal relationship between these two disorders has not been proved. That is also true for the comorbidity of ADHD and dyscalculia. Whereas in some cases there may be a causal relationship, there is also some evidence that ADHD and dyscalculia are independently transmitted in families.

It has been thought that the combination of DD with reading disability is a specific subtype of DD. These children with comorbid mathematics and reading difficulties tend to be more impaired than children with DD only.

Nonverbal learning disability is characterized by visuospatial difficulties, visuomotor coordination, and reasoning problems. In this syndrome, dyscalculia is the most frequent academic problem (Gross-Tsur, 1995). People with certain genetic conditions, like fragile X syndrome, Williams syndrome, and Turner syndrome, have more learning problems in mathematics, compared with reading.

GERSTMANN SYNDROME

Josef Gerstmann, an Austrian neurologist, described (1940) a few patients with concomitant impairment in discrimination of their own fingers (finger agnosia), writing by hand (dysgraphia), distinguishing left from right (right-left disorientation), and performing calculations (dyscalculia). Constructional apraxia can be another finding in Gerstmann syndrome. He claimed that it constitutes a syndrome and all these symptoms have a common functional denominator, which is a lesion of the dominant parietal lobe. Neuroimaging showed a correlation between the syndrome and lesions in the left posterior parietal area.

There are reports of developmental Gerstmann syndrome in children who are otherwise apparently normal (Kinsborne & Warrington, 1963; Temple, 1987), with no history of an insult or of other symptoms and signs suggesting a previous brain insult. The children described by Kinsborne and Warrington did not have difficulties with number concept but had difficulties in using place values in representing and manipulating numbers. The site of pathology in developmental Gerstmann syndrome is not known.

Over the years there have been many discussions regarding this syndrome, with the main obstacle being lack of ability to find one anatomical or physiological lesion that will explain all its symptoms. Also, because the four symptoms can appear individually and in any combination, and are frequently associated with other conditions such as reading disability, it is unlikely that the symptoms are related in terms of a single underlying deficit. Similar questions are also present for developmental Gerstmann syndrome, namely, is this combination of symptoms specific and unique. Kinsbourne and Warrington hypothesized that it is a learning disorder. Some think it is not specific (Miller et al., 2004).

Anatomically, it was argued that it is unlikely that all these symptoms will be caused by damage to one same population of neurons. It is more likely that Gerstmann syndrome is a disconnection syndrome, caused by a lesion to separate but co-localized fiber tracts in the subcortical parietal white matter. A functional magnetic resonance imaging (fMRI) study using diffusion tensor imaging mapped brain responses to the four symptoms of Gerstmann syndrome—calculations, left-right orientation, writing, and finger agnosia— and found that brain activation for these different task-related functions did not overlap, but fiber tracts from these four domain-related networks consistently travelled through a certain locus of white matter in the parietal lobe. A lesion to this locus can result in a Gerstmann syndrome (Rusconi et al., 2010; Kleinschmidt, 2011).

In essence, this suggests that the abnormalities in Gerstmann syndrome are the result of white matter damage.

COGNITIVE STRUCTURE OF MATHEMATICS

Mathematical competence is complex and reflects both procedural and conceptual knowledge. The conceptual knowledge that is needed is the understanding of the basic principles of the mathematical domain (counting; the concept of cardinality; estimation; and number sense, which involves understanding quantity). Procedural knowledge includes the understanding of algorithms or step by step procedures needed to perform calculations and mathematical operations. Learning the relationship between numbers represented by Arabic numeric, spoken language, written verbal forms, and internal numeric representations involves language ability. During normal development, as procedures become more familiar they may be represented by explicit knowledge of overlearned arithmetic facts retrieved from long-term memory (e.g., 3 + 2 = 5) (Ardila & Rosselli, 2002).

McCloskey et al. (1985) proposed a cognitive model of numerical processing based on three basic abilities: Number processing, which needs number comprehension (understanding of the number, comprehension of quantities, number symbols); production of a number; and processing the mathematical procedures.

There are many cognitive processes involved in learning mathematics. Learning numbers represents a language that involves a system of symbols. We need to recognize the numbers and be able to name them. Numerical recognition involves visuospatial discrimination ability. One also has to perceive the spatial organization of the quantities, and the relationship among them. Beyond the recognition of numbers, the solution of a numerical problem demands understanding the meaning of mathematical symbols (like + or X) and knowing the steps needed for adding, subtracting, etc. The central neural mechanisms employed in the recognition of numbers is different from the one employed in solving arithmetic problems, which involves other verbal and conceptual abilities, and therefore requires the participation of numerous cerebral structures.

In addition, to be able to handle all of the these processes, there is a need for good working memory. In addition, retrieving previously learned mathematical facts from memory involves good long-term memory skills. Working memory is comprised of three components: the phonological loop for the temporary storage of phonological information; the visual spatial sketch pad for the temporary storage of visual spatial information; and the central executive, a modality free supervisory system responsible for a range of regulatory functions including control of both the phonological loop and the visual spatial sketch pad and the incorporation of information from long-term memory. The importance of working memory for arithmetic has been long recognized (Adams & Hitch, 1997).

The protoquantitative schema (Resnick, 1989)—is the comprehension of the concept of quantities and their increase or decrease after addition and subtraction of amounts. This schema forms the basis of the mental imaginary needed for rapid comparison and approximation of numerical quantities (Resnick, 1989; von Aster, 1994).

Human infants have some biological primary "numerosity" abilities at birth (Geary, 1993), meaning the ability to perceive and compare nonsymbolic quantities of items. They can respond, without formal training, to increases and decreases in objects and events (up to 4) in their immediate surroundings. They can discriminate between two displays on the basis of numerosity and can match numerosity across modalities. This basic approximate number system, which is nonverbal, exists also in nonhuman species (Butterworth, 2010) and may be the foundation for arithmetic learning. Later, Younger children use fingers to assist the numerosity code—oneness is represented by one element, twoness by two elements, etc. There is a correlation between the child's ability to do these tasks and mathematical attainment (Halberda et al., 2008; Piazza et al., 2010). Symbolic numerical representations build on these basic abilities. The range of numerical ability widens as soon as children acquire language, and enable older children and adults to use precise number words, symbols, and linguistic quantifiers. Acquisition of language allows them to associate verbal labels to any previously defined quality. Language is important in the symbolization of numerosities. It can be used to think about numbers and to communicate numerical facts. So the development of arithmetic skills can be affected by abnormal language. It may cause a failure to link intact number concepts with their symbolic representation. This can also be an underlying factor in dyscalculia.

The skills affected in mathematical disorders can be linguistic skills, perceptual skills, attentional skills, or unique "mathematical skills"—following sequences of mathematical steps, counting objects, or learning mathematical skills like multiplication tables. Abnormal language skills may cause a failure to link intact number concepts with their symbolic representation. This can also be an underlying factor in dyscalculia. Others include a basic failure to name, read, or write numbers, sequencing deficits, visual-spatial difficulties, or a general problem with speed of processing. Clinically one can, therefore, expect that subjects with dyscalculia will have deficits in one or more of these many cognitive processes involved in mathematical competence. For instance, there may be subjects with deficits in basic recognition of numbers, or there can be patients with an exclusive problem in the analysis of mathematical signs. Indeed, the neuropsychological abnormalities found are variable and include abnormalities in using numerical reasoning, solving arithmetic problems, and performing numerical operations, in spatial organization, visual attention, procedural motor, judgment, reasoning, and memory.

There is a group of patients with independent, very basic deficiencies that underlie DD (Ansari & Karmiloff, 2002; Henik et al., 2011). Otherwise, investigating the cognitive neuropsychological substrates of dyscalculia could gain from studying its comorbidities. Dyscalculia is frequently found in combination with reading disorders, attentional problems, ADHD, poor hand-eye coordination, poor working memory span, epilepsy, fragile X syndrome, Williams syndrome, and Turner syndrome, although causal relationships between these disorders and dyscalculia have not been established.

Over the years, there have been attempts to understand the cognitive abnormalities underlying dyscalculia and classify different variants of this condition including by Kos, Rourke, Dehaene, and Von Aster.

Kos (1974) distinguished types of dyscalculia: verbal (affects the verbal designation of mathematical terms), apractognostic(difficulty manipulating objects in a mathematical way), lexical (difficulty in reading the symbols of mathematics), graphic (difficulty in writing the symbols), ideognostic (difficulty in understanding mathematical ideas), and operational (difficulties in execution). Somewhat similar classifications are between disorders of number processing, disorders in establishing mathematical facts and disorders of arithmetical procedures.

Rourke proposed that dyscalculia is secondary either to visuospatial or verbal and auditory perceptual dysfunction (Rourke, 1993).

Dehaene's model contains three modules: auditory verbal word frame (skills founded on general language processing), the visual Arabic number form (numerical operations in the Arabic notation system), and analog magnitude representation (skills comparing and approximating numerical quantities).

THE NEUROPSYCHOLOGICAL BASES OF DYSCALCULIA

What are the cognitive/neuropsychological deficits which underlie developmental dyscalculia? Is the numerosity deficit the only problem in dyscalculia, which means it is the only process which needs to be tested in order to make a diagnosis of dyscalculia, or do we need to test other multiple cognitive traits?

A number of cognitive deficits have been described in developmental dyscalculia. Working memory has a central role in mathematical achievements. Geary (1993) suggests that poor working memory resources not only lead to difficulty in executing calculation procedures, but may also affect learning of arithmetic facts. He suggested that cognitive causes of dyscalculia include abnormal representations in semantic memory and difficulty with working memory, and that semantic memory difficulties may underlie the problems experienced by developmental dyscalculics in learning number facts (Geary et al., 2000). Several studies show a relationship between DD and spatial working memory (Camus, 2008; Rotzer et al., 2009). Memory abnormalities may also underlie the comorbid reading difficulties frequently found with dyscalculia. A study of memory abilities in children with dyscalculia and children with dyscalculia and reading disability had the same pattern of mathematical impairment, and both groups had lower scores than controls on working memory skills (Rosseli et al., 2006). Working memory is frequently assessed by the number of spoken items (generally digits) that can be remembered in the correct sequence. However, there is no clear evidence for a correlation between reduced digit span and developmental dyscalculia. So although various forms of working memory difficulty may co-occur with mathematics difficulties, there is no convincing evidence that a deficit in working memory as a cause of dyscalculia.

A study by Landerl et al. (2004) included 54 participants who were selected from a larger group of 8- to 9-year-old children from 11 middle schools in the London area. The dyscalculic children identified in this study demonstrated general deficits in number processing, including accessing verbal and semantic numerical information, counting dots, reciting number sequences, and writing numbers. Dyscalculic children without reading disability were normal or above average on tasks involving phonological working memory, accessing nonnumerical verbal information, nonverbal intelligence, language abilities, and psychomotor abilities. Children with reading disability were slower than controls in reciting number sequences (although less so than dyscalculic children), and there were non-significant trends toward slowness in number reading and number naming. However, unlike with the dyscalculic groups, the number naming trend disappeared once general naming ability was controlled for. Dyslexic children were also identical to controls on nonverbal (or nonphonological) tasks such as number writing and number comparison. This pattern of results suggests that children with only reading difficulties do not have number processing deficits, although difficulties with verbal or phonological aspects of some of these tasks may have affected their performance (Landerl, Bevan, & Butterworth, 2004). The patterns of performance of the two dyscalculic groups on the numerical tasks were very similar. This study has found no evidence for a qualitative difference in the numerical abilities of dyscalculic children with and without reading disabilities (Landerl, Bevan, Butterworth, 2004). In many tasks, the double deficit group's performance was slower or more error prone than that of the dyscalculic group, suggesting that their difficulties may be more severe, as suggested by other works (Jordan & Montani, 1997). However, the pattern of impairment was the same for both groups: They had difficulties with every aspect of numerical processing tested in this study (Landerl, Bevan, & Butterworth, 2004).

Reading disabled children may have difficulties in reading math problems, because of their reading difficulties, but no problems with simple calculations (Shapiro & Gallico, 1986). It was found that the evoked potentials of children who manifest impaired arithmetic performance in addition to impaired reading and spelling differ from those whose impaired arithmetic performance is not accompanied by reading and spelling disability (Rourke, 1993). It is, therefore, less likely that dyscalculia is, like most reading disorders, an abnormality of language processing.

Another study measured short-term memory, processing speed, sequencing ability, and retrieval of information from long-term memory in 7-year-old children. After controlling for reading ability, arithmetic ability was best predicted by processing speed, with short-term memory accounting for no further unique variance (Bull and Johnston, 1997). Other studies found indications that an abnormality of working memory is a factor in some cases of DD. An Event Related Potentials (ERP) study (Soltesz, 2007) found difference between individuals with DD and controls at 400 to 440 ms after the onset of the numerical stimuli. At that time the right parietal lobe of the DD subjects was no longer involved with the numerical difference effect. This suggests that the processes involved are the more complex processes such as executive functions or working memory and not the simple mental operations.

One of the main deficits of DD subjects is difficulty in retrieving arithmetic facts. This difficulty is more related to attentional deficits, working memory and executive functions deficits, or long-term memory deficits.

DYSCALCULIA AND ATTENTION DEFICIT HYPERACTIVITY DISORDERS

There are reports of decreased or abnormal attention variables in dyscalculia but it is not clear whether attention deficit is a comorbidity of some dyscalculic children or it contributes to the pathogenesis of the condition. Early work by Rosenberger (1989) found that when a group of students with low mathematics achievement was compared with a group of students with low reading achievements, the low mathematics achievement group had lower scores on a Bender Visuomotor Gestalt test and on "freedom from distractibility quotient" (considered a reflection of attention).

Independence of the Ability to Calculate

The studies just described have attempted to get at the root of dyscalculia by examining various abilities not directly related to number processing, but which are hypothesized to effect dyscalculia. This approach involves an implicit assumption that the representation and manipulation of numerical information is dependent upon other higher-order traits, including attention. However, there has been neuropsychological evidence that the ability to understand numbers and to calculate is dissociable from language, from semantic memory, and from working memory (Butterworth, Cipolotti, & Warrington, 1996; Cohen et al., 2000), and that impaired arithmetic skills result from selective deficits in cognitive processes that are unique to calculation, appear to be "hardwired" and are manifested even in infants (Wynn, 1995), and may be independent of other abilities.

A number of studies have found numerical processing abilities in animals (see Gallistel, 1990 for a review). Thus, number processing appears to be a function that emerges in infants at a very early age, and is independent of other abilities. There is evidence that children are born with a capacity for recognizing and even mentally manipulating small numerosities (Wynn, 1995), and seem able to carry out judgements on small numerosities. This argues against a role for language-related abilities such as semantic or working memory in developmental dyscalculia. There is evidence that dyscalculic children have problems with even the most basic functions involving numbers such as subitizing, counting small numbers of objects, using number names, and comparing numerical magnitudes, as well as more advanced arithmetical skills (Kirby & Becker, 1988; Koontz & Berch, 1996). Basic numerical functions, such as comprehension of numerical symbols, counting, and simple calculation, are built primarily upon early mechanisms for processing small numerosities which are independent of other abilities. These mechanisms may be the basic deficit underlying dyscalculia: a congenital failure to understand basic numerical concepts, to represent and process numerosity in a normal way. This is revealed by deficits in very basic numerical capacities, dot counting, and number comparison; lack of understanding of numerosity; and a poor capacity to recognize and discriminate small numerosities. These may prevent dyscalculics from developing the normal meanings for numerical expressions and lead to their difficulties in learning and retaining information regarding numbers (Landrel et al., 2004). Failure to develop normal representations may also account for the difficulty experienced by dyscalculic children in memorizing arithmetical facts, which do not have the same meanings for them.

The underlying cause of dyscalculia is likely to be related to dysfunction of a "number module" based in the parietal lobe that deals with numerical representations. It was suggested (Cantlon, Platt, & Brannon, 2009) that number representation depends on an innate approximate number system, which represents the number of objects, events, and time as continuous (analogue) mental magnitudes. This system involves the intraparietal sulcus (IPS) and is compromised in those with DD.

In other words, the pathophysiology of dyscalculia can be explained by the presence of a fundamental deficit specific to dyscalculia, which is a deficit in the representation of numerosities—the number of objects in a set (Piazza et al., 2010). Some researchers of DD claim that this core deficit relates to impairment in the mental and neural representations of fingers (Butterworth et al., 2011). Fingers are used in acquiring arithmetical competence. It involves understanding the mapping between the set of fingers and the set of objects to be enumerated. If the mental representation of fingers is weak, this representation is difficult. Weakness in finger representation is a predictor of arithmetic ability (Noel NP, 2005). The brain area involved is located in the intraparietal sulcus.

One of the difficulties with explaining all DD by one core deficit is that it occurs frequently together with reading disorders and ADHD and that a relationship exists between arithmetic and working memory. There is also a relationship between mathematical ability and the amount of arithmetic instruction time. This means that there may be other subtypes of DD. In an article called "Developmental dyscalculia: heterogeneity might not mean different mechanisms," Orly Rubinstein and Avishai Henik (2009) suggest that the behavioral deficits are heterogeneous; there are comorbidities in most cases; and also: different aspects of intact number processing are represented in different brain areas as shown by functional brain imaging. They define two different terms: developmental dyscalculia (DD), which is a deficit in core numerical abilities (e.g., difficulty in processing quantities), a relatively specific malfunction at the behavioral level; and Mathematical Learning Disability MLD caused by several possible cognitive deficits such as deficient working memory, visual-spatial processing, or attention.

When children and adolescents with unilateral left- or right-hemisphere lesions were administered a standardized test of mathematics ability and a battery of experimental tests that examined the components of numerical and arithmetic processing, both groups performed lower than control. Left-lesioned subjects (ages 7–12) had deficits on the verbal counting, digit matching, speeded addition, and written subtraction tasks. Deficits among younger right-lesioned subjects were similar in nature, yet less pronounced than in the left-hemisphere group. Older left-lesioned subjects showed differences from their controls only on complex verbal counting and speeded addition. The conclusions of this study were that earlier onset of left-hemisphere lesion is associated with more serious disruption of mathematical processing. Also, these disruptions are not well assessed by a typical standardized test of mathematical performance, but are clearly in evidence with more precise, focused tasks. This has implications on research in DD. The extent of the deficits and the underlying pathophysiology may differ, depending on the age of the subjects and on the depth of investigation (Ardila & Rosselli, 2002).

THE BRAIN DURING CALCULATIONS

One of the best mathematical brains of our time was that of Albert Einstein, the devisor of the law of general equivalence of mass and energy and the 1921 Nobel Prize laureate. When Einstein died of a ruptured abdominal aneurysm in 1955, at the age of 76, a postmortem study of his brain was carried out (Witelson, Kigar, & Harvey, 1999). The brain was compared with the brains of a large control group consisting of 35 male and 56 female brains. The examination showed that in Einstein's brain the parietal lobes were relatively wider and the brain was more spherical than the control group. His parietal lobes were also symmetrical, due mainly to his left parietal lobe being larger than usual. The posterior end of the Sylvian fissure had a relatively anterior position resulting in the absence of the parietal operculum and in a larger expanse of the inferior parietal lobule. It was suggested that, in Einstein's brain, "extensive development of the posterior parietal lobes occurred early, constraining the posterior expansion of the Sylvian fissure and the development of the parietal operculum but resulting in a larger expanse of the inferior parietal lobule" (Witelson et al., 1999). The inferior parietal lobule is involved in cognitive faculties including mathematics and visuospatial cognition. Expansion of the inferior parietal lobule was noted in the brains of other physicists and mathematicians. These suggest that mathematics have a tangible substrate in the brain.

Biological Source for Numerosity

Recent studies in human neuroimaging, indicate that the human ability for arithmetic has a tangible cerebral substrate and that brain areas important in relation to arithmetics as well as dyscalculia, are in the parietal areas. This is evident in cases with brain damage to this area, in particular to the left angular gyrus (Cipolotti & van Harskamp, 2001). Both human and monkey studies relate the processing of numerical quantity information to the posterior parietal cortex, including the IPS (Dehaene et al., 2004; Nieder, Miller, 2004). It was proposed that "number sense" is a basic capacity of the human brain (Dehaene et al., 1998), and that a number sense is built in with dedicated brain circuits and specialized neural networks for number processing engaged in recognizing numerosity—the number of objects in a set.

In humans a specific neural substrate, located in the parietal lobes, is involved with a cortical network for number processing. There are other areas in this cortical network that are active when people do math. Those include left frontal areas. This suggests that neurons in the posterior parietal and prefrontal cortices are linked to form a functional network for the representation of numerical information across space and time (Nieder et al., 2002, 2006). Dehaene and Cohen (1997) proposed the hypothesis that "number sense" is a basic capacity of the human brain built in with dedicated brain circuits that are engaged in recognizing numerosity (the number of objects in a set) (Dehaene et al., 2004). Pathology within this system can lead to acalculia in adults or to developmental dyscalculia in children (Dehaene et al., 2004).

A monkey analogue of these parietal-frontal regions has recently been identified, suggesting an earlier evolution of these areas, and a neuronal population that codes for numbers has been characterized.

Electrophysiological recordings from monkey parietal cortex reveal that neurons in the lateral intraparietal cortex respond more when more objects are presented to the monkey. These neurons are in areas in which neurons also respond to space, time and object size, and it is possible that numerical responses are not distinct from responses to these dimensions. Neurons in the lateral prefrontal cortex of the monkey are also selectively tuned to numerical rank and numerical quantity but typically later than IPS neurons (Nieder et al., 2004; Nieder et al., 2006).

The Intraparietal Sulcus

The IPS is part of an extensive network of brain areas that support human arithmetics. It is involved in the representation of the quantity and magnitude of symbolic numbers (Piazza et al., 2007), and its activation varies with the number of operants involved. It is not completely clear whether it is specific for numbers or would be engaged by quantitative processing of other nonnumerical dimensions such as physical size.

Checking activation of the IPS in response to multiple tasks including pointing, attention, or phoneme detection, the depth of the intraparietal sulcus was active solely during calculation. The human IPS is activated in most neuroimaging studies of number processing and may constitute a central amodal representation of quantity (Dehaene et al., 2003). It reacts identically whether numerals are spoken or written in different manners (Naccache & Dehaene

2001; Eger et al., 2003). Functional neuroimaging studies demonstrate that the IPS is involved in various aspects of calculation including processing of numerical quantities, number detection, magnitude comparison, number comparison, and simple quantity manipulations (Dehaene et al., 1998, Dehaene et al., 2003). This brain region is selectively implicated in most neuroimaging studies of number processing (Dehaene et al., 2003) as opposed to letters or colors, and can be activated by spoken and written input (Eger et al., 2003).

In very simple experiments, which involve number detection or comparison rather than more complex calculation, the IPS is sometimes the only region specifically engaged. Neither calculation nor working memory is needed to obtain parietal number-related activations (Eger et al., 2003). This demonstrates that the IPS region plays a central role in basic quantity representation and manipulation. When it is disturbed, the ability to estimate discrete magnitude is affected. Other prefrontal areas might serve a more supportive role in the management of successive operations in working memory (Dehaene et al., 2004).

There is a difference between the brain areas involved in exact or approximate calculation. Exact calculation like doing a sum lights up mostly language areas, The angular gyrus, which is also activated during some arithmetic tasks such as multiplication, and tasks that might relate more to linguistic, including digit naming, than to quantity processing (Cohen et al., 2000; Zago et al., 2001; Dehaene et al., 2003; van Harskamp, Rudge, & Cipolotti, 2002; Dehaene et al., 2003; Garcia-Orza, Leon-Carrion, & Vega, 2003). In addition, areas of the precentral and inferior prefrontal cortex also activate when subjects engage in mental calculation (Stanescu-Cosson et al., 2000). In a PET study, multiplication activated a number of other brain areas including the left and right inferior parietal gyri, the left fusiform and lingual gyri, and the right cuneus (as well as preferentially left lenticular nucleus and precentral and inferior frontal gyri; Dehaene et al., 1996), suggesting that multiplication and comparison may rest on distinct networks.

Impaired arithmetic skills may result from selective deficits that are unique to calculation. The evoked potentials of children who manifest impaired arithmetic performance in addition to impaired reading and spelling differ from those whose impaired arithmetic performance is seen within the context of normal reading and spelling (Rourke, 1993). Clinically, reading-disabled children may have difficulties in reading math problems because of their reading difficulties, but may not have problems with simple calculations (Shapiro & Gallico, 1986).

Angular Gyrus

There are a number of hypotheses for the function of the angular gyrus (AG) in mathematics. The AG, which is activated during some arithmetic tasks such as multiplication, belongs to the language system and relates more to linguistic tasks including digit naming than to quantity processing (Zago et al., 2001; Dehaene et al., 2003).

It was proposed that the left AG belongs to the language system, supporting the retrieval of verbally stored arithmetic facts (such as a multiplication table) from memory (Dehaene, 2003; Grabner et al., 2011). Some arithmetic operations are more dependent on language-based fact retrieval (and thus more on the angular gyrus) and others on quantity processing (and thus on the IPS).

There may also be an effect of training, in which left AG activation is seen in the untrained but no longer in the trained individual (Dehaene et al., 2003).

Mathematical competence involves the ability to extract information from different representation formats (e.g., equations, tables, diagrams). An fMRI study of a matching task in which the subjects had to evaluate whether the numerical information of a symbolic equation matches that of a bar chart was performed with adults with higher and lower mathematical competence. Angular gyrus activation was consistently stronger in the more competent individuals, independent of whether the task requires cognitive processes (Grabner, 2011). The left AG activation level was linearly related to individuals' score in the mathematical competence test. It is argued that stronger angular gyrus activation in the more competent adults may reflect their higher proficiency in processing mathematical symbols.

The right AG may be involved in rapid enumeration (Warrington & James, 1967), and in retrieval of arithmetic facts (Grabner et al., 2009), whereas the left angular gyrus and left prefrontal regions are mainly implicated in exact, verbal memory- based, language-dependent calculation (Dehaene & Cohen, 1997; Dehaene et al., 1999).

Van Eimeren et al. (2010) studied structure–function relationship in the left AG during mathematical calculation. They studied the correlations between cortical activated regions and their underlying white matter structures by collecting data generated by activated fMRI and fractional anisotropy (FA) of defined white matter regions, measured by diffusion tensor imaging. The results indicate structure–function relationships, including a link between the integrity of the left superior corona radiate and neural activity in the left AG during calculations, particularly strong for problems that have a high probability of being solved via the retrieval of arithmetic facts (problems with a relatively small problem size).

In addition to participation in arithmetic fact retrieval, the left AG may also support more fundamental cognitive function including a function in symbol processing, digit naming, and phoneme detection.

Inferior Prefrontal Cortex

There are other cortical areas that activate when subjects engage in more complex mathematical calculation, including the inferior prefrontal cortex

(Stanescu-Cosson et al., 2000). The task of the inferior prefrontal cortex during more complex mathematical calculations can be for reasoning and working memory.

When learning to solve complex arithmetic problems, solving new problems requires more activation in the inferior frontal gyrus for reasoning and working memory, and in the IPS for the representation of the magnitudes of the number involved and comparing them to previously learned facts (Delazar et al., 2005). Functional MRI study of the neural basis of integral calculus in healthy young subjects demonstrated activation of a left lateralized cortical network, which includes the horizontal IPS, posterior superior parietal lobe, posterior cingulated gyrus, and dorsolateral prefrontal cortex (Krueger et al., 2008). The IPS, which represents the magnitude of the numbers involved and compares them to previously learned facts (Delazar et al., 2005), is always activated and in simple experiments, which involve number detection or comparison rather than more complex calculation, the IPS is sometimes the only region specifically engaged. This suggests that the IPS region plays a central role, whereas other areas including prefrontal areas might serve a more supportive role in the management of successive operations in working memory (Dehaene et al., 2004). Neither calculation nor working memory is needed to obtain parietal number-related activations (Eger et al., 2003). Doing more complex mathematical calculations involves the inferior frontal gyrus (for reasoning and working memory) in addition to the IPS, which represents the magnitude of the number involved. The basic representations of magnitude are always activated.

Some work strongly supports the notion of an internal number-line and of quantity- versus language-dependent operations (Cohen et al., 2000), whereas others present challenges to this view (van Harskamp, Rudge, & Cipolotti, 2002; Dehaene et al., 2003; Garcia-Orza, Leon-Carrion, & Vega, 2003). To summarize, three parietal circuits are involved in number processing: One circuit—bilateral horizontal intraparietal sulci—is thought to be domain specific for numerical processing. The other two—posterior parietal attention system and left AG verbal system—are most probably shared with other cognitive domains. The IPS bilaterally is the crucial area for the representation of quantities (Piazza et al., 2007). The IPS is more strongly activated in approximate calculation than in exact calculation and more strongly activated in subtraction than in multiplication (Stanescu-Cosson, 2000). The third parietal region includes the superior parietal lobule and supports visuospatial processes, attention, and spatial working memory related to numerical processing. There is evidence of the involvement of the IPS, AG, and superior parietal lobule in different aspects of numerical processing, but some of the triple code models are controversial (Zamarian, Ischebeck, & Delazer, 2009).

When faced with exceptional, nonroutine problems, students had to extend an algorithm they knew so they could solve the problem. The exceptional problems were associated with different pattern of brain activation. Some brain regions showed a cognitive pattern of being active only until the problem was solved—with no difference between regular and exceptional problems. Other regions showed a metacognitive pattern of greater activity for exceptional problems and activity that extended into the postsolution period, particularly when an error was made. There are multiple separate modules that perform different functions when the problem involves metacognition (Anderson et al., 2011).

Dehaene and Cohen suggested a neuroanatomical circuit for arithmetic under the "triple code model" (1997). The model suggests that basic numerical knowledge is distributed over three brain regions that code for different aspects of number knowledge: the horizontal intraparietal sulcus (HIPS) that processes numerical quantities, a left perisylvian language network that is involved in the verbal processing of numbers, and a ventral occipital-parietal region that processes visual representations of digits. Two other parietal areas, in addition to HIPS, are the angular gyrus (part of the perisylvian language network) and the posterior superior parietal lobule, which processes visual representation of digits. In the prefrontal cortex, the region of the lateral inferior prefrontal cortex (LIPFC) is involved in more advanced tasks involving topics like algebra, geometry, or calculus, and in retrieval of arithmetic facts. Dehaene et al. showed, using PET, MRI, and ERP, that different brain systems are activated in mental multiplications. In a variety of arithmetic tasks, involving algebra and geometry, the posterior parietal cortex was the best correlate of problem complexity, and activity in the LIPFC was the best correlate of student proficiency.

Patients with acquired IPS lesions particularly failed numerical problems for which approximation, numerical comparison tasks, or subtraction were necessary, whereas simple multiplication might be unaffected, presumably because it can still be retrieved from intact verbal memory (Dehaene & Cohen, 1997), and patients with acalculia following a perisylvian lesion exhibited greater impairment in the verbal processing of numbers needed for multiplication tables rather than for quantity-based operations (Cohen, 2000). This dissociation could not be systematically replicated in normal and disabled calculators (Venkatruman et al., 2005).

Developmental Aspects

Basic foundations of arithmetic emerge early in childhood. There is a system of approximate numerosity representation capable of coding a broad range of numerosities in the first year of life. Preschool children already have some knowledge of arithmetic. These are based on the presence of cerebral circuits devoted to the processing of magnitudes or quantities.

In tasks involving numerical symbols, children rely more than adults on prefrontal regions (Kucian, 2008). Developmental changes in the way routine calculations are done include the shifting from frontal areas to parietal and temporal-occipital areas. As children grow up, the IPS and the left temporal-parietal cortex become more specialized for numerical magnitude processing and calculation (Ansari, 2008), with a concomitant decrease of reliance on general purpose (frontal) areas. An increase in brain activation in correlation with age was found in the left supramarginal gyrus and anterior IPS, as well as in the left lateral-temporal-occipital cortex (Rivera, Reiss, Eckert, & Menon, 2005).

Holoway and Ansari (2010) examined the development of the brain regions involved in representations of numerical magnitude. They reported changes seen in normally developing children that coincide with gain of arithmetic competence. Their conclusion was that the "format independent" representation of numerical magnitude in the right inferior parietal lobe is the result of a developmental processes and cortical specialization. The right inferior parietal lobe near the intraparietal sulcus showed increased fMRI activation to both symbolic and nonsymbolic magnitudes. There may also be a functional specialization within the parietal cortex with age. A shift of activation was observed within the parietal lobe from the intraparietal sulci to the left angular gyrus. Again, these changes, seen in normally developing children, coincide with gain of arithmetic competence. It is possible that growing mathematical expertise is related to a greater involvement of specific parietal areas. Left angular gyrus activation is modulated by interindividual differences in arithmetic performance (Zamarian, Ischebeck, & Delazer, 2009). Increases in angular gyrus activation with gaining of expertise have also been documented in other cognitive domains.

The fact that brain areas dealing with mathematics change with development also suggests interaction between the brain and experience.

Learning Effects

Arithmetic expertise consists of the shift from slow and effortful processing to skilled and fast retrieval. The neural organization during this process consists of shifts from one neural network to the other. Learning new arithmetic facts (e.g., solving a new multiplication problem) involve the IPS to represent the magnitude of the numbers in the problem and the frontal lobes - for control of goal setting, working memory, and attention. Dealing with the same problem the second time elicits activity in the angular gyrus in the left parietal area which manages the access of previously learned mathematical facts from memory us (Delazar et al., 2005). Functional MRI monitoring demonstrates a shift that occur during a short arithmetic training session, from the intraparietal sulcus to the left angular gyrus.

There are similar training effects in the AG for arithmetic and nonarithmetic conditions (Zamarian et al., 2009). Several morphometric studies have also shown that experience can alter the anatomical structure of the human brain, such as the gray matter density. Significantly higher gray matter densities were observed in mathematicians than in nonmathematicians within the inferior parietal lobule bilaterally and the inferior frontal gyrus. An MRI study to assess whether there are brain correlates of competency differences found consistently stronger left AG activation in the mathematically more competent subjects (Grabner et al., 2011).

THE DYSCALCULIC BRAIN

There is a multitude of aberrations in the normal central nervous system development that can be the basis of impaired arithmetic abilities, which includes genetic and environmental factors or can be acquired, like perinatal hypoxia-ischemia and brain trauma.

There is speculation that in developmental dyscalculia, there may be a developmental anatomical abnormality or deficiency in the brain "mathematical" areas or an abnormal connectivity with other areas. it is possible that a child will have an abnormal "number sense" area in the IPS causing him or her to have DD. Alternately, the IPS may be normal but the connectivity other brain areas involved in the mathematical process is poorly developed.

What are the brain areas/networks of the developmentally dyscalculic subject that are different from the typically developing controls (Kucian et al., 2006)?

As previously discussed, the IPS is part of an extensive network of brain areas that is involved with arithmetics. The central part of this network is in the parietal lobes that are activated in almost all numerical tasks. In particular, the IPS is activated whenever numerical magnitude (verbal, visual, auditory) is involved. Learning new arithmetic facts (e.g., solving a new multiplication problem), involves the IPS as well as the frontal lobes, whereas dealing with the same problem the second time causes activity in the angular gyrus in the left parietal area.

If the basis of learning disability in mathematics is impaired numerical magnitude processing (the core deficit in processing numerosities), then abnormalities should be found in the parietal network (in particular the IPS) and, depending on the type of mathematical problem, in additional brain areas.

Dyscalculia—Brain Imaging Studies

Multiple brain imaging techniques have been conducted in patients with dyscalculia in order to elucidate the correlation of dyscalculia with neuronal processing, morphology, and metabolism. These include structural, morphometric (Isaacs et al., 2001; Molko et al., 2004), functional (Rivera et al., 2002; Molko et al., 2003), and spectroscopic MRI techniques.

Studies revealed abnormal brain function and structure in the parietal cortex, especially in the interparietal sulcus (Rubinstein & Henik 2009; Butterworth et al., 2011).

Because it is thought that the IPS holds an amodal and format-independent representation of numerical magnitude and is therefore systematically engaged in any task drawing on magnitude manipulations—from basic number comparison to complex calculations (Dehaene et al., 2003, 2004)—the different activation pattern of the IPS in dyscalculics supports an opinion that at least one basis of developmental dyscalculia is impaired numerical magnitude processing (Grabner et al., 2011).

Brain activation studies in developmentally dyscalculic people revealed reduced brain activation during comparison of numerosities, comparison of number symbols, and during arithmetics (Kucian et al., 2006; Price et al., 2007; Mussolin et al., 2010). Price et al. found that distance between numbers in a simple number comparison task less strongly modulated right IPS activation in dyscalculics compared with control children. When asked to judge whether pairs of numerical stimuli were close or far on the relevant dimension, fMRI of children 9 to 11 years old showed brain activation in the bilateral IPS which was modulated by numerical distance in controls but not in children with DD. In addition, the right IPS in the dyscalculic children responded to numerical distance only. It was concluded that dyscalculia is associated with impairments in areas involved in number magnitude processing and, to a lesser degree, in areas dedicated to domain-general magnitude processing (Mussolin et al., 2010).

Price, Holoway, and Rasanen, et al. (2007) found reduced right intraparietal activity in MD children.

Kucian, et al. (2006) studied 18 children with DD aged 11.2 ± 1.3 years. Their diagnosis of dyscalculia was based on the definition of the ICD-10, which uses the discrepancy between the individual's general intelligence and his or her mathematical performance that cannot be explained by inadequate schooling, sensory deficits, or other neurological, psychiatric, or medical disorders alone. Twenty age-matched typically achieving school children were used as controls. The study consisted of fMRI during the performance of approximate and exact mathematical calculation, and magnitude comparison. The calculation task consisted of three cycles of alternating approximate and exact calculation blocks. The magnitude comparison task involved comparing two sets of different objects (pictures of fruits or vegetables) and selecting the set with the larger number of objects. Dyscalculic and typically achieving children activated, in general, similar neural networks during number processing. Children with DD showed greater interindividual variability and had weaker activation in almost the entire neuronal network for approximate calculation, including the intraparietal sulcus, and the middle and inferior frontal gyrus of both hemispheres. Brain activation correlated with accuracy rate in the left intraparietal sulcus, the left inferior frontal gyrus, and the right middle frontal gyrus. In contrast, no differences in brain activation could be detected for exact calculation mediated by arithmetic fact retrieval and for nonsymbolic magnitude comparison. There were no differences between children with DD and control children in accuracy and response time.

The researchers concluded that there are differences between children with DD and controls in approximate calculation, with dyscalculic children exhibiting weaker activation in almost the entire neural network, suggesting a deficient recruitment of neural resources in children with DD when processing analog magnitudes of numbers. These results may indicate a difficulty in establishing an abstract spatial number representation. The observed differences in brain activation could be attributed to differences in cerebral organization.

In a later study, examination of brain activation related to nonsymbolic distance effects in children with and without DD again revealed differences in brain activation, in particular in the supplementary motor area and the right fusiform gyrus, with the DD children demonstrating stronger activation. This was attributed to greater difficulty in response selection, possibly due to a deficient development of a spatial number representation in DD (Kucian et al., 2011).

Functional Magnetic Resonance Imaging of Spatial Working Memory in Developmental Dyscalculia

Functional brain activation studies in children with DD focus mainly on number- and counting-related tasks. There is a paucity of studies on more general cognitive domains that are involved in arithmetics, such as working memory. Using fMRI, a study compared brain activity associated with spatial working memory processes in 8- to 10-year-old children with DD and normally achieving controls. The children with DD showed weaker neural activation compared with the control group during a spatial memory task in the right IPS, the right insula, and the right inferior frontal lobe. A significant correlation was found between right IPS activity and performance on the verbal digit span forward and the spatial Corsi Block Tapping Test (Rotzer et al., 2009).

Electrophysiological Studies

Electrophysiological recordings from monkey parietal cortex show that there are neurons in the lateral IPS that respond more when more objects are presented, and neurons in the fundus of the IPS are coarsely tuned to specific numerosities. These neurons are in areas that also respond to space, time, and object size.

Visual spatial processing deficits are associated with MLD and impede visuospatial orientation on the mental number line. The right fusiform gyrus might be implicated in the identification of Arabic numerals and may be involved in MLD.

An event-related potential study did not find differences between individuals with DD and controls during the initial stages of processing, but found differences at a later stage of 400 to 440 ms after onset of numerical stimuli (Soltesz et al., 2007). That suggested to the authors of this study that individuals with DD have problems with the more complex processes such as executive functions or working memory, rather than with simple mental operations that appear early in processing and may be performed in the parietal lobe.

A magnetoencephalography study was performed in students with math difficulties and average or above average reading skills during simple addition and numerosity judgments. This type study can give information on the relative degree as well as timing of cortical number processing. Compared with controls with normal mathematical ability, the students with DD had an increased degree of neurophysiological activity in inferior and superior parietal regions in the right hemisphere, and increased early engagement of prefrontal cortices, whereas the left hemisphere activity was delayed and did not show the expected task-related changes. These findings were interpreted as "increased reliance on a network of right hemisphere parietal and possibly frontal areas for simple math calculations in students who experience specific math difficulties" (Simos et al., 2008).

Neuropathology

Cohen et al. (2000) reported a case of a woman who suffered from aphasia, deep dyslexia, and acalculia following a lesion in her left perisylvian area. She showed a severe impairment in all tasks involving numbers in a verbal format, such as reading aloud, writing to dictation, or responding verbally to questions of numerical knowledge. In contrast, her ability to manipulate nonverbal representations of numbers (i.e., Arabic numerals and quantities), was comparatively well preserved, as evidenced for instance in number comparison or number bisection tasks. The explanation of her differential pattern of difficulty is that her brain lesion affected the classical language areas but spared a subset of the left inferior parietal lobule that was active during calculation tasks, as demonstrated with functional MRI. This example, taken from a case of an acquired lesion, points to the anatomical substrates of calculation and may project also to cases of developmental dyscalculia. The relative preservation of subtraction versus multiplication may be related to the fact that subtraction involves the intact right parietal lobe, whereas multiplication involves predominantly left-sided areas.

Developmentally dyscalculic subjects had reduced grey matter in brain areas involved in basic numerical processing—the left, right, and bilateral IPS (Isaacs et al., 2001; Mazzocco, 2007; Rotzer et al., 2009). Using voxel-based morphometry, Isaacs et al. (2001), found a region of grey matter in the left inferior parietal lobe that was significantly reduced in size in children who had low birth weight and had calculation difficulties. Rotzer et al. (2009) examined structural brain differences between children with DD and typically achieving children. Children with DD had reduced grey matter volume in the right IPS, the anterior cingulate gyrus, the left inferior frontal gyrus, and the bilateral middle frontal gyri. White matter comparison demonstrated clusters with significantly less volume in the left frontal lobe and in the right parahippocampal gyrus in DD children. Reduced connectivity between parietal areas involved in numerosity and occipital-temporal areas involved in the processing of symbolic number forms was demonstrated using techniques such as diffusion tensor imaging.

GENETIC ABNORMALITIES IN DEVELOPMENTAL DYSCALCULIA

Dyscalculia in Specific Genetic Syndromes

Differences in the IPS region, in isolation or as a part of a more extensive brain abnormality, are found in a number of genetic conditions associated with mathematical dysfunction, including Turner syndrome, fragile X syndrome, and valocardiofacial syndrome (Eliaz et al., 2001; Rivera et al., 2002).

Turner syndrome is a genetic syndrome resulting from a partial or complete absence of one of two X chromosomes in a phenotypic female. Women with Turner syndrome typically experience visuospatial and number processing deficits. An fMRI study of patients with Turner Syndrome, impaired in number processing during exact and approximate calculations, demonstrated an abnormal modulation of intraparietal activation as a function of number size. Intraparietal activation did not increase with number size in exact calculation, and was not larger in small approximate relative to small exact calculations. In addition, a morphological analysis revealed an abnormal length, depth, and sulcal geometry of the right intraparietal sulcus. Molco et al. (2003) reported that the right IPS of patients with Turner syndrome was shorter than the left, and smaller and more variable than in a control group. Also, the gray matter of the right fusiform gyrus, considered to be involved with perceiving written numbers, was significantly reduced in those with TS compared with controls. These results indicate that in this genetic syndrome, which includes mathematical disability, there is a functional brain correlate of the arithmetic impairment manifested by insufficient recruitment of the intraparietal sulcus, as well as an anatomical structural abnormality (Molko et al., 2003).

Similar dysfunction was found in a study of fragile-X subjects who, compared with controls, failed to show an increase in activation with increased mathematical difficulty, in brain areas including both frontal and parietal regions (Rivera et al., 2002).

Williams syndrome (WS) is a neurodevelopmental disorder caused by a hemizygous deletion on chromosome 7q11.23 (Hillier et al., 2003). Cognitive hallmarks of WS include severe visuospatial deficits and relative strengths in face and object processing (Meyer-Lindenberg et al., 2006).

Hoeft et al. (2007) used diffusion tensor imaging to examine white matter integrity in the dorsal and ventral streams among individuals with WS compared with two control groups (typically developing and developmentally delayed) and using three separate analysis methods (whole brain, region of interest, and fiber tractography) and demonstrated that the visuospatial deficits in WS were associated with a significant increase in the FA—a measure of microstructural integrity—in the right superior longitudinal fasciculus (SLF) in WS compared with both control groups. Together, these findings suggest a specific role of right SLF abnormality in visuospatial construction deficits in WS. The cellular mechanisms underlying the increased FA in right SLF for WS are unknown but may involve abberations in myelination or in branching. The study demonstrates how a genetic abnormality can cause aberrant brain connectivity and provide the link between the genetic and the cognitive visuospatial abnormalities in WS.

Conclusions: Neural Correlates of Mathematical Competence

- Brain areas in the posterior parietal cortex, including the IPS are important in the processing of numbers, in both human and monkey studies.
- Functional neuroimaging has revealed that the IPS plays a major role in number processing. It is systematically activated in all number tasks and probably hosts a central amodal representation of quantity. In adults, the IPS seems to be mainly involved in the processing of numericals (Dehaene et al., 2003, 2004). It is present early in evolution, is shared by humans and animals, is under genetic control, and plays a significant role in early numerical development. Its disorganization can create impairment in arithmetic.
- The left angular gyrus and left prefrontal regions are mainly implicated in exact, verbal, memory-based, language-dependent calculation, and in retrieval of learned arithmetic facts, such as multiplication tables.

- Areas of precentral and inferior prefrontal cortex are also activated when subjects are engaged in mental calculation. The dorsolateral prefrontal cortex has a more supporting role, including sequential ordering of operations, control over their execution, and inhibiting verbal response. Neurons in the lateral prefrontal cortex of the monkey are selectively responsive to numerical rank and quantity but typically later than IPS neurons.
- The posterior superior parietal lobe is activated in tasks requiring number manipulation but is not specific to number domain.
- Neurons in the posterior parietal and prefrontal cortices are linked to form a functional network for the representation of numerical information.
- The neural organization involved with arithmetics shifts from one network to the other during the process of learning. Learning new arithmetic facts involves primarily the frontal lobes and the IPS. Using previously learned facts involves the left angular gyrus.
- Three parietal circuits are involved in number processing: One circuit, bilateral horizontal intraparietal sulci, is domain specific for numerical processing. The other two, posterior parietal system and left angular gyrus verbal system, are most probably shared with other cognitive domains. The third parietal region includes the superior parietal lobule and supports visuospatial processes, attention, and spatial working memory related to numerical processing.
- Patients with IPS lesions particularly fail to comprehend numerical quantities that are required in approximation, numerical comparison tasks, or solving subtraction trials, whereas simple multiplication might be unaffected, because it can still be retrieved from intact verbal memory. Patients with acalculia following a perisylvian lesion exhibited greater impairment in the verbal processing of numbers needed for multiplication tables rather than for quantity-based operations.
- Developmentally, the organization of routine number activity shifts with age from frontal and temporal areas to parietal and occipital-temporal areas. An increase in brain activation in correlation with age was found in the left supramarginal gyrus and anterior IPS, as well as in the left lateral temporal-occipital cortex. This suggests that the neural specialization for arithmetical processing may arise from a developmental interaction between the brain and experience.
- Developmental dyscalculia is likely to be the result of the failure of these brain areas to develop normally, whether because of injury or because of genetic factors. There is evidence for a genetic basis for mathematics as evidenced in studies of Turner syndrome. Research in mathematical learning disabilities (dyscalculia) revealed abnormal brain function and structure in the parietal cortex, especially in the interparietal sulcus. Activation in the IPS for approximate calculation differed between dyscalculic children and controls.

Dyscalculia Therapy

Deficiency in calculation and mathematics constitute a significant handicap in school. Without intervention, most dyscalculic students are symptomatic in secondary school.

The "core deficit" theory previously discussed in this chapter is fundamental to all aspects of elementary school mathematics and to the remedial approach to dyscalculia. Neurobiological studies in normal subjects demonstrate that active manipulation of numbers, for instance during calculation or number comparison tasks, systematically activates the horizontal segment of the intraparietal sulci, independent of the notation used for the numbers. Even the simple presentation of numbers without explicit magnitude processing appears sufficient to specifically activate the intraparietal sulci (Eger et al., 2003).

This knowledge can be applied to the teaching of calculation to regular students and for remedial therapy in mathematically disabled students. One role of the therapy is, at least in principle, to stimulate, "train," and hopefully normalize these affected brain areas.

The practical principles that should guide math education from kindergarten through high school include building number sense, and strengthening the meaningfulness of numbers and the link between math facts and their meanings. In addition, students need to learn automatic recall of basic facts and acquire mastery of key algorithms. Teaching also needs to encourage abstract reasoning. It is agreed that the inclusion of calculators and real-world problems is important.

In terms of methods, concrete manipulation of numbers is used. Examples include using games with physical manipulables (e.g., Cuisenaire rods, number tracks, playing cards). Many of these methods require specialty trained teachers working with a single learner or a small group, which is costly.

There is adaptive software for math education: Some focuses on exact numerosities (Butterworth & Laurillard, 2010). Piazza et al. suggested programs that include exercise aimed at training the core nonsymbolic sense of numbers and their connection to numbers. There are board games using small exact numerosities based on dice.

The Number Race Game is a digital environment effective in promoting basic number skills. It attracts the numerosity system in the IPS. The task is to assess the difference between two arrays of dots. The difference between the two arrays becomes gradually smaller, as the learners' performance improves, and provides feedback to the learner (Wilson et al., 2006). Another learning game is Graphogame-maths. The game targets the system for representing and manipulating sets in the IPS, which is impaired in dyscalculia. The task is to identify the link between the number of objects in the set and their verbal numerical label (Butterworth, 2005).

Training children 8 to 10 years old, using a computer based training program aimed to improve the construction and access to the mental number line, improved the spatial representation of numbers as well as the number of correctly solved arithmetical problems. Functional MRI testing demonstrated reduced recruitment of brain regions for number processing in both dyscalculic and control children trained with this program, after the training, which can be attributed to automatization of cognitive processes necessary for mathematical reasoning (Kucian et al., 2011).

It is thought that informational feedback provides intrinsic motivation in a task, and it is of greater value than extrinsic motivation. In general, it is not yet clear whether these programs provide long-lasting improvement that generalizes to mathematical proficiency.

It has to be remembered that the numerosity deficit may not be the only problem in children with dyscalculia. That means it is not the only process that needs to be tested in order to make a diagnosis of dyscalculia. Similarly, it is a question of whether numerosity should be the only focus of remediation. Depending on the cognitive and behavioral issues, other types of assessments and therapy may be required.

CHAPTER 13

Nonverbal Learning Disabilities

INTRODUCTION

Ever since the time of Broca (1861) and Wernicke (1874), neurobiologists have been trying to map different functions to one or both cerebral hemispheres, mainly through the study of patients with acquired lesions, head traumas, and strokes, and later by intracarotid injections, cortical stimulation, and more recently by functional magnetic resonance imaging (MRI).

The observation that some individuals present signs suggestive of cerebral involvement in absence of known lesions gave rise in the 1960s and 1970s to the widespread acceptance of the concept of minimal brain damage or minimal brain dysfunction (MBD). This entity comprised a variety of disabilities, such as developmental dyslexia (Galaburda & Kemper, 1979) and attention deficit hyperactivity disorder (ADHD). The concept of MBD was not liked in part because there was no evidence of brain damage. autopsy and no conclusive link between anatomical abnormalities and specific symptoms, and in part because diagnostic terminology found more use for descriptive, syndrome-based denominations (like Specific Learning Disabilities or Attention Deficit hyperactivity Disorder) than for a specific etiologically based labels.

Learning disabilities involving a verbal component (e.g., developmental dyslexia) are ascribed to anomalies principally located in the left cerebral hemisphere. Other learning disabilities not primarily involving a verbal component are attributed to dysfunctions of the right cerebral hemisphere (Voeller, 1986, 1991; Rourke, 1987).

Indications of the presence of possible dysfunctions can be obtained through such tests of general intellectual functioning as the Wechsler Intelligence Scales, in which IQ scales separately measure the verbal (i.e., mainly left hemisphere) and nonverbal (i.e., predominantly right hemisphere) components of intellectual capacity. A significant asymmetry of verbal IQ (VIQ) and performance IQ (PIQ) scores may be a signal, if not explained by other elements, of language-based or of nonverbal learning difficulties.

Reading disability is the most common and the best investigated type of SLD. The underlying cognitive deficit in this type of SLD frequently involves language processing. There are other types of SLDs in which the underlying cognitive abnormality is not in the language-verbal domain. and the main academic problem is in arithmetic, geometry, or science, rather than reading. Ten percent of learning disabilities are of this type (Beitchman & Young, 1997). The main manifestations are deficits in arithmetic, visuospatial-constructive abilities, and social skills (Weintraub & Mesulam, 1983; Semrud-Clikeman & Hynd, 1990). Academically they may have more difficulties with math. Although reading disabled subjects may have trouble memorizing math facts and understanding math "word" problems because of their reading disability, they usually do not have basic conceptual problems with mathematical understanding. In contrast, nondyslexic children with poor math performance have fundamental conceptual problems in understanding mathematics.

Nonverbal learning disability (NWLD), is sometimes referred to as "right hemisphere" LD, and was also known as right hemisphere developmental learning disability (Rourke, 1987) and as developmental right hemisphere dysfunction (Tranel et al., 1987). Using the term "right hemisphere learning disability" implies that cognitive functions reside in specific brain areas, namely, that verbal functions are located in the left hemisphere, whereas nonverbal functions are located in the right hemisphere. According to this scheme, the phrase right hemisphere learning disabilities suggests that the clinical problems that exist in people with this condition are caused by right hemisphere dysfunction. The more current name for these types of learning disabilities, "nonverbal learning disabilities," is more appropriate and does not imply that the abnormality is specifically in the right hemisphere, although the syndrome may present features reminiscent of acquired right hemisphere lesions in absence of overt cerebral insult (e.g., trauma, anoxia, hypoxia, vascular accidents).

While the concept of language-based learning difficulty is readily understood by most to include dyslexia and dysnomia, the concept of a nonverbal learning disability (NVLD) is relatively new and not well understood. The term "nonverbal learning disability" is sometimes used as a general concept under which several highly specific but extremely varied neuropsychological syndromes are discussed, including autism and Asperger syndrome. Spreen, Risser, and Edgell use the term in the more traditional manner to refer to individuals with combined deficits in mathematics skills acquisition and social behavior.

UNDERLYING BRAIN ABNORMALITIES IN NONVERBAL LEARNING DISABILITY

Is there evidence that nonverbal cognitive functions originate exclusively in the right hemisphere, and is there evidence of right hemisphere pathology in this condition? What is the neurological basis of the functions impaired in NVLD? Knowledge of the functions of the right hemisphere was obtained in the past from acquired lesions or circumscribed brain damage, and more recently from functional neuroimaging studies. Neurobehavioral abnormalities following unilateral right hemisphere strokes include symptoms such as anosognosia, prosopagnosia, constructional apraxia, poor performance in drawing, copying designs, and putting blocks together, spatial neglect, and motor impersistence. Factor analysis suggested that the behavioral patterns that result from right hemisphere stroke can be grouped into three major clusters: "inattentional" signs (motor impersistence, denial of illness, and extinction), "paretic" signs (arm and leg weakness), and "visuospatial" deficits (constructional apraxia, hemianopia) with no significant abnormalities of language (Hier, Mondlock, & Caplan, 1983).

Neural Circuits That Underlie Aspects of Social-Emotional Processing

The neural circuits underlying social-emotional processing are complex and involve subcortical and mesial cortical structures, including the cingulate cortex. Social-emotional behaviors are facilitated by sensory input mechanisms. Human faces provide an important source of social information. Our ability to recognize facial expressions allows us to make inferences about moods and feelings, and in some cases it also may significantly influence our comprehension of language. Little is known of the neural basis of the recognition of facial expression. Neural structures involved in responding to facial expression are present in the temporal cortex, hippocampus, and amygdala. Several lesion studies have shown that damage to the right hemisphere or to either frontal lobes results in impairment in matching facial expressions. These patients exhibit various abnormalities in social interaction. Another way by which affective information is conveyed is by the speaker's voice. The auditory-vocal analog of facial expression is prosody, the pitch, tempo, and tonal contours of the voice. Like the recognition of facial affective expression, emotional prosody appears to be selectively processed by the right hemisphere (Ross, 1981). Patients with right hemisphere lesions had difficulty interpreting facial expressions, compared with those with left hemisphere lesions and normal controls. Such patients may also have difficulties with comprehending and discriminating emotional prosody. The same may apply to developmental right-hemisphere abnormalities in childhood (Voeller, 1991).

In general, brain lesions disrupting neural circuits involved with social-emotional processing impair the ability to process information of a social-emotional nature. Adult patients with more anterior lesions (involving the motor system) may generate affective signals poorly but comprehend well, whereas those with temporal-parietal lesions (involving processing of incoming information) have difficulty with comprehension but expression is preserved.

Social perception has a developmental timetable. Laughter is understood by children at age 3 years. They perceive that a person is in pain by age 6 to 7 years. Anger is understood at 7, fear at 10, and surprise at 11 years. Scorn is described by 11+-year-old children. A study of the perception and comprehension of facial expression showed an advance in the perception of facial expression between the ages of 6 and 8 years, little further change until about 13 years, and then a second advance to adult performance at about 14 years (Kolb, Wilson, & Taylor, 1992).

It is possible that right hemisphere abnormalities affecting specific brain areas in children would result in deficits similar to those seen in adults with right hemisphere lesions. Indeed, children with right hemisphere lesions confirmed by computed tomography (CT) demonstrated a lower PIQ and a normal VIQ relative to normal controls regardless of whether their brain lesion occurred before or after age 1 year. Children with early injury to the right hemisphere, including those with infantile hemiplegia affecting the left side of the body, have problems with functions that depend on visuospatial skills, directed attention, modulation of affect, and paralinguistic aspects of communication. These abnormalities can be recognized at a young age. For instance, toddlers with right hemisphere dysfunction were found to have behavioral characteristics that predisposed them to interpersonal difficulties by 2 to 3 years of age.

How does all this apply to NVLD? In most children with NVLD there is no evidence of a right hemisphere structural lesion. However, the concept of a "lesion" can be expanded. The neuronal circuits underlying social–emotional behaviors potentially can be disrupted by aberrant development of the central nervous system without evidence of a focal structural lesion. Factors giving rise to such disruption could be genetic, with a disturbance of normal intrauterine brain development or insults to the brain in early postnatal life. The clinical symptoms seen in these cases may be similar to those of an early structural lesion of the right hemisphere, with deficits in arithmetic, visuospatial constructive, and social skills. Initially, the term "social (emotional) learning disabilities" was suggested for this triad.

THE SYMPTOMS AND SIGNS OF NONVERBAL LEARNING DISABILITIES: HISTORICAL REVIEW

The scope of abnormalities seen in people with NVLD is large and includes academic, social, behavioral, neurological, and cognitive deficits. Although reports were published in the early 1970s (Rudel, Tauber, & Twitchell, 1974), the one that brought attention to this syndrome was published by Weintraub and Mesulam in 1983. They presented a detailed description of 14 such patients who had a developmental syndrome, which began in early life and consisted of emotional and interpersonal difficulties, visuospatial abnormalities, and academic failure, especially in math, all within the context of normal intelligence. In this article, they describe a group of patients in whom they:

> . . . encountered a behavioral syndrome which begins early in life and is characterized by emotional and interpersonal difficulties, shyness, visuospatial disturbances, and inadequate paralinguistic communicative abilities. All . . . patients had at least average intellectual capacity, but each had demonstrated some academic failure, particularly in arithmetic. . . . Most of the patients avoided eye contact and lacked the gestures and prosody that normally accompany and accentuate speech. . . . [There] was no evidence that they were unable to experience affect. (Weintraub & Mesulam, 1983)

Their examination revealed neurological and neuropsychological signs frequently seen with right hemisphere dysfunction. Neurological abnormalities found in some of these patients included left extensor plantar response and posturing of the left arm. Neuropsychological testing revealed a significant discrepancy between an average or above average verbal score and a much lower performance score. Most had average (scaled score = 10) or above-average scores on the vocabulary subtest of the Wechsler Intelligence Test, whereas only few had scores in the normal range on the block design or object assembly subtests. They had significant differences between good recall of verbal information and poor recall of geometric design, and difficulty with constructional tasks.

In addition, they had significant behavioral problems. They avoided eye contact and lacked gestures and prosody. Shyness, social isolation, and chronic depression were frequent. Several of the patients had been identified in elementary school as having "adjustment problems," and three of them had been labeled "schizoid." Eight of them had a family history of similar symptoms. The authors postulated that this clinical picture, which is similar to the clinical picture caused by right hemisphere brain damage in adults, could be caused by an abnormality of right hemisphere development. They suggested that "there is a syndrome of early right-hemisphere dysfunction that may be genetically determined and that is associated with introversion, poor social perception, chronic emotional difficulties, inability to display affect, and impairments in visuospatial representation." This may be analogous to the genetic factors that predominate in dyslexia (Weintraub & Mesulam, 1983).

A later series of cases described 11 patients with a similar constellation of symptomatology marked by chronic emotional and social maladjustment and defective nonverbal visuospatial cognitive functioning, but normal verbal skills, including verbal intellect, verbal memory, and propositional speech and language. They had academic failure in arithmetic but not reading or spelling, and paralinguistic deficits, such as impaired prosody and eye contact. It was again suggested that this constellation of symptomatology represents a developmental learning disability of the right hemisphere (Tranel et al., 1987). These and others have confirmed the existence of a clinical syndrome, now named NVLD, which has a wide scope of symptomatology in the cognitive, behavioral, social, and academic spheres.

Rourke (1987, 1989), who described this triad, suggested that it represents a developmental disorder of right hemispheric capacities and noted that these children have numerous cognitive, academic, and social deficits, including deficiencies in visual perceptions, problem solving (especially of novel material), and pragmatic language usage, including difficulty in utilizing nonverbal cues in conversational contexts. Academically, they have difficulties with arithmetic computation and mathematical reasoning. They are inept in adapting to novel situations and social competence. Emotionally, they differ from nonaffected children in negative emotions, mostly anger.

He later adopted the designation "nonverbal learning disabilities" (NLDs) for these syndromes. Brumback and colleagues suggested the presence of chronic depression, extreme shyness, and social isolation as part of these syndromes (Brumback & Staton, 1982).

THE CLINICAL FEATURES OF NONVERBAL LEARNING DISABILITY

Nonverbal learning disability is manifested by academic difficulties, neuropsychological abnormalities, problems with attention, and social interaction (Myklebust, 1975). It is estimated that the gender ratio is 1:1.

History given by parents includes physical clumsiness and awkwardness. The neurological examination may reveal difficulties with complex motor coordination skills and oral motor apraxia.

Intellectual Functioning

There is in most patients a marked disparity between the verbal and performance components of the Wechsler Intelligence Scales in which VIQ is higher than PIQ (Weintraub & Mesulam, 1983; Tranel et al., 1987).

Neuropsychological Characteristics

In addition to the V>P discrepancy, there is an impairment in visuospatial processing and constructional praxis. Memory for temporal visuospatial sequences and face recognition may be impaired. Similarly attentional flexibility, (the ability to switch visual and auditory attention) may be impaired.

According to Weintraub and Mesulam (1983), patients commonly have below-average performance in the Block Design and/or Object Assembly subtests of the Wechsler Intelligence Scales. Tranel et al. (1987) found varying degrees of impairment in visuospatial judgment and visual construction tests. In the latter test, delayed reproduction capacities seem to be more impaired than copying (Weintraub & Mesulam, 1983). Left-sided spatial neglect is described in some patients (Weintraub & Mesulam, 1983; Voeller, 1986). In their study of learning-disabled children, Bloom et al. (1986) concluded that all nine subjects with lower PIQs presented deficits in copying ability and visuomotor coordination that were tied to cognitive or visuoperceptive problems, not to motor or visual problems.

Lower reading comprehension scores may be caused by deficits in recall capacity. Weintraub and Mesulam (1983) found that memory for verbally presented material is lower in the Digit Span subtest of the Wechsler and in a memory for prose task. The authors felt that attentional factors are not involved, even though these are frequently impaired in NVLD. There may be other specific memory deficits. Tranel et al. (1987) found impairment in the Benton Visual Retention Test but not in the Wechsler Memory Scale.

Academic Functioning

Performance at school can be impaired. Common academic problems are deficiency in math calculations, graphomotor skills, and difficulty manipulating complex concepts, especially nonverbal problem solving such as those encountered in science. Other problems are encountered in reading comprehension and, in general, learning novel information and the capacity to benefit from positive and negative informational feedback in novel or otherwise complex situations (Gross-Tsur et al., 1995).

The deficit in visuospatial cognition may be the cause for specific problems in math and handwriting, and possibly for the social and behavioral problems present in children with this syndrome. Several studies demonstrated that visual perceptual measures accounted for more variance in mathematical achievement than did IQ. In a study conducted by Bloom et al. (1986) on schoolchildren with VIQ–PIQ discrepancies of at least 25 points, eight of the nine subjects with lower PIQs presented learning difficulties involving both reading and mathematics, and were at least two school years behind. In each of these nine, the VIQ was greater than 85. Standardized tests of achievement show that mathematical skills are generally below reading skills; spelling capacities also seem to be affected, although less frequently (Voeller, 1986; Tranel et al., 1987). Specifically, the concept of number is described as uncertain, the ability to align columns properly is impaired, and mathematical signs are often misread. This finding is paralleled by the scores obtained on the Wechsler Intelligence Scales, in which patients generally perform poorly on the arithmetic subtest (Weintraub & Mesulam, 1983).

Communicative Abilities

Although linguistic abilities and reading may be normal, paralinguistic abilities, including prosody, eye contact, and gesturing, are not normal.

Communicative disturbances have been described involving deficits in affective language or prosody (Weintraub & Mesulam, 1983; Voeller, 1986). The capacity to decode facial expressions and to understand contradictions is reduced. Eye contact is frequently diminished (Weintraub & Mesulam, 1983; Voeller, 1986; Tranel et al., 1987). Gesturing is atypical (Tranel et al., 1987).

Social and Behavioral Correlates

Children with NVLD have significant deficits in social perception, social judgment, and social interaction skills. Their social competence and ability to adapt to novel situations are impaired. They are described as shy and isolated (Weintraub & Mesulam, 1983; Voeller, 1986; Tranel et al., 1987). They have difficulty relating to other people, are sometimes considered "weird" by their peers, and have few friends. In elementary school, children with NVLD are sometimes labeled as being schizoid or having adjustment problems (Tranel et al., 1987). Their behavior is often inappropriate, and the nuances of social situations are difficult for them to grasp.

There is a tendency toward social withdrawal and isolation as age increases (Voeller, 1990). They are very much at risk for the development of socio-emotional disturbance, especially "internalized" forms of psychopathology, including depression. Studies have reported significant problems with shyness, depression, and social isolation, and abnormalities on measures of eye contact, gestures, and prosody (Trane et al., 1987). Similarly, the presence of chronic depression, extreme shyness, and social isolation has been described (Brumback & Staton, 1982). There is a correlation between deficits in visuospatial, executive, and social skills and depression.

There are attentional deficits, specifically to visual and tactile stimuli, which have a potentially important comorbid relationship with NVLD and ADHD (Pennington, 1991, (Voeller, 1986). Bloom et al. (1986) found that seven of their nine children with lower PIQs had associated attention deficits, some with hyperactivity or impulsiveness. Among adults, the most commonly reported comorbidity consists of depression (Weintraub & Mesulam, 1983; Tranel et al., 1987).

Neurological Signs

NVLD subjects are frequently described as being clumsy (Tranel et al., 1987) and have a stronger R>L motor preference compared with normal R>L difference (Weintraub & Mesulam, 1983).

Left-sided neurological motor signs have been described, including hyperreflexia, increased muscular tone (Weintraub & Mesulam, 1983), asymmetry of the face, posturing of the upper limb on toe-walking, and extensor (Babinski) signs (Voeller, 1986). Among Voeller's patients, about one-third also had parietal sensory signs (deficits in graphesthesia, astereognosis, extinction of left stimuli on double simultaneous stimulation) and/or opticokinetic nystagmus. Bloom et al. (1986) found that all nine subjects with lower PIQs presented some deficit on neurological examination.

Electrophysiological and Neuroradiological Correlates

Electroencephalograph abnormalities have been described in proportions that vary from 25% (Voeller, 1986) to 70% (Tranel et al., 1987) of different samples. Other electrophysilogical anomalies may be found on Evoked Potential tests. Duane (1993) found increased P300 and N100 latencies in one-half a group of adult patients with NVLD.

Neuroimaging has yielded conflicting results. Although Voeller (1986) found a specific computed tomography anomalies in about two-thirds of the children in her sample, Tranel et al. (1987) did not find radiological abnormalities in their group of adolescents and adults. It should be said that 60% of Voeller's (1986) patients presented left-sided motor signs, whereas this was the case in only 18% of Tranel's patients.

Functional magnetic resonance imaging (fMRI) performed in a case of early right brain injury that resulted in both dyscalculia and dyslexia demonstrated predominantly left hemisphere activation involving the frontal and posterior parietal regions. The same task produced bilateral activation of the supramarginal gyrus in seven of nine normal subjects. It was concluded that these fMRI findings are consistent with early interhemispheric transfer of visuospatial skills normally committed to the right and left parietal regions, possibly similar to the postulated interhemispheric reorganization of function, which explains the development of relatively normal speech and language in children who sustained early left hemisphere insult (Levin et al., 1996).

ETIOLOGY AND PATHOPHYSIOLOGY

Neither the etiology nor the pathophysiology of NVLD is known. Rourke found a similarity between the neurobehavioral profile of children with developmental NVLD and the neurobehavioral profile of groups of children with head injuries, hydrocephalus, Turner syndrome, neurofibromatosis, congenital abnormalities of the corpus callosum, and children with cancer who have received large doses of radiation over a prolonged period of time (Rourke, 1987). One patient in Trenel et al.'s series had a history of carbon monoxide poisoning. An association has also been found with another specific genetic syndrome, the fragile-X in females (Hagerman, Ahmed, & Mariner, 1986).

The spectrum of behaviors seen in RHLD overlaps with autism, Asperger syndrome, and schizophrenia. Asperger syndrome has clinical features in common with NVLD more than high functioning autism, including high V>P ratio.

McKelvey et al. (1995) described three patients with Asperger syndrome: One patient's CT and MRI revealed enlargement of the right lateral ventricle, reflecting right hemisphere atrophy. A single photon emission computed tomography scan (SPECT) demonstrated right temporal hypoperfusion with a central area of increased perfusion and frontal polar hyperperfusion, as well as a smaller right cerebellar hemisphere with increased uptake. The second patient had a normal MRI and CT but an abnormal SPECT with decreased right hemisphere perfusion and decreased uptake in the cerebellar vermis and right hemisphere. The third patient had a normal MRI and CT but an abnormal SPECT with a decreased frontal and occipital uptake, and cerebellar vermis uptake. Asperger syndrome has been postulated to arise from a developmental dysfunction of the right hemisphere.

Although these three subjects had involvement of the right hemisphere, clinically they had different cognitive profiles and none had the clinical features of NVLD.

Children with Tourette syndrome may have of an "output" subtype of learning disability, reduced performance on visuomotor and expressive language measures as well as measures of complex cognition, but not generalized nonverbal difficulties (Brookshire et al., 1994). Similarly, features of NVLD may also be found in ADHD, depression, over focused attention, and overanxious disorder. Therefore, it seems that the cognitive, social, behavioral, and academic abnormalities observed in NVLD are seen in children with a large variety of brain abnormalities and developmental problems. It is suggested that a possible common denominator for all these lesions and insults is that they all affect white matter (Rourke, 1987). According to this suggestion, nonverbal learning disability occurs when there is destruction or dysfunction of white matter that is necessary for intermodal integration. The ratio of gray matter (neuronal mass and short nonmyelinated fibers) to white matter (long myelinated fibers) is higher in the left than the right hemisphere; therefore, there is relatively more white matter than gray matter in the right than the left hemisphere. In addition, cortical areas of intermodal associative zones are larger in the right than the left hemisphere; therefore, the right cerebral hemisphere is particularly geared to the handling of tasks involving intermodal integration, whereas the left cerebral hemisphere is particularly adept at processing an intramodal variety.

Clinically the syndrome evolves developmentally with age. It is less apparent at the age of 7 to 8 years than at 10 to 14 years, and becomes progressively more apparent (and more debilitating) as adulthood approaches. In other words, it becomes more apparent when there is need for a higher degree of intermodal integration.

A CASE STUDY OF NONVERBAL LEARNING DISABILITY

Patient E.R. was seen in our pediatric neurology office at the age of 8 years. His parents were concerned about his "writing ability and incoordination." He was "an excellent reader," reading above grade level, but had difficulty with arithmetic and performing writing assignments. He did not have significant behavioral problems but sometimes "gets upset and cries." He was clumsy with motor activities, including throwing a ball, running, and buttoning. His developmental milestones were mostly normal. He walked at 12 months, spoke his first words at 1 year, and had good sentence structure at 2 years. He was toilet trained at 3 years, but had nocturnal enuresis until the age of 5.

He had no significant chronic medical problems, had a normal eye examination, and a hearing test at the age of 5 years. His father was a college graduate, who reportedly was left back in the first or second grade and "is not an athletic person." The mother did not have significant school or behavioral problems.

His examination revealed normal weight and head circumference. He was right-handed. Tone and strength were normal and symmetrical in the upper and lower extremities. Deep tendon reflexes were obtained symmetrically, +2 in the upper and lower extremities. There was no clonus. The Babinski sign was not elicited. The sensory examination was normal for touch, pain, and position sensation. The Romberg test was negative.

The cranial nerve examination was normal. Funduscopic examination did not reveal abnormalities. The coordination examination showed no ataxia or tremor. The finger-to-nose test was normal. He could perform tandem gait forward and backward appropriately. He could perform finger sequential movements and heel-toe taping, but made some mistakes.

He was attentive, had good (normal) communication, could answer questions, and followed instructions well. He had right–left disorientation.

Psychological tests revealed superior verbal ability, significantly better than an average nonverbal ability (VIQ 112, PIQ 94, FSIQ 105). The arithmetic subtest was lower than all the other verbal subtests. Picture completion scaled score and block design score were low, 6 and 7, respectively (average 10).

On the achievement tests, math was the lowest score, consistent with the history of arithmetic problems but there was no evidence of a reading difficulty.

His written sample revealed poor letter and word formation, and inconsistent letter size and spacing.

On behavioral DSM-4 compatible behavioral questionnaires completed by parents and teachers, he did not fulfill the criteria for ADHD. On a continuous performance test, he did not have abnormalities on measure of inattention or impulsivity, but his reaction time was slower than normal and his variability was higher than normal.

Academic achievement tests revealed that "he did extremely well on those tasks that required him to analyze and use his ability to reason things out."

In summary, this boy had an asymmetry of cognitive functioning, with verbal functioning being significantly better than performance functioning, although both were normal. In his case, asymmetry of cognitive functioning, manifesting as a visuospatial cognition abnormality, was associated with a nonverbal learning disorder in which both mathematics and handwriting were affected, more in settings in which he was required to respond nonverbally within a limited time, as well as with motor clumsiness. He had some positive measures of ADHD, but did not have independent behavioral evidence for this condition. Similarly, in his case there was no evidence of significant psychological–social adaptation dysfunction, as found in NVLD.

THERAPY

Children with NVLD should get help in school for organizational skills, have more time to complete assignments and unlimited time for tests.

Occupational therapy may be helpful, especially at a younger age. Adaptive physical education instead of the regular physical education is suggested when the children are very clumsy. Psychological counseling is very important to help these children adapt to their difficulties, so that their self-esteem will not be hurt. Social training programs may help.

SUMMARY

Nonverbal learning disability is sometimes referred to as "right hemisphere" LD, also known as right hemisphere developmental learning disability, and as developmental right hemisphere dysfunction.

It is a complex syndrome rather than only a specific learning disability, and is manifested by difficulties in various areas of functioning, including the cognitive, learning, social, and emotional domains.

Neuropsychologically it has been highlighted by IQ "asymmetry" (VIQ>PIQ); that is, asymmetry between higher verbal comprehension versus lower perceptual organization. There is impairment in visuospatial processing and constructional praxis, memory for temporal visuospatial sequences, and face recognition.

Common academic problems are a deficiency in mathematic calculations and graphomotor skills, and difficulty manipulating complex concepts, especially nonverbal problem solving such as those encountered in science. Other problems are encountered in reading comprehension and, in general, in learning novel information and the capacity to benefit from positive and negative informational feedback in novel or otherwise complex situations.

Children with NVLD have significant deficits in social perception, judgment, and interaction skills. There is a tendency toward social withdrawal and isolation as age increases. The presence of chronic depression, extreme shyness, and social isolation has been described (Brumback & Staton, 1982). They have attentional deficits.

Neither the etiology nor the pathophysiology of NVLD is known. Similarity was found between the neurobehavioral profile of children with developmental NVLD and that of groups of children with head injuries, hydrocephalus, Turner syndrome, neurofibromatosis, those with congenital abnormalities of the corpus callosum, and children with cancer who have received large doses of irradiation over a prolonged period of time.

It is suggested that a possible common denominator for all these lesions and insults is that they all affect white matter. Nonverbal learning disability occurs when there is destruction or dysfunction of white matter that is necessary for intermodal integration.

Therapy consists of recognition and diagnosis of the syndrome, providing appropriate special education and modifications, including more time to complete assignments and unlimited time for tests, as well as modifications in academic demands in mathematics and geometry, organizational skills, and occupational therapy, especially for younger children. Adaptive physical education instead of regular physical education is suggested when these children are very clumsy. Psychological counseling is important, and social training programs may help as well.

Despite detailed descriptions of the syndrome, NVLD has not been adequately validated. There is still no evidence to localize any academic ability (e.g., reading or calculation) in one hemisphere. Some studies of children with NVLD do not find the proposed relationship between neuropsychological abnormalities and learning and academic difficulties.

If the pathophysiology of NVLD is an early brain abnormality localized to one hemisphere, it may be expected that the other hemisphere can compensate for it. A study of two groups of children with learning disabilities and a group of nondisabled children provided support for the hypothesis that the right hemisphere subserves attention and concentration, but no support was found for the hypothesis that right hemisphere deficits are more frequently associated with deficient arithmetic calculation, as opposed to reading and spelling performance (Branch, Cohen, & Hynd, 1995).

CHAPTER 14

Not Simply a Learning Problem

Behavioral, Social, and Emotional Aspects of Specific Learning Disabilities

INTRODUCTION

Although the major manifestation of specific Learning Disabilities (SLDs) is the disturbance of school performance, these conditions are not simply academic handicaps. Specific Learning Disabilities encompass almost all aspects of a chronic neurological disorder, and affect all aspects of the youngster's life, in and out of school. Beyond academic difficulties, social and emotional manifestations may be the most important manifestations of SLD.

Children with learning disabilities exhibit a wide range of possible emotional and behavioral disturbances. In addition to the frequent comorbidity of Attention Deficit Hyperactivity Disorder (ADHD), children with SLD are more likely to exhibit increased levels of anxiety, withdrawal, depression, and low self-esteem compared with their nondisabled peers (Shapiro & Gallico, 1993; Beitchman & Young, 1997). Some learning disabled children may also have social skill deficits, may be less socially competent than their normally achieving classmates, and have difficulty understanding others' affective states, especially in complex or ambiguous situations. Social, behavioral, and emotional problems may persist into adulthood, and many adults with a history of SLD need to continue to receive counseling or psychotherapy for low self-esteem, social isolation, anxiety, or depression.

INTERACTION BETWEEN BEHAVIORAL AND ACADEMIC ASPECTS OF SPECIFIC LEARNING DISABILITIES

Contrary to what is frequently told to and understood by parents, behavioral and social abnormalities in children and adolescents with SLD are usually not the primary cause of academic difficulties and learning disabilities, although treatment of behavioral problems will have a positive effect on academic learning (Yasutake & Bryan, 1995). Nevertheless, there is a question as to whether social and emotional manifestations are secondary and result from academic difficulties or are independent manifestations of SLD (Johnson, 1995; Beitchman & Young, 1997).

One theory regarding this issue is the school failure hypothesis, which argues that a lack of educational success produces low self-esteem, frustration, and acting-out behavior. This hypothesis claims that the child's awareness of his or her inadequacy, which is repeatedly confirmed by continuing academic failure, results in the development of a poor self-concept, which leads to emotional and behavioral abnormalities. Cognitive deficits underlying SLD may impair the child's ability to adapt and to build defenses against these feelings of inadequacy. Children with a language disorder as well as those with NVLD and social skills deficits do not have effective defense strategies and likely respond to their poor self-concept with acting-out behaviors.

The second theory is the susceptibility hypothesis, which argues that certain brain-based personality characteristics are an integral biological part of the complex entity of SLD. These personality characteristics predispose the individual to abnormal and delinquent behaviors. In other words, the academic problems result from a much larger basic neuropsychological dysfunction of the central nervous system, which emerges when these children start their formal education. The same basic neuropsychological dysfunction that leads to learning abnormalities can result in dysfunction of neuroanatomical substrates underlying behavior and emotion, including modulation of anxiety, depression, impulsivity, pleasure, and relatedness. The neuropsychological dysfunction also limits coping mechanisms and puts these children at even higher risk of frustration and failure.

With respect to this hypothesis, it is important to remember that brain lesions in adults can cause behavioral and emotional symptomatology along with classical neurological symptomatology. Depression is frequent in people who suffered a stroke. Post-stroke depression is associated with the location of the brain infarct. With a left hemisphere stroke, proximity to the frontal pole is frequently associated with depression, and an opposite relationship is seen with injury to the right hemisphere (Sinyor et al., 1986).

Similarly, SLD, ADHD, anxiety, and depression may be a shared result of early encephalopathic events, which cause all or some of these problems in different subjects.

A third theory is the differential treatment (or detection) hypothesis, which suggests that students with learning disabilities have the same number of affective and antisocial traits as students without learning disabilities, but are treated differently from non–SLD youths by the educational and later the justice system.

There is evidence for the susceptibility hypothesis. Language-based learning disabilities are associated with delinquent behavior (Beitchman & Young, 1997), and language factors, especially in figurative language, are responsible for this relationship (Vallance & Wintre, 1997). In nonverbal learning disabilities (NVLDs), social difficulties appear to be a strong inherent component of the syndrome. In addition, longitudinal research finds relationships between academic achievement patterns and personality subtypes, with no increase in psychopathology with advancing age, which supports the susceptibility hypothesis (Tsatsanis, Fuerst, & Rourke, 1997).

It is possible that more than one of these hypotheses is correct. In some individuals with learning disabilities, especially NVLDs, social skills deficit is an underlying brain-based insufficiency, whereas in other types of SLDs (e.g., language-based SLDs) language processing problems that underlie the learning disability lead to impaired social interactions. In still other patients there may be emotional and behavioral abnormalities resulting from chronic lack of success and reduced self-esteem.

Neural Mechanisms Responsible for the Association Between Learning and Behavioral Abnormalities in Specific Learning Disabilities

What is the reason for this association between learning and behavioral problems in this population? Specifically, what is the neural mechanism responsible for the association?

The answer to this question is not completely known. One theory is the susceptibility hypothesis, which suggests that LDs are biologically accompanied by personality characteristics that predispose the individual to behavioral abnormalities.

The susceptibility hypothesis is neurologically logical because both behavior and learning are brain functions. It is common that learning as well as behavior can be affected by a brain abnormality. Brain damage, especially in the cerebrum, frequently causes learning as well as behavioral problems because it frequently disrupts brain networks controlling both learning and behavior. A seminal case, described in 1848, demonstrated how brain damage can cause behavioral abnormalities. This was the case of Phineas P. Gage, a 25-year-old foreman for a New England railroad who was accidentally injured by a rod, which hit his face under his left cheek, went through his brain, and exited at the back of his skull. He recovered from his wound but his behavior and personality changed remarkably. Before the accident, he had been a socially responsible person, who was well-liked by those who knew him. Following his brain injury his behavior changed and he could no longer make appropriate decisions, could not be trusted to honor his commitments, became a liar, and began using profane language. These abnormal behaviors were the result of damage to his frontal lobes, which are involved with planning behaviors, control of impulsivity, behavioral feedback, and judging the consequences of actions (Macmillan, 1992). Similarly, a developmental brain abnormality that affects brain pathways involved in learning is likely to also interfere with brain networks controlling behavior. Consequently, children with neurodevelopmental abnormalities, including those with SLD, frequently have associated behavioral problems that further interfere with their functioning both at home and school. The association of learning and behavioral problems in these children may be, like in the case of Mr. Gage, the result of abnormality of brain areas or systems controlling both learning and behavior. The associated behavioral problems may include deficits of "executive functions," impulsivity, hyperactivity, and a short attention span, and other emotional and social problems.

Unlike the case of Mr. Gage, brain abnormality in SLD is developmental (possibly genetic), not acquired. Susceptibility in this case may stem from the possibility that genes that govern the development of networks associated with learning are in some way related or are in close proximity to genes that govern the development of certain behaviors.

There is experimental evidence supporting this hypothesis. For example, children who have had both reading disabilities and behavioral problems since infancy differed in their behavior and temperament from children who only have reading problems. This indicates that there is a group of children with a biologically determined pattern that includes learning and behavioral problems (Smart, Sanson, & Prior, 1996). The underlying biological entities that determine the association in this group of children are not known. The common factor giving rise to learning and behavioral abnormalities may be specific cognitive factors underlying both SLDs and behavioral abnormalities. There is evidence that antisocial behavior in adolescence and adulthood can be linked with variables related to verbal deficits. There is a high prevalence of language impairments and reading disabilities in children with behavioral disorders, including ADHD (Purvis & Tannock, 1997). Primarily depressed school-refusing adolescents who were hospitalized in a psychiatric unit were found to have significantly lower WISC-R verbal intelligence scores, and a significantly higher incidence of both language impairments and LDs compared with controls. Therefore, it is possible that the biological factor associated with behavioral problems in people with SLDs is the underlying language processing disorder.

The common presence of a reading disability (RD), a common type of SLD, and ADHD, comorbidity raises the possibility that although ADHD and RD can be present independently, speech and language disorders such as phonological deficits may be important in the etiology of both hyperactivity and reading disability (Cantwell & Baker, 1991).

There may be a higher risk of other significant behavioral problems in those children who have both ADHD and LDs, compared with the risk of a behavioral disorder in any one of these alone. Children with RDs and ADHD have significantly more antisocial behaviors than children who have RDs or ADHD alone.

There are other hypotheses for the frequent co-occurrence of behavioral and learning abnormalities in patients with SLDs. These suggest that behavioral abnormalities of children with SLDs may have an emotional origin, reflecting adjustment difficulties to the academic failure, which produces low self-esteem, frustration, and acting-out behavior. Although this hypothesis is intuitively valid, because frustration and low self-esteem are frequently seen in children and adolescents with SLDs, a causal relationship needs to be proved, and some studies do not support this hypothesis. For instance, a study of poor readers revealed high rates of inattentiveness in mid childhood, but did not demonstrate increased risk of aggression or an antisocial personality disorder in early adulthood (Maughan et al., 1996).

The most common behavioral disorder associated with SLDs is ADHD. Because it is a common comorbidity to SLDs, when other behavioral abnormalities are present, it is difficult to assert whether those are related to SLDs or the comorbid ADHD. For instance, when an antisocial behavior appears in an adolescent or a young adult with SLDs, it may not be clear whether it is related to their SLDs or to a comorbid ADHD.

Specific learning disabilities frequently go undiagnosed because parents and teachers may not be able to differentiate between the symptoms and signs of SLDs and those of associated comorbid behavioral disorders. In particular, they tend to "blame" attention deficits and other behavioral abnormalities for academic problems (which may, in fact, be manifestations of an SLD). Attention deficit hyperactivity disorder may cause classroom disturbances, but does not cause specific deficits in reading or other learning achievements. Academic problems, especially when present in the first 2 to 3 years of school, are usually caused by an SLD. Confusion between ADHD and SLDs may also occur because children with SLDs who cannot keep up with the class frequently seem inattentive and are identified by their teachers as having ADHD inattentive type. Last, when ADHD is present in a child with SLDs, it is not uncommon that the ADHD, which is better recognized by parents and educators, is treated, whereas the SLD, which is the more important disability interfering with academic success, is not recognized until much later.

It is important to recognize SLDs as a different entity from ADHD, understand the different clinical characteristics of ADHD and SLDs, and become acquainted with the different diagnostic tools used to diagnose these entities (Shaywitz, Fletcher, & Shaywitz, 1995). In a study demonstrating the differences between the manifestations of ADHD and SLD, children with and without RDs were asked to perform tasks requiring recall of a narrative, and assessing knowledge of the semantic aspects of language. While children with ADHD exhibited difficulties in organizing and monitoring story recall—difficulties consistent with higher-order executive function deficits—they did not have language processing difficulties. Those children with RD had deficits in tests of language processing, consistent with deficits in the basic semantics of language. There was a comorbid group (ADHD + RD) that exhibited both types of deficits (Purvis & Tannock, 1997). The study demonstrates, therefore, that although both groups—ADHD and DR—may manifest similar academic difficulties, there are basic neuropsychological and cognitive differences between them, which are very important to detect.

ATTENTION DEFICIT HYPERACTIVITY DISORDER

Attention deficit hyperactivity disorder is a very common comorbidity of SLD. It is characterized by developmentally inappropriate degrees of inattention, impulsivity, and hyperactivity. Symptoms need to be present by age 7. Historically, the disorder has been known for a century, although the name Attention Deficit Hyperactivity Disorder is relatively new—given in 1994. In the past, this behavioral disorder has had other names, including minimal brain dysfunction (MBD) and Attention Deficit Disorder (ADD). One of the first reports in the medical literature that may fit this disorder is by Sir George Frederic Still, who in 1902 described a group of children that were aggressive, defiant, resistant to discipline, and showed no inhibitions. Some of the children who had encephalitis during the epidemic of 1917–1918 and sustained brain damage had behavioral problems characterized by short attention span, hyperactivity, and poor impulse control as part of their neurological abnormalities. It was recognized that these behavioral symptoms are manifestations of brain damage. It was also thought that hyperactivity, impulsivity, and a short attention span can be manifestations of brain abnormality, even though many children with such symptoms have no evidence of an insult to their brain and no other neurological signs (see Pennington's 1991 book on learning disabilities). Hence, the diagnosis "minimal brain damage" was given to these children initially. This term was later replaced by the term "minimal brain dysfunction," suggesting that these abnormalities result from faulty brain functioning in the absence of a structural brain abnormality. The core symptoms of ADHD are hyperactivity, impulsivity, and inattention, in a degree and fashion inappropriate for the subject's age. The guide to ADHD diagnosis has been *The Diagnostic and Statistical Manual* (the DSM), published by the American Psychiatric Association. The criteria for ADHD diagnosis have been revised over the years in subsequent editions of the DSM.

Criteria set forward in the DSM-III demanded the presence of three core dysfunctions: hyperactivity, short attention span, and impulsivity. The DSM-III-R (1987), made another change in the name of the syndrome, now called "Attention Deficit-Hyperactivity Disorder." A diagnosis of ADHD could be made if the patient had any 8 out of a given list of 14 symptoms of hyperactivity, impulsivity (inability to inhibit inappropriate responses), or inattention (disturbance of vigilance or sustained attention). The DSM-IV (1994) did not change the name of the disorder, but changed the way ADHD diagnosis was made. It divided ADHD into two types with different diagnostic criteria: ADHD-inattentive type and ADHD-hyperactive/impulsive type. A third, combined type (ADHD-C) had subjects who achieved criteria for both types—ADHD-I and ADHD-HI. When a child has six out of nine possible symptoms in a category (e.g., inattention), he or she achieves criteria for this type of ADHD.

Attention deficit hyperactivity disorder is a condition that may evolve over the subject's life span, and symptoms may change (increase or decrease) as the child grows. In preschool, hyperactivity and impulsivity are the most disturbing symptoms; in grade school, inattention may become prominent. Later, disorganization and inability to plan become major symptoms. Clinically, the diagnosis of ADHD is made by obtaining a detailed medical, behavioral, and developmental history during an interview with the child's parent or guardian, and by scoring validated behavioral questionnaires completed by parents and teachers. "Laboratory" tests, including Continuous Performance Tests and other measures of executive function such as the Wisconsin Card Sorting Test, are infrequently used and do not always correlate with the scores of the behavioral questionnaires. Therapy includes classroom modifications with allowance for more time to complete assignments and tests, special education teaching learning strategies, stimulant medications, and behavior therapy. Attention Deficit Hyperactivity Disorder symptoms may continue into adolescence and adulthood. The adult outcome of ADHD includes an increased risk of antisocial personality and substance abuse, but no significantly increased risk for major psychiatric illnesses.

The differential diagnosis includes other conditions with attentional deficits and sometime hyperactivity, such as schizophrenia, early treated PKU, exposure to lead, neurofibromatosis, Turner syndrome, fragile-X syndrome, and the syndrome of generalized resistance to thyroid hormone, a condition caused by mutations in the thyroid receptor gene and characterized by reduced responsiveness of peripheral and pituitary tissues to the actions of thyroid hormone. There is evidence of a familial and genetic predisposition to ADHD. Family studies have found increased rates of hyperactivity among first and second degree relatives of hyperactive children compared to the rates among relatives of controls. There are no identified genes for ADHD.

Children with ADHD were found to differ from non affected children on certain electrophysiological measures, including electroencephalography and event related potentials, on regional cerebral blood flow, and some biochemical measures of catecholamines (dopamine and norepinephrine) metabolism. Lower levels of the dopamine metabolite homovanillic acid (HVA) were found in the cerebrospinal fluid of children with ADHD.

Magnetic resonance imaging (MRI) scans of some ADHD subjects demonstrates absence of the usual R>L frontal asymmetry, supporting a hypothesis of an abnormal brain development lacking the appropriate "pruning" of brain tissue. Other MRI and functional imaging studies of patients with ADHD revealed a larger right caudate nucleus and hypoperfusion of the right striatum (Mataro et al., 1997). A positron emission tomography study found that brain glucose metabolism in adults who had been hyperactive since childhood, was reduced, mostly in the frontal cortex. These findings support a frontal-striatal system dysfunction in this disorder (Zametkin et al., 1990).

SPECIFIC LEARNING DISABILITIES AND ATTENTION DEFICIT HYPERACTIVITY DISORDER

Attention deficit hyperactivity disorder is the behavioral disorder most commonly associated with SLDs (Semrud-Clikeman et al., 1992). The important ADHD symptom accounting for this relationship is the attentional problem. Estimates of the frequency of ADHD behaviors in children with learning disabilities range from 15% to 80%, depending on the criteria used for the diagnosis (Shapiro & Gallico, 1993). In the cases of comorbidity of ADHD and SLDs it is difficult to assess the relative contribution of the two conditions to the cognitive and academic achievement abnormalities. It seems that when children with reading disabilities also manifest attention deficit disorder, their reading deficits are more severe and resistant to intervention. Learning difficulties may be more common in children with ADHD, although this is debatable.

Although the precise reasons for the comorbidity between SLDs and ADHD are not known, the overlap between these two entities may be due to heritable influences, at least in part. It is not clear whether ADHD and SLD are transmitted independently in families, or there is a shared genetic origin. A study of the influence of genetic factors in the comorbidity of spelling disability and hyperactivity in two samples of same-sex twin pairs estimated that approximately 75% of the co-occurrence of these two conditions was due to shared genetic influences. Another examination of the shared genetic variation in ADHD and reading disabilities reported that up to 70% of the observed covariance between reading and hyperactivity is accounted for by heritable variation. Other studies of ADHD and SLD concluded that the two disorders are transmitted independently in families, and their co-occurrence may be due to nonrandom mating (Faraone et al., 1993; Shaywitz, Fletcher, & Shaywitz, 1995).

As noted in the Introduction, parents and educators may find it difficult to differentiate between SLD and ADHD, or to observe the presence of both conditions in the same person (Cavanaugh, Tervo, & Fogas, 1997). Children with ADHD only are not impaired on tasks of a particular information processing domain, which is the main abnormality in SLD. But because of the common comorbidity of both conditions, it is frequently necessary to test for both conditions. On DSM IV behavioral questionnaires children with SLD may score similarly to those with ADHD-I; therefore, in the presence of academic difficulties, one should not look at the diagnosis of ADHD-I as exclusive. The appropriate testing for learning disabilities should be performed. Children with pure ADHD may only be impaired on executive functions, whereas children with pure dyslexia, for example, may be impaired only on phonological processing. Children with both conditions show combined deficiencies.

THE FRONTAL LOBES

Subjects with ADHD symptomatology who achieve criteria for the disorder, as well as some who do not achieve criteria, sometimes have other important symptoms, including abnormal organizational skills. On cognitive testing they may have "working memory" deficits. This gave rise to another related dysfunction known as "executive dysfunction." The ability to plan activities and later execute them in the right order and time is one of the most complex activities of the brain and is known as "executive functions." Frontal systems play an important role in executive control of the planning, flexibility, organization, and regulation necessary for the planning and execution of appropriate behaviors. To that end one needs the flexibility and ability to shift from one concept to another, relate and integrate isolated details into a coherent whole, and manage simultaneous or multiple sources of information. Cognitive components that are necessary for these and for which the frontal lobes may be essential include working memory (temporary storage and manipulation of information). The frontal lobes are the most uniquely "human" of all the parts of the human brain (Goldberg, 2001) and are late in evolution. It is thought that the normal development of organization of attentional, executive, and self-reflexive processes depends on the normal development of the frontal lobes.

Lehrmite, a French neurologist, has demonstrated functions of the frontal lobes in a series of interesting investigational interviews with adult patients who had a lesion in their frontal lobes, and have lost the ability to plan and organize their activities. They had a tendency to imitate the examiner's gestures and behaviors, and became "environmentally dependent." Children with ADHD have a similar type of deficiency—an inability to organize their activities and inhibit their impulses, and may primarily respond to environmental activities around them.

Although ADHD is defined by the three main symptoms of inattention, hyperactivity, and impulsivity, its pathophysiology may involve a fundamental deficit in self-regulatory mechanisms that includes regulation of arousal and alertness, and deficits in planning, the ability to inhibit impulses and set maintenance and self-monitoring. Children with ADHD have been found to be impaired on monitoring and search tasks such as the continuous performance test and the Rey Osterrieth Complex Figure, and on other measures of prefrontal function, including the Wisconsin Card Sorting test, and the Tower of Hanoi planning task (Pennington, 1991). Problems of attention span and executive functions are associated with low functioning on tests of working memory. Children with such problems of attention and executive functions show difficulties on these tests, similar to the difficulties exhibited by subjects who have brain damage affecting the frontal lobes. There is evidence from blood flow and other studies that the underlying neuroanatomical deficit in ADHD is in the frontal lobes and their connections to the striatum. Case studies of two children with frontal lobe injury at different ages showed that the early important symptoms were behavioral, manifested by lack of goal direction and self regulation. Other manifestations including the ability to inhibit and modulate response, mental control and flexibility, direction and maintenance of attention, and organization of effort became evident later when the children were in situations requiring formal reading.

The relationship between executive functions and SLD may be through the relation of executive functions to the phonological loop and the cognitive model of phonological loop—central executor—visual spatial sketch pad (Baddeley Hitch model). So the relationship between SLD and executive functions can be independent of the comorbidity of ADHD.

Although SLD and ADHD frequently comorbid, the profiles of ADHD and reading disability are different. Specific learning disabilities involving reading and word recognition are associated with phonological awareness deficits regardless of the presence or absence of ADHD. Attention Deficit Hyperactivity Disorder may have an effect on cognitive functioning but is mostly associated with executive functions (Fletcher et al., 2007). There may be a difference between dyslexia and dyscalculia in that the profile of variables in dyscalculia may include difficulty with sustained attention. So ADHD and Dyscalculia may overlap. The presence of ADHD in patients with mathematical disability results in more severe mathematical disability.

BEHAVIORAL AND EMOTIONAL PROBLEMS OF LEARNING DISABLED CHILDREN

Children with academic disabilities may have in addition to possible ADHD, social and emotional difficulties (Bryan, Sullivan-Burstein & Mathur, 1998. Estimates of the prevalence of social problems in students with SLD in the United States are 38% to 75% (Baum, Duffelmeyer, & Greenlan, 2001). Learning disabled children frequently rate themselves lower than their non-disabled peers in academic domains, and sometimes also in social competence. Problems of self-esteem appear frequently in learning disabled adolescents and adults, but not necessarily among elementary school children. This loss of self-esteem over time may reflect the accumulated effect of repeated failure encountered by some learning disabled individuals within both academic and social domains. In addition, learning disabled children are less popular compared with the non–learning disabled, suffer more rejection, are looked on as shy, and are victims of bullying significantly more than non–LD children, and fewer are nominated as leaders.

The psychological effects on these children and their families is sometimes more pronounce than the effects of physical handicaps, because physical handicaps are obvious, and easily recognized, whereas SLD are not. There is a frequent lack of understanding of these conditions and the feeling of helplessness that accompanies them.

Emotional difficulties include low self-esteem, social isolation, anxiety, and depression. Students with SLD may also have more stress in dealing with the usual transitions of school, and have to find ways of dealing with stressful events (e.g., avoidance, less reliance on peer help). Improved achievement leads to improved behavior. Reading and math instruction to young children, in programs that provide positive behavioral support, and subsequent improvement in reading and math, lead to improvement in behavioral problems.

Contrary to the above, Margalit (1998) found that preschool children experience loneliness that preceeded their school learning difficulties, and raises the possibility that negative affect may predate academic difficulties and social rejection. Tur-Kaspa and Bryan (1994) presented third to fourth and seventh to eighth grade students with social dilemmas followed by probe questions (Dodge's (1994) model of social information processing). Students with learning disabilities performed less well than low achieving students on a number of steps.

Bryan, Sullivan-Burstein, and Mathur (1998) found that students with and without learning disabilities in a self-induced positive affect condition

generated more problem solutions than did students in a neutral condition. Thus, social problem solving can be improved, at least temporarily, by
self-inducing positive affect.

Although learning disabled children tend to see themselves as less able in
areas involving school achievement, this view does not spread to areas involving extracurricular activities. It is possible that reduced self-esteem related
to academic failure may cause students with SLD to try to distinguish themselves in other positive as well as negative areas. A study of a group of adolescent mothers and their infants showed that a majority of the girls for whom
Achievement test scores (CAT) were available scored one or more years below
grade level in reading and language skills, and it was suggested that early moth-
erhood may represent an alternative avenue to experiencing success for these
girls who are having academic difficulties. Although there may be additional
explanations to these findings, it seems that reduced self-esteem in learning disabled children stems mainly from their academic failure, whereas they
may not have a reduced self-concept in other areas. Therefore, a therapeutic
approach for reduced self-esteem may be promoting nonacademic activities in
which children with SLDs may see themselves as successful. This is in contrast
to the common situation in which learning disabled children spend more time
than nondisabled children doing their homework and preparing for tests, and
the practice of punishing them for their lack of academic success by restricting
their nonacademic activities.

It is possible that there are more emotional behavioral problems in children
with mathematical disabilities.

Children with the NVLDs tend to have a specific pattern of behavioral
problems, including social skills deficits, which are considered a part of this
syndrome. These children tend to be socially isolated, have few close friends
and limited social activity, and are in danger of developing depression. It
is hypothesized that their deficits in social skills are perceptually based
(Shapiro & Gallico, 1993). Teachers are more motivated to participate in social
skills interventions that are embedded in academic instructional activities.

EXTERNALIZING AND INTERNALIZING
ABNORMALITIES

Reading disabled people have a higher frequency of conduct disorder, including aggression and delinquency. Similarly, there is evidence that learning disabilities are prevalent among those who are delinquent. There is not much
evidence to support a distinct comorbid subtype of SLD and conduct disorder,
and this association can be partially explained through the comorbidity of
reading disability and ADHD. Discriminant analysis revealed that certain personality characteristics, such as impulsivity and poor judgment, discriminate

between persisting and nonpersisting delinquency in youth with learning disabilities. The association also can be explained in part by language-related difficulties, which is frequently present in children with learning disabilities, and by their underachievement.

Children with SLD also have a higher frequency of anxiety symptoms compared with non–SLD children (Fisher, Allen, & Kose, 1996). Other important but less common overlapping psychiatric conditions are depression and bipolar affective disorder.

Adolescents with learning disabilities experience higher levels of trait anxiety and have a significantly higher prevalence of minor somatic complaints than nondisabled peers. There are also higher than normal rates of depression on self-report measures (Beitchman & Young, 1997). The psychiatric conditions seen in conjunction with learning disabilities include depression and bipolar disorders (Stanley, Dai, & Nolan, 1997). There are reports suggesting an association of dyslexia with positive schizotypal traits, and particularly with unusual perceptual experiences.

Several studies have found that students with SLDs are more depressed and lonely in comparison with those without SLDs (Margalit & Al-Yagon, 2002). It is possible that difficulty making friends and loneliness produce negative effects, including depression.

In an early monograph on learning disabilities, Critchley wrote: "All children with difficulty in learning to read, tend quite early to develop neurotic reactions. Sometimes those are severe and may lead to a striking personality change. . . . The dyslexic is apt to find himself an alien in a critical, if not hostile, milieu; mocked, misunderstood, or penalized, cut off from opportunities for advancement" (1970).

Do students with learning disabilities engage in more drug addiction than nondisabled students? Risk factors that were found to influence the use of minor substances by learning disabled as opposed to non–LD students include use of substances by close friends and susceptibility to peer pressure. Risk factors that affect the use of major substances by students identified as learning disabled, as opposed to non–LD students include stressful life events.

SUMMARY

Attention deficit hyperactivity disorder is a very common but not the only behavioral comorbidity of learning disabilities. Children with learning disabilities exhibit a wide range of behavioral and emotional disturbances, including anxiety, withdrawal, depression, and low self-esteem (Shapiro & Gallico, 1993). Children with SLD may also have social skills deficits; they may be less socially competent than their normally achieving classmates and have difficulty understanding others' affective states, especially in complex or ambiguous situations. Social, behavioral, and emotional problems may persist into adulthood, and many learning disabled adults continue to receive counseling or psychotherapy for low self-esteem, social isolation, anxiety, or depression. Treatment of the child and adolescent with SLD should not focus only on the academic part of the disability, but also on the social, emotional, and behavioral parts. These, equally and sometimes more than the educational part, depend on the strengths of the child and the support system, including the child's parents, school, and immediate social circle.

CHAPTER 15

Diagnosing Specific Learning Disabilities

The Process

INTRODUCTION

The purpose of the evaluation is to confirm a Specific Learning disability (SLD) diagnosis, identify a possible behavioral comorbidity, and find an etiology for the condition. Comorbidity between SLD and other behavioral disorders, including pervasive developmental disorder and attention deficit hyperactivity disorder (ADHD), is common. Depression, obsessive compulsive disorder, and conduct disorder may also co-occur with SLD. A behavioral screening should, therefore, be part of the evaluation of every child with an SLD. The clinician needs to be acquainted with the symptoms and signs of these behavioral disorders. A careful review of the child's symptoms and the use of validated behavioral forms may detect these comorbid behavioral conditions.

In addition to making a diagnosis, the physician also attempts to find an etiology for the learning disability. SLD can be caused by a neurodevelopmental condition (e.g., neurofibromatosis, chromosomal anomaly, cortical dysplasia), a neurological disease (i.e., temporal lobe epilepsy), or rarely be a manifestation of a progressive neurological disorder. A careful neurodevelopmental intake, neurological examination, and, if indicated, laboratory tests, including magnetic resonance imaging (MRI), electroencephalogram (EEG), and genetic evaluations may identify those infrequent patients in whom an SLD is the a component of such a condition.

The specific tools used in the diagnostic process of SLD are a careful comprehensive history, academic achievement tests, cognitive testing, behavioral affective assessment, and a neurological examination.

MODELS OF DIAGNOSIS

There are different diagnostic approaches, from a more confined one consisting of documenting low academic achievement, and using response to intervention (RTI) as a test—to measuring aptitude/achievement discrepancy, or a complete neuropsychological profile.

Classification Based on IQ/Achievement Discrepancy Measure

The role of intelligence (IQ) measure and IQ/achievement discrepancy measure in the evaluation of SLD has been debated. A study by Share et al. (1989) of a large longitudinal cohort (ages 7, 9, 11, and 13) in New Zealand found no relation between IQ and reading achievements. IQ was also not predictive of change of reading skills over time, and was not the determinant of the effect of intervention. Other studies point to some relationship between I.Q. and reading comprehension. In one study children with reading comprehension abnormalities had lower verbal IQs than typically achieving children (but similar phonological skills and nonverbal IQs) (Stothard & Hulme, 1996).

Studies that try to assess whether an I.Q./achievement discrepancy measure differentiates between reading disabled children and poor readers who do not have a specific reading disability, demonstrated only a small, although statistically significant, difference between these two groups (see reviews, Stanovich, 1991; Aaron, 1997). Hoskins and Swanson (2000) conducted a metaanalysis of 19 studies and concluded that most cognitive abilities assessed by those studies, especially the ones related to reading, showed a considerable overlap of the two groups. The core cognitive skills closely related to reading disability did not significantly discriminate between the two groups. Therefore, they questioned the validity of the IQ/achievement discrepancy in diagnosing reading disability.

In summary, models based on aptitude–achievement discrepancy do no clearly identify a unique group of reading disabled. There is, therefore, no clear value in using this model for the diagnosis of specific reading disability.

Classification Based on Individual Differences

One can use an individual difference model with an individual strength and weakness cognitive profile to identify unexpected underachievement. The person with an SLD has strengths in many areas but weaknesses in some core cognitive processes that lead to underachievement. In a reading achievement test, reading impaired subjects differed from non–reading impaired and from mathematically impaired subjects in their achievement tests. The groups also had different cognitive patterns consisting of strengths or weaknesses in tests of phonological awareness, rapid naming, or visual motor tests), a finding that gave validity to the use of the concept of reading or math disability. As described later, these groups are also distinguished by neural correlates and heredity factors (Plomin & Kovas, 2005).

Cognitive deficits are an inherent part of SLDs, and knowledge of cognitive strengths and weaknesses can facilitate treatment planning. This appears to be an attractive proposal for diagnosis, but only a few studies show that such assessment is either necessary or sufficient to identify SLDs (Reschly & Tilly, 1999). There is little evidence that instruction addressing a "recipe" of strengths and weaknesses in cognitive skills is related to intervention outcome

Response to Intervention Model

There is a difference in baseline preintervention achievement and cognitive tasks scores between responders to intervention and nonresponders. At least a partial definition of SLDs can be based on an inadequate response to instruction that is effective with most individuals (Fuchs & Fuchs, 1998; Gresham, 2002). That is a basis for the model of diagnosis based on response to intervention (Fletcher et al., 2005, 2007). Extensive assessment of cognitive, neuropsychological, or intellectual skills is not needed, at least initially, in order to identify children as learning disabled. They hold the following views: (a) SLDs cannot be diagnosed on the basis of a battery of psychometric tests administered on a single occasion. (b) There is no good evidence that these assessments contribute to intervention and remediation. (c) People should not be identified as learning disabled until a proper attempt at instruction has been made.

They suggest the following practical approach to the diagnosis of SLDs: When a learning problem is suspected, a diagnosis is needed to assess the extent and degree of under achievement. Achievement tests will identify the academic area in which there is underachievement, the student should be given specific directed instruction, and progress should be monitored by achievement test battery in that academic area. The main issue is that as soon as it is apparent that a person has an achievement problem, intervention should begin. Students should not be identified as having an SLD until a proper attempt of instruction is carried out. An SLD is diagnosed only after a period of specific systematic instruction.

Student who need a comprehensive evaluation at the initial evaluation are those in whom mental retardation is suspected. Others may have it late, if necessary. If a language disorder is considered, language testing needs to be done. Attention needs to be paid to comorbidities and associated conditions. To that end, teacher and parent rating scales can be used.

A Suggested Model of Specific LD Diagnosis

Although the diagnostic model of RTI (response to intervention) may work in some places and schools, in the rest of this chapter I will outlines a comprehensive evaluation sequence for a student with a possible SLD.

HISTORY AND INTAKE

The history is a comprehensive review of the problem or problems that initiated the visit to the diagnostic team. This intake involves the parents and sometimes the child, and is done by the physician, a psychologist, or a social worker. Although the parent needs to be allowed a spontaneous description of the problem the way she sees it, the professional should then follow with a "structured" interview. Even though the problem that is frequently presented is academic failure or reduced attention span, the interviewer needs to get a full history of the student's academic, behavioral, affective, and social status.

The academic history includes the time of onset, type and severity of any academic difficulty, whether the student has received academic help at school or at home, and whether he or she responded favorably to it. A detailed school history, starting from nursery school, is obtained and includes the student's achievements and grades, the amount of time she or he spends doing homework, and whether they has been involved in other school activities.

The presence of behavioral problems should be assessed. Attentional difficulties, inability to complete tasks, distractibility, hyperactivity, and impulsiveness—the core symptoms of ADHD—may be a cause of academic difficulties or a comorbidity of SLD. Other behavioral problems, including discipline problems, school avoidance, and oppositional or aggressive behaviors need to be explored.

Specific questions should be directed toward the student's affective/emotional status. Low self-esteem, sadness, depression, or frequent somatic complaints (mostly headaches or stomachaches) and anxiety are frequent comorbidities or possible consequences of SLD, and may significantly contribute to the student's disability.

Other issues that need to be explored during the initial interview are the student's social participation, popularity, and leisure activities. Social skills issues may be a cause or a consequence of an academic problem.

Motor skills, excessive clumsiness, and participation in group sport activities are important and are sometime an indication of the student's social skills and motor talents, which are frequently areas of weakness for children with academic learning problems.

The next step in the history taking is past medical history, which includes information on any past illness, trauma, toxins, or metabolic abnormalities with a potential effect on the brain and development (sometimes named "encephalopathic events," meaning insults or events that could have damaged the brain or affected its development). Examples are exposure to medications or drugs during pregnancy, prematurity, perinatal abnormalities, significant head trauma, encephalitis, meningitis, or sickle cell anemia.

A review of developmental milestones follows. It may reveal a delay in the achievement of gross or fine motor, speech or language milestones, late onset of handedness, difficulty with coordinated motor acts such as cutting or coloring, or buttoning or tieing shoes—especially when compared with unaffected family members. A difficulty with language processing is the most consistent feature in the history of children with reading difficulties, and is a strong predictor of dyslexia. A quite typical chronology of a child with dyslexia is a delayed speech, inability to learn nursery rhymes or letters, and no mastery of reading by first grade.

Family history is a very important part of the intake and history. Learning disabilities are frequently genetically transmitted; therefore, evidence of an difficulty in reading, calculating, or writing in close family members should be noted. Similarly, a family history of pervasive developmental disorder, mental retardation, or ADHD should be noted. The family socioeconomic status is also important.

Whenever appropriate, it is important to obtain a history from the student. Here, one of the aims is to get an insight into how students view their problems and difficulties, what they see as their strengths and weaknesses, and how they view their social successes or failures. However, we need to understand that youngsters with SLD may view us with distrust. Many have the perception that the outside world, including their teachers and parents, does not understand their problems. Often, they have had previous investigations and tests, and have a great deal of suspicion toward more tests and examinations. Mostly, they have a long experience of repeated failure and low self-esteem, and may not want to admit to any difficulties, particularly not in front of their parents.

PHYSICAL AND NEUROLOGICAL EXAMINATION

A physical examination performed by a physician aims to assess whether the child or adolescent has any physical abnormalities or conditions that may affect his or her learning or behavior. The examiner gives specific attention to physical characteristics of disorders that may be associated with learning abnormalities. These include dysmorphic features, particularly craniofacial abnormalities, which may be present in genetic syndromes, abnormal head size (including macrocephaly and microcephaly), neurocutaneous abnormalities (including café-au-lait or depigmented skin areas), protruding ears and large scrotum (physical abnormalities found in children with the fragile X syndrome), liver or spleen enlargement and retinal lesions (which are suggestive of certain storage diseases). Such abnormalities may indicate genetic and systemic conditions that can cause learning abnormalities and are therefore important to include or exclude. Hearing and vision should be screened as part of the physical examination.

A neurological examination should be performed. It typically includes the examination of the motor system, sensory system, the cranial nerves, gait, motor coordination, and mental status. This section discusses parts of the examination that have specific relevance to patients with SLD.

The motor part of the neurological examination measures tone, strength, and gait, and the presence of abnormal movements, and records abnormalities or asymmetries. Motor coordination testing includes tandem gait (heel to toe on a straight line), hopping in place on each foot, standing on each foot, and skipping. Fine motor coordination can be assessed by asking the child to perform repetitive sequential movements of the fingers such as rapidly touching each of the fingers in turn to the thumb. The examiner assesses the regularity, accuracy, and fluency with which the task is performed, as well as the presence of excessive mirror movements on the nonperforming hand. Motor coordination difficulties, hypotonia, and dyskinesia are common among children with learning and behavioral problems and are statistically related to cognitive and behavioral problems (Soorani-Lunsing et al., 1993). Motor coordination ability is age dependent, reaching maturity at about 10 years, and the examiner needs to be acquainted with the norms for each age. Timed motor coordination batteries can assist in detecting motor abnormalities. The Physical and Neurological Examination for Soft Signs (PANESS) has norms for the timed performance of a number of fine and gross motor tasks (Denckla, 1973). Children with SLDs may have difficulty performing various fine and gross motor tasks, known also as "soft neurological signs," which include difficulties with alternating hand movements (dysdiadochokinesis), mirror or overflow movements, and dyskinesias (pseudo choreoathetosis). Such motor abnormalities are also present in children and adolescents with attentional deficits (Schoenfeld, Shaffer, Barmack, 1989), and therefore, are not specific to SLDs. Although seen frequently in children with SLDs and providing information about the functional integrity of the central nervous system, the presence of "soft signs" does not, by itself, determine or predict SLD. And treatment of these developmental abnormalities does not, by itself, improve the SLD.

The neurological examination also includes measures of handedness, the ability for right/left discrimination, and graphomotor coordination. The sensory examination includes tests that require the child to identify numbers, letters, and forms drawn on his or her fingertips, and with eyes closed to detect whether one or two of his or her fingers are being touched, as well as the number of fingers between the fingers touched (Kinsbourne & Warrington, 1963).

Motor coordination difficulties, hypotonia, and dyskinesia are common among children with learning and behavioral problems and are statistically related to cognitive and behavioral problems (Soorani-Lunsing et al., 1993).

It is possible to quantify some of these abilities (see neurological exam by Weinberg), by using, for instance, the Edinburgh Laterality Quotient to quantify the extent of right-or left-handedness (Duane, 1993; Frank, 2000), the Benton test of visual retention to quantify graphomotor coordination (Mattis, French, & Rapin, 1975), the Halstead-Reitan sensory-perceptual tasks to identify numbers, letters, and forms drawn on fingertips, and the Kinsbourne-Warrington (1963) test of finger order and differentiation as a measure of finger agnosia. Weak lateralization and poor graphomotor coordination are common in SLD. Similarly, finger agnosia and abnormalities on sensory-perceptual tasks are found in subjects with SLD.

PSYCHOEDUCATIONAL EVALUATION

Academic achievements can be measured for reading and reading comprehension, spelling, arithmetic, and other academic abilities. Standardized measures of academic achievements are assessments of academic achievements of students using tests with normative data derived from large numbers of same age and same grade peers. These tests are an essential component in the assessment of SLDs, providing an objective estimate of the student's ability compared with other children of the same age, and independent of the subjective estimates offered by teachers and parents. These tests may prove the presence of SLDs by demonstrating that the student's achievements in one or more of these academic subjects is below normal for his or her age or grade.

An evaluation for learning abilities or disabilities is commonly done by school psychologists (or through the Committee on Special Education), separately or together with intelligence testing ("psychoeducational testing").

Assessing academic ability is a complex task (Shapiro & Gallico, 1993). For example, how would we assess reading? Reading ability has a number of components, including the abilities to decode print and understand its meaning. Some children can decode well, but have difficulty understanding what they have read. Reading comprehension may also influence reading accuracy via the use of contextual cues to facilitate word recognition. Therefore, reading tests need to also include reading comprehension (Nation & Snowling, 1997). School children with reading disability may have difficulty with one or both aspects of the reading skill, as well as with other aspects of reading, including speed or complexity of reading. Although decoding difficulties are usually noted early in school life, reading comprehension problems may be noted later, and these children are in some ways more disadvantaged than dyslexic children whose difficulties are documented earlier. Different reading tests measure different aspects of the reading process. In light of these children's academic difficulties, selection of reading tests and understanding the results are important.

Psychologists use a variety of academic achievement tests. They may use individual tests as well as complete batteries of academic achievement tests. Examples of achievement batteries are the Kaufman Test of Educational Achievement; Peabody Individual Achievement Test-Revised (PIAT-R); and Woodcock-Johnson Test of Achievement-Revised (WJ-R). The last, for example, covers the subjects of writing, reading, mathematics, science, social studies, and the humanities. The WJ and WIAT include tests that measure word recognition, reading fluency, reading comprehension, math computation and problem solving, and spelling.

Achievement batteries that yield standard scores are available. Examples include the Kaufman Test of Educational Achievement-Comprehensive Form (K-TEA); Peabody Individual Achievement Test-Revised (PIAT-R); Woodcock-Johnson Tests of Achievement-Revised (WJ-R, now in a third edition); and the Wide Range Achievement Test-Revised (WRAT-R).

The major disadvantage to the use of a battery approach is that it has to be administered in full, including parts that may be irrelevant to the problem of the individual student, and less depth of analysis can be undertaken. Individual subject area tests are more likely to be used when a child is experiencing difficulty in only a single academic area. Many school districts offer periodic assessments of the academic achievement of their students. These achievement test scores are readily available to the practitioner who is evaluating a student with school-related difficulties.

Many students with SLD have disabilities in more than one academic area; therefore, the pattern of academic strengths and weaknesses is important (Fletcher, 2005) In nonverbal learning disabilities (NVLD), one of the best indicators is the discrepancy in word recognition versus math skills (Pelletier, Ahmed, & Rourke, 2001).

PSYCHOLOGICAL TESTING

There have been recent changes in public policy involving education, including the No Child Left Behind Act of 2001 and the 2004 reauthorization of the Individual with Disabilities Education Act (IDEA, 2004). In the 2004 reauthorization of IDEA, the US Congress passed statutes that permitted alteration of the 1977 regulations indicating that states could not require districts to use IQ tests for the identification of students for special education in the category of LD and also permit districts to implement different identification models including the incorporation of RTI (IDEA, 2004). That was at least partially based on the evidence of the limited value of the IQ test–achievement discrepancy in identifying students with LDs.

Although, as discussed, a full neuropsychological examination is not immediately needed for the diagnosis of SLD, such testing can be very valuable in assessing the type of cognitive dysfunction and cognitive strengths and weaknesses. Full neuropsychological testing examines the many cognitive functions involved in the different areas of academic learning, may uncover underlying cognitive abnormalities responsible for the SLD, and may assist in the selection of the appropriate type of intervention (Nation & Snowling, 1998). Neuropsychological testing includes a standard test of intelligence (i.e., Wechsler Intelligence Scale for Children [WISC-IV] or the Stanford Binet Intelligence Scale, fourth ed.), and tests for language, memory, visuomotor skills, and construction, as well as executive functions such as attention, working memory, and learning strategies. As in achievement tests, standardized test batteries are available, such as the NEPSY and Halstead Reitan, but pediatric neuropsychologists more commonly use a combination of individual tests for the evaluation rather than one of the standard batteries.

General Intelligence

The most frequently used intelligence tests for school-aged children are the WISC and the Stanford Binet Intelligence Scale.

It is important that parents and educators understand that intelligence tests are not the determining tests for learning disabilities. Standing alone, intelligence testing is inadequate and sometimes misleading. Children with possible SLD are sometimes administered intelligence tests with no other cognitive or achievement testing. The parents are then reassured that the child was tested and no abnormality was found, leading them to believe there is no LD. Strictly speaking, traditional IQ tests do not directly indicate the presence of SLD and may not delineate the underlying pathophysiology (Fennell, 1995). As an example, the key abnormality in many cases of reading disability is a problem with phonological processing, which may be independent of intelligence (Naglieri & Reardon, 1993). The first goal of intelligence tests is to rule out mental retardation when this is an issue. A significant variability of scores on the different subtests of the WISC, for instance, verbal performance IQ discrepancies, means that specific measures of intellectual abilities do not correlate in the usual manner, and raises suspicion that the central nervous system may not be well integrated. Specific variability in IQ subtests may be associated also with the underlying cognitive abnormalities responsible for a SLD. Abnormalities of verbal comprehension may be related to language processing deficits, interfering with reading, whereas perceptual organization difficulties suggest abnormal visuospatial processing, which may cause other types of SLD, including mathematical LDs.

Another factor that can be derived from the WISC subscales is the "freedom from distractibility" measure, which is composed of the subtests of arithmetic, coding, and digit span. Although school psychologists sometimes use this measure as an indication for attentional deficits, other behavioral measures (i.e., DSM-IV compatible questionnaires) are better used for this purpose. Last, the outcome in many cases of SLD does depend on general intelligence, so the assessment of intelligence is helpful in projecting prognosis.

Cognitive Testing

The cognitive (neuropsychological) evaluation of children usually includes the following domains: arousal, attention, affect, language, memory, perceptual skills, reasoning, judgment and insight; spatial-construction, executive, and motor skills (Cognitive Assessment, Drake Duane). It may vary according to the child's age.

The aim of this comprehensive examination in the context of SLD is to identify the cognitive abnormalities underlying these disabilities. For instance, neuropsychological abnormalities frequently found in children with reading disabilities include language processing and verbal learning impairments (Frank, 2000).

An important part of the examination of the child with suspected SLD is the search for behavioral comorbidities. The most common comorbid behavioral abnormality is ADHD, with its core symptoms of hyperactivity, impulsivity, inattention, and oppositional behavior. Functions related to attention include vigilance, attention span, perseverance, response inhibition, and distractibility. Neuropsychological tests of attention may include continuous performance tests (CPT), available on computers (Halperican et al., 1988).

Executive functions, which are frequently impaired in subjects with ADHD, can be assessed by tests that examine the ability to strategize conceptual flexibility (e.g., the Wisconsin card sorting test categories test; and measures of verbal learning and memory (Frank, 2000).

Language skills assessment is important in the evaluation of SLD because a language processing abnormality is responsible for reading abnormalities in a large number of cases. Language testing needs to include all the elements of language and speech.

Tests of spatial constructional skills, visual perception, and visual motor integration are important components of neuropsychological testing. The ability to copy specific symbols such as a cross, a circle, and a diamond (and more complex geometrical shapes) follows a developmental pattern. The Beery-Buktenica Developmental Test of Visual Motor Integration is a drawing test that requires the child to copy geometric designs. Another is the Benton Test of Visual Retention (Mattis, French, & Rapin, 1975) in which the adequacy of construction is not highly skewed by graphomotor factors. Other visual perceptual tests include the Raven coloured progressive matrices, which utilizes patterned visual stimuli and requires no constructional or skilled motor output, the Benton line orientation test (Benton, Hannay, & Varney, 1975), and the facial recognition test.

Motor coordination is tested by the neurologist or developmental pediatrician as part of the clinical neurological examination, but can also be tested by the neuropsychologist in a more quantitative way. Neuropsychological tests commonly used for fine motor tasks are the grooved pegboard Purdue pegboard (Costa, Scarola, & Rapin, 1964), and the finger tapping test (Klonoff & Low, 1974).

Although the cognitive factors that underlie reading disabilities have been well assessed, cognitive deficits that underlie mathematical learning disabilities are less well known., These may include difficulties with procedural knowledge, attentional difficulties, and language processing abnormalities. The extent and direction of testing in these cases are assessed by a neuropsychologist.

Emotional and social factors should be taken into consideration when cognitive tests are interpreted, and a primary major psychiatric disorder should be excluded. It should also be remembered that learning disabled children are more likely to have fear of failure and thus tend to exhibit more test anxiety than their nondisabled peers (Bryan & Smiley, 1983). Test scores may be artificially depressed as a result of such anxiety.

BEHAVIORAL ASSESSMENT

Behavioral and emotional abnormalities are frequent comorbidities of SLD and can cause or exacerbate learning difficulties. A detailed history of any behavioral or emotional problems should be taken in the initial medical interview. Affect is examined at the same time by looking at the child's appearance (animated, flat), by the content of his or her conversation, speech prosody, and vegetative signs. In addition, a number of screening questionnaires can be used for this purpose.

The Achenbach Child Behavior Checklist (CBCL) and Teacher Report Form provide parent and teacher behavioral observations. These questionnaires are scored by scales reflecting internalized emotional symptoms such as anxiety and depression, and externalizing symptomatology, such as hyperactivity, aggressiveness, and delinquency. DSM-IV checklists for disruptive behavioral disorders (e.g., SNAP-IV or the Conners scale for hyperactivity) completed by teachers or parents provide data on inattention, hyperactivity-impulsivity, and oppositional behavior. The Diagnostic Inventory for Children and Adolescents-Revised (DICA-R) is given as an interview, and can be used for the diagnosis of a number of behavioral conditions, including ADHD and depression. Specific depression scales, for instance the Children's Depression Index (CDI), provide information of depressive symptomatology, but their reliability is limited by the language skill and truthfulness of the patient (Duane, 1993). In my opinion, general behavioral questionnaires such as the Achenbach, and a DSM-IV compatible questionnaire for ADHD should be completed by the parents and teachers of every child evaluated for a SLD. Other, more specific tools, including questionnaires for depression, can be used as clinically indicated.

Certain guidelines can be helpful in deciding whether to refer the child for a psychiatric consultation. These include a thought disorder, severe depression, obsessive compulsive disorder, preoccupation with fantasies, or uncontrollable aggression. It is sometime difficult to distinguish between very low self-esteem and depression. It has been our convention that when a child has any expression of despair ("I wish I were dead" or similar expressions), we suggest an urgent psychiatric consultation.

In a child with learning difficulties and emotional–behavioral difficulties, referring him or her for educational intervention only without treating the emotional–behavioral difficulties will diminish RTI. Both the academic and emotional–behavioral areas of difficulty need intervention.

Social skills, communication skills, adaptive behavior, and daily living abilities are important domains of the student's life both in and out of school. Social skills and communication issues may be the main areas of difficulty in children with high grade autism or Asperger syndrome who present with school difficulties, but these issues can be important also in other children with SLD. Assessing social and communication skills and adaptive behavior is, in some cases, as important as the measurement of academic functions, but is rarely done in school age children. The team evaluating children with school difficulties needs to include these functions along with academic achievements.

LABORATORY TESTS

There are no specific laboratory tests for the diagnosis of SLD. Medical diagnostic tests are done to rule out a number of systemic conditions that may cause learning abnormalities. That includes blood tests for anemia, glucose, kidney, liver, and thyroid functions screen for metabolic–toxic abnormalities, including hypothyroidism and lead toxicity. Genetic tests such as chromosomes, fragile X DNA, and arrays are considered when there is a strong family history of learning difficulties or other genetic abnormalities, or when the child has dysmorphic features. Dysmorphic features specific to fragile

X syndrome are elongated face, large protruding ears, and a large scrotum. (Corrigan et al., 1997).

It is uncommon that a significant hearing loss responsible for a SLD is not detected before school age. If not previously done, audiometry is recommended in children with a history of developmental speech and language disorder or repeated ear infections. Similarly, ophthalmological abnormalities are only rarely responsible for SLD, but school learning can be affected when visual acuity is impaired. Therefore, ophthalmological examination should be done to rule out abnormalities of visual acuity (Latvala, Korhonen, Penttinen, & Laippala, 1994).

In some children with school problems, the presenting symptom is that the student seems to be intermittently inattentive, does not respond when spoken to, or has to be physically touched before responding. Although these problems can be caused by inattentiveness (part of ADHD) or language processing difficulties, a non–motor type of epilepsy (e.g., petit mal) is rarely a cause. An electroencephalogram (EEG) should be considered, and if there is a diagnostic question, prolonged video EEG monitoring can be used to correlate unusual behavior with EEG changes. In most children with SLD, the EEG is normal or reveals nonspecific abnormalities, mostly mild slowing or disorganization of background activity. Rarely, it will demonstrate epileptiform activity.

Quantitative EEG or brain mapping techniques may demonstrate a pattern different than normal, but do not help to make a diagnosis of SLD because of lack of adequate specificity and validity. Event-related potentials tests (N-100/P-300) of subjects with ADHD or SLD may reveal a prolonged response latency or decrease of amplitude. Again, lack of specificity and validity of the results prevents broad clinical use. Consistency of test paradigms and improved norms may allow the use of these tools for clinical testing in the future.

Continuous performance tests may demonstrate abnormalities in children with LDs, especially those with comorbid ADHD, usually in the form of a slower response speed, but do not contribute to the diagnosis of SLD.

Electrooculographic (EOG) recordings were suggested as a clinical diagnostic method for reading disability. Although some differences were found between eye movement pattern of learning disabled and typical readers, it is not substantiated that such abnormalities can diagnose or explain reading disability (Poblano et al., 1996).

Neuroimaging studies are generally not helpful in the diagnosis of SLDs, but can be used for the differential diagnosis of children with learning disorders if an underlying structural abnormality is suspected by the history, the physical or neurological examination. Thus, neuroimaging may be diagnostically useful in patients with neurofibromatosis or tuberous sclerosis when a history of a perinatal or other encephalopathic event is present, or in cases of an acute deterioration of learning ability. Research studies using quantitative or functional neuroimaging, including positron emission tomography and functional MRI, have shown group differences between learning disabled people and controls on various measures. However, none has as yet achieved the degree of specificity and reliability needed to become a diagnostic tool (Duane, 1993).

SCREENING FOR SPECIFIC LEARNING DISABILITIES

There is no specific uniform screen for SLDs. A general screen of a child's cognitive and learning abilities, which can be done by an experienced physician in his or her office, should include age-appropriate reading (including reading of nonwords), writing and spelling, a memory test, and copying geometrical shapes.

A psychoeducational screening battery for the school age child with a possible SLD needs, in my opinion, to have an estimate of (a) general verbal and nonverbal intellectual abilities (using the WISC-IV), (b) tests of academic achievement, (c) tests of motor coordination, and (d) a naming test. Developmental language disorders are very prevalent in learning disabled children. The naming test is included in the screening battery because naming of objects is a highly sensitive index of language ability and disability. The Boston Naming Test is a commonly used naming test.

The Mini-Mental State Examination for children has been tested, and results are promising for detecting abnormalities in children older than age 4 years. The test covers a range of mental functions, including orientation, attention–concentration, memory, language, and constructional ability, and takes a short time to administer. Its value for the diagnosis of SLD has not yet been assessed (Ouvrier et al., 1993). In general, the definitive diagnosis of SLD should be done only after a formal psychoeducational battery and neurobehavioral tests, as delineated earlier in this chapter.

INFORMATIVE SESSION

Informing parents that their child has an SLD is a difficult task. In general parents are frequently dissatisfied with communication with physicians who inform them that their child has a significant mental or physical disability (Quine & Rutter, 1994). Although this has a number of reasons, not all of them related to the physician, it is important to conduct the informative session in a way that leaves the parents with the clearest possible understanding of their child's condition, and a plan of therapy and prognosis. In the case of

SLD, this is a difficult task. Understanding how the brain works and the intricate systems of cognition is a difficult task, even for physicians and scientists, as is explaining to parents that although their child is adequately intelligent, he or she has a selective cognitive abnormality making it difficult for him or her learn to read or calculate is even more difficult (Pennington, 1991). We usually cannot provide laboratory or blood tests to demonstrate the brain abnormality. We then talk about "processing problems" or "abnormalities in the wiring of the brain," although we cannot demonstrate those on any imaging testing. We can only point to the abnormalities found in the psychoeducational and neuropsychological tests and suggest that those are responsible for the child's academic problems. We also need to consider the fact that a diagnosis of SLD is frequently not made until the beginning of school and sometimes later, in the third of fourth grade, and this informative session takes place at about that time. Parents frequently ask why, if there is some abnormality in the way the brain is wired, did their child appear normal and intelligent until that time? In effect, children with SLD frequently have some signs of learning difficulties before the beginning school, including difficulties learning to speak and perform fine or complex motor activities, but as those are not severe and the child is otherwise developing normally, the parents and even educators usually do not associate them with a risk for a learning problem. Therefore, SLDs are hard to diagnose before the beginning of formal learning in school (Shapiro & Gallico, 1993).

When parents understand that their child has a SLD, they are usually stunned. "Will he or she be able to go to college?" and "Can he or she live a normal life?" are frequently asked questions. The informative session has to address all these issues (Pennington, 1991).

It is advisable that the diagnostic team have a discussion of the results of the tests and diagnosis before the meeting with parents, so there is a uniform presentation of the results. The outline of the informative session should include the following: (a) a description of the diagnostic process, (b) a review the biological basis of the SLD, and (c) an explanation how the child's symptoms and signs are explained by the SLD and associated behavioral problems. We can explain how a language processing deficit can cause a reading disability, visuospatial abnormality can lead to problems learning geometrical shapes, or how difficulties with attention span can interfere with writing and completing homework. The last part of the informative session consists of the recommendations for treatment and interventions.

Many terms used in behavioral–cognitive diagnoses are terms unknown to nonprofessionals and are certainly new to the parents. Therefore, the discussion should be conducted in plain language so the parents can understand it. At the first follow up after the informative session I usually try to find out the parents' understanding of the content of that session. Frequently they understand only part of the discussion, and may miss or change important parts. For instance, in patients in whom SLD is accompanied by a comorbidity of ADHD, they may remember only the ADHD diagnosis. They may disregard the diagnosis of SLD, which may be the most important part of the diagnosis, because it is less known and harder to understand.

Part of the informative session can be looked on, in some way, as a psychotherapy process. Parents of learning disabled children are frequently perplexed because their child, who seems intelligent, keeps failing in school. They may have tried to find what is keeping him or her from succeeding academically, and have received confusing information from different sources—family, friends, therapists, or the Internet. In many cases they would prefer to hear that their children are lazy rather than that they have a neurologically based disability. At times there is guilt, and they may be angry with their child as well as the diagnostic team. It is clear that "any learning disorder, however mild, represents the loss of the perfect child, a fantasy all parents have at some level" (Pennington, 1991, p. 38). An attempt should be made to alleviate some of these anxieties. The difficulties associated with SLD should not be minimized, but it can be stressed that it does not mean low intelligence, and when appropriately handled, is compatible with a normal, productive, and successful life. Therefore, it is important to discuss the child's cognitive and behavioral strengths along with his or her weaknesses.

Children with SLD encounter professionals from various disciplines, some of whom will be involved in their diagnostic process and treatment, including teachers, school psychologists, and sometimes physical, occupational, and speech and language therapists. These professionals may generate competing explanations for the child's learning problems, and may have different recommendations, both conventional and unconventional, for therapy, some of which may be are conflicting. This can be quite confusing to parents. It is the task of the physician to ascertain that the diagnostic process is appropriate, the therapies recommended are evidence based, and to advise the parents to avoid unnecessary therapies that may also be expensive.

HOW TO EXPLAIN THE DIAGNOSIS TO THE CHILD

Children with SLD often recognize that they have a problem and are different from other children. When they undergo psychological evaluations they understand that they are being evaluated because of their school-related difficulties. Therefore, it is important that they will be informed about the results of the evaluation. Most younger children may not benefit from participating in the parent-informing conference. They do not understand the discussion, which may be intimidating and make them anxious. In my experience most parents prefer that their children not be present in the informative session, and ask us to advise them how to convey the information to the child. The exception may be older adolescents. A decision about the participation of older children in the conference should be taken after consultation with the parents. In all other cases, children need to be informed separately. Many learning disabled children think they are "stupid" or, as frequently pointed out to them, "lazy." They, and sometimes their parents, are constantly told that "they can do better if they try harder." This is one of the myths repeated by teachers or parents, and is frequently applied to children who are actually trying their best. Many children with SLD initially work harder than non–learning disabled children. They may later lose motivation, however, as a result of constant failure. It is therefore very important that children with SLD have their condition explained to them in a developmentally appropriate manner, a task that is hard to accomplish during a short session. We usually try to assure children that they are intelligent, not lazy and not "crazy," and tell them the reason for and the nature of the evaluation. We explain that people usually have strengths and weaknesses in different areas—some excel in sports, whereas others excel in music. Similarly, they may have weaknesses in some academic areas, but may have strength in others. However, it cannot be expected that such a short explanation will suffice. It is important to continue the process of explanation and reassurance and suggest psychological therapy if it is evident that they have low self-esteem.

WRITING A COMPREHENSIVE REPORT

A comprehensive written report is an important part of the diagnostic process. We usually send the report to the pediatrician with a copy to the parents. It is very important for the pediatrician to know the results of the evaluation, and recognize that the child has a LD that may interfere with his or her emotional as well as physical well-being. Learning disabled children are under daily stress trying to keep up with the academic school demands and face failure constantly. Some develop headaches, stomachaches, and sleep disturbances. They may visit the school nurse frequently. The parents can use the report to further understand the diagnosis and be able review the recommendations. They can also use it to advocate for their child's needs at school.

THE ROLE OF DIFFERENT PROFESSIONALS

Different disciplines play a role in the diagnosis and treatment of SLDs. Physicians, psychologists, and neuropsychologists are involved in the diagnostic process. Special education teachers plan and implement appropriate educational assistance, and therapists provide the support and help that the child and family need. The physician has a central and continuous role in the care of the child with SLDs because they are biological neurodevelopmental disorders, not merely learning disorders. Affected children have academic learning problems, but may also have neurological, physical, and other developmental and psychological problems. The physician has an understanding of the differential diagnosis of the learning disorder and can decide on the need for further neurodiagnostic tests, as well as the possible advantage of medications for the treatment of associated behavioral disorders. Physicians need to participate in early identification and the diagnostic process, discuss the diagnosis with the parent and child, and be involved in long-term management. These tasks demand appropriate expertise. Not all pediatricians choose to be actively involved with the diagnosis and treatment of this condition. Even more important, many are not adequately informed. Therefore, it is important to educate pediatricians, neurologists, and psychiatrists in issues related to SLD.

CHAPTER 16

Treatment of Specific Learning Disabilities

INTRODUCTION

Generally, the treatment of medical conditions follows one of a number of patterns. The first is prevention, taking measures to prevent the condition from happening. A second pattern is a curative treatment that will eradicate the condition. A third pattern, the least desirable but probably most common, is symptomatic treatment.

The previous chapters discussed the fact that Specific Learning Disabilities (SLD) are the result of an abnormality in a specific brain cognitive network (e.g., phonological processing), caused by an aberration that occurred during brain development, a process that starts early in utero and continues throughout infancy and childhood.

Can such a brain abnormality be prevented? There are some preventive measures that can reduce the risk of SLD. These apply more to nongenetic SLD. Reducing prematurity, providing good prenatal care, and ensuring infant stimulation will, no doubt, reduce the occurrence of SLD. But, as previously discussed, many cases are genetically determined and cannot be prevented unless the responsible genes are identified and modified. The second mode of therapy—a curative treatment—is hard to achieve because of the complex nature of SLD. What follows is that, like many neurodevelopmental conditions, SLD do not have a complete cure, and follow the pattern of "static encephalopathy," namely, a condition that is non-deteriorating and usually steadily improves, although without total cure. Therefore, we should look upon SLD as an ongoing disorder, which frequently cannot be cured, can be treated but needs ongoing attention.

Another important fact is that SLD involve more than difficulties with academic learning. Children with these conditions encounter emotional, motor, behavioral, and social as well as academic difficulties. Their treatment, therefore, should include academic, psychological, and at times pharmacological measures. The short-term treatment goals are improving academic and social competence, and preventing adverse behavioral symptoms. The long-term goal is that the person with SLD emerges from the school years academically successful, and emotionally and socially intact. With timely remediation, the prognosis is usually good. Children with SLD improve, learn, and have a productive life. Without intervention, the prognosis of SLD is guarded. Therefore, it is very important to intervene as early as possible both academically and psychologically.

A word of caution: At the present time there is no form of therapy that offers a cure for SLD. There are no special diets or special therapies that offer a complete cure. Legitimate suggestions for remediation should aim to enhance learning ability, retrain brain systems, help store or use information, or develop "bypass" learning techniques.

CAN THE BRAIN BE TRAINED?

The parallel goals of treatment of SLD are to stimulate and retrain the impaired brain networks responsible for the SLD (i.e., phonological processing in the case of reading) and at the same time encourage the development of other "bypass" pathways of acquiring knowledge. To achieve the first goal there is a need for rehabilitation of a faulty brain system. The second, "bypass" goal, is achieved by training other, hopefully unaffected, brain systems. Ideally, we should try to achieve both goals.

There is evidence that the brain can change as a result of experience or practice (Petersen et al., 1998; Karni et al., 1998; Raichle, 1998). A short practice of a task alters the brain areas involved in this task. For the developing brain, some areas are active early in practice and then drop away, whereas the activity of other areas increases (Petersen, 1998).

The method of remediation is mainly through practice, repeated training and education, done with an underlying understanding that experience can cause gain in performance.

Supporting this understanding is evidence that sensory experience, obtained by practice, induces gains in basic perceptual skills through brain mechanisms facilitating the encoding aspects of a learned motor and possibly other behaviors. In other words, there is an experience-dependent plasticity by which discrete changes can occur within sensory and motor neuronal groups in the cortex as a result of repeated performance of a task. The learning of the task induces long-lasting changes in those sensory or motor representations that are critical for the performance of that task. For instance, training rats to reach for bits of cookies resulted in a selective increase in dendritic length and branching complexity in the apical branches of layer V pyramidal cells within the motor-sensory forelimb cortex. This demonstrates a selective alteration of brain structures, occurring as a result of training the animal to perform a certain task, and possibly representing a brain correlate of this type of learning (Withers & Greenough, 1989).

It is possible that this may only apply to training of perceptual but not cognitive tasks. It may also apply to a normal brain but not when anatomical or "network" abnormalities are present. The nature and possibly the location of these abnormalities may be important in relation to the types of remediation, rehabilitation, and training used. We know that for adults, recovery from aphasia after a stroke depends on etiology, initial severity, and type of aphasia. Conduction and transcortical aphasia may have a better prognosis for recovery compared with global aphasia or Wernicke's aphasia. This may be true for SLDs, although the underlying brain abnormalities in SLD are very different from those present after acquired brain damage in the adult; consequently, rehabilitation of function in the brain may take different pathways.

It is possible that normal neurons or neuronal connections are reassigned to tasks of the abnormal neurons or networks. Future developments in brain sciences may also make it possible that brain cells containing appropriate neurotransmitters will be implanted or grafted into the brain and will produce missing neurotransmitters, with an improved ability to learn (Li, Field, & Raisman, 1997; Clarkson et al., 1998). The effects of various nerve growth factors on restoration of neurological function are being tested.

EDUCATIONAL REMEDIATION

The cornerstone of treatment of SLD is educational remediation. The primary treatment is special education, which should be school based, include slower and repetitive teaching, individually or in small groups, and be administered by special education teachers using special techniques and teaching aids. After-school tutoring is usually effective only in less severe cases or for treatment during the summer vacation. In addition, individual skills differences should be accommodated, and traditional education may need to be supplemented with functional curricula, computers, vocational training, or work study.

Grade retention is not a valid method of treatment of SLD. Grade retention may frequently delay the recognition of SLDs, thus delaying the onset of appropriate treatment, and worsen the prognosis. Students recognized as having an SLD need special education.

The intensity of special education and the extent of "mainstreaming" of the individual child with SLD depends on the degree of the disability. Special education can be of different forms, starting within the regular classroom with bypass-compensatory strategies implemented by regular classroom teachers. Some children with SLD may be recommended for an inclusionary program, which means that the child spends the full day in a regular classroom, and the regular education teacher is supported by a special education teacher to provide services within the regular class and individualize the child's program (Fleischner, 1995). Other forms of special education include a resource room, in which the student goes out of the classroom for a period of time and is taught, usually in a small group, by a special education teacher. In more difficult cases a special class placement may be needed. The more severely affected student may need a special class (self-contained class) in a regular school, a separate special school, or a residential school or homebound instruction. The usual approach is to find the least restrictive placement for the student. The greatest number of students receive special education in a resource room for an hour or more a day (20%-60% of the day), which includes basic academic skills and instruction in learning strategies. Resource room services do not seem to be associated with diminished self-esteem and may even enhance the student's confidence and signal to him or her that there is understanding and support for his or her difficulties. Self-contained classes provide students with special education outside of the general education classroom for more than 60% of the school day. This suits students with very deficient academic achievement or who also have significant behavioral problems.

The needs of each student may be different. There is increasing pressure to reduce the numbers of students placed in more restrictive settings such as special classes and increase the number of students who receive all their education in the regular classroom, and the inclusionary form of special education has become increasingly popular (Zigmond, 1995).

INDIVIDUALIZED TREATMENT

Special education for children with SLD should be tailored to the needs of each student. It should distinguish between different forms of SLD so that mathematical disability is treated in a different way from reading disability. The best approach is to prepare an individual educational plan according to the student's neuropsychological deficits. However, in practice, mixed types of SLD are common. Therefore, treating each area of difficulty separately may not be useful and one has to find a more generalized way of helping the child acquire knowledge (Johnson, 1995). There are a number of principles guiding the approach to treatment.

It should be remembered that the purpose of school is to help children acquire knowledge. Individual differences in the way a child acquires knowledge should be accommodated and bypass systems should be used. The bypass-compensatory strategies helpful to children with SLD include multimedia (movies, filmstrips, tapes, and talking books) for input and oral or written multiple choice examinations, and designated writers, calculators, computers, and other assistive technologies—for output. Homework is frequently difficult for the learning disabled child and can become an area of conflict between students and parents and between students and teachers. A large volume of homework does not necessarily improve the child's academic abilities, and may have an adverse impact by increasing stress; therefore, it should be modified. A systematic program to train parents in effective homework practices can be initiated (Jenson, Sheridan, Olympia, & Andrews, 1994). Homework policies and practices for students with SLD need to emphasize (a) simple, short assignments, (b) careful monitoring by and rewards from teachers, and (c) parental involvement, especially to provide structure, conducive environments, and immediate rewards (Cooper & Nye, 1994). In addition, the traditional education for children with SLD may need to be supplemented with teaching of functional skills, including computers and vocational or work study. Last, learning disabled students with reading or math difficulties may have other talents (athletics, art, music) and should be encouraged to pursue their own individual assets, talents, and interests, in which they can excel.

The fact that a student receives a diagnosis of SLD has a therapeutic value, because it signals school understanding and recognition of the student's problem, explains the student's academic difficulties to the school personnel, and removes the notion that he or she is lazy, unmotivated, and oppositional. Once this recognition is achieved by school personnel and parents, accepting the need for a more individual approach is easier. It is, therefore, important to explain the diagnosis of learning disability, and the student's specific difficulties, to the teachers and parents.

GUIDELINES TO EDUCATIONAL THERAPY

Classroom modifications are an important part of therapy. These include extra time or untimed written examinations, and additional time to complete assignments. Extended time for tests can be of significant value to students with SLD. A study of the effects of extended time on the algebra test performance of community college students with and without learning disabilities found that although the students with learning disabilities scored significantly lower than the regular students under timed conditions, their scores under extended-time conditions did not differ significantly from the timed or extended-time scores of the students without learning disabilities (Alster, 1997).

Other accommodations include modifications of the curriculum. Specific learning disabilities, particularly reading disabilities, are frequently language based. Second language courses are notoriously difficult for students with SLD. In such cases they should be excused from second foreign language requirements. Oral exams should be permitted for severely impaired dyslexics. They should not be panelized for spelling errors.

Technical help includes keyboards with word processors for writing assignments, the use of a tape recorder, and emerging computer technologies. For instance, reading disabled children were able to profit from instructional procedures that segment the printed word into units. A training that employed a "talking" computer system that provides synthesized speech feedback during the course of learning can be used (Lovett et al., 1994).

Educational considerations may change with age. In high school a major consideration should be long-term planning, and it is important to tailor students' course choices and career goals to bypass areas of weakness. For instance, geometry, trigonometry, and calculus are likely to be extremely difficult for children with mathematical disabilities or nonverbal learning disabilities, as are physics and possibly the other sciences.

TREATMENT OF DYSLEXIA

Five to ten percent of school age children have a reading disability. The pathophysiology of dyslexia largely involves a deficit in the phonological component of language—the ability to identify and mentally manipulate the constituent speech sounds. Phonological awareness has been found to predict much of the variance in reading skills starting at a very young age (Eden & Moates, 2002). A confluence of anatomical, physiological, and genetic evidence points to the neural origin of this disability. Other language processing abnormalities are the cause of reading disability in some cases.

Anatomically, functional magnetic resonance imaging (fMRI) studies have shown a deficit in the neural mechanisms underlying phonological processing in children and adults with dyslexia. The abnormalities seen in dyslexia involve a number of brain areas in the left more than right hemispheres (Galaburda et al., 1985; Eden & Zeffiro, 1998). The anomalous brain activity seen in dyslexics is quite consistent across different cultures (Paulesu et al., 2000; Grigorenco, 2001).

Multiple genes may be involved in dyslexia, and environmental factors and experience are also involved (Peterson, Reis, & Ingvar, 2001).

The abnormalities that cause reading disability are common to poor readers of normal as well as abnormal intelligence. There is frequently a delay in diagnosis, sometimes until the third grade, by which time remediation is more difficult, and secondary emotional problems are common.

The way to use neuroscience knowledge to help treat dyslexia (Eden & Moats, 2002) is first through diagnosis and early identification—the essential first step in the process of treatment. Early testing of phonological awareness can be used to identify children with phonological processing problems. Phonological awareness–based instruction significantly improves reading performance of poor readers in the first grade (National Reading Panel [NRP], 2000). Treatment programs should start early and include the teaching of phonological awareness (orally identifying and manipulating syllables and speech sounds), phonics (making associations between sounds and letters), fluency, and vocabulary. Although the instructional approaches for students with dyslexia include the same strategies as recommended by the NRP for the general classroom, the teaching of phonological awareness to dyslexic children needs to be more explicit, the amount of practice given—greater, and teachers should use multisensory techniques to link speaking, reading, and writing. (Torgesen et al., 2001; Swanson, 1999).

It is essential that treatment for a reading disability start early, before or in first grade, in order to achieve better reading results and prevent secondary emotional abnormalities.

Because subjects with dyslexia may have abnormal rapid temporal processing, they may require longer time intervals between successive auditory stimuli in order to discriminate between them or sequence them (Tallal et al., 1996). Computer-based programs to address this problem and extend acoustic speech stimuli are available (including commercial programs like Fast ForWord), although it is not clear that their use has a long-term advantage compared with other reading programs.

TREATMENT METHODS FOR READING DISORDERS

Treatment methods for reading disability may attempt to teach reading or remediate the underlying cognitive deficit. Although attempts have been made to classify dyslexia to distinct types with the hope of having specific types of remedial programs tailored to each type, these attempts have not been successful. In addition, many students have a mixed type of underlying difficulties with reading, spelling, and mathematics, and difficulties may change with age. Therefore, there is a need for individual educational plans, rather than one remedy that will fit all (Shapiro, 1993).

It is not clear that there is one best classroom technique for teaching reading, and the advantage of any one specific remedial reading program for reading disability (i.e., the Orton-Gillingham, Distar, or Stevenson reading programs) over the others, is questionable.

Spelling problems, which are common to many reading disabled students, appear to be less remediable than reading problems (Pennington,

1991). A common deficit in dyslexia is the inability to acquire the alphabetic code due to deficits in phonological processing. Therefore, disabled readers need to be provided with programs that explicitly teach phonological awareness, application of phonological rules to reading, word recognition, and a phonics-based approach to reading. Longitudinal data indicate that systematic phonics instruction results in more favorable outcomes for disabled readers than does a context emphasis (whole language) approach. Instructions and interventions for reading failure that focus primarily on context and reading comprehension without commensurate attention paid to phonological awareness, decoding, and word recognition, show limited results. Phonological awareness develops before reading ability and independently of it, and the phonological awareness facilitates subsequent reading acquisition (Schneider, Kuspert, & Roth, et al., 1997). Identifying children at risk for reading difficulties and providing them with phonological-processing intervention significantly improves their phonological processing and reading abilities. Instruction in phonological awareness at the kindergarten level has significant positive effects on reading development during the first grade (Blachman, Ball, & Black, 1994; Gillon & Dodd, 1997).

It is possible that a combined program of structured reading in a phonics-based approach, training in phonological awareness, and language intervention, is an effective form of treatment for poor readers and produces greater gains than training in either reading or phonological awareness alone. Effective classroom-based programs should include several components: structured phonemic awareness (orally identifying and manipulating syllables and speech sounds), phonics (making associations between sounds and letters), fluency (developing speed and automaticity in accurate letter, word and text reading), vocabulary expansion and, last, text comprehension.

Perceptual Training

Studies of individuals with specific language impairment (defined by poor oral language and frequently accompanied by reading problems) show that they can discriminate between successive auditory inputs if the interval between them is longer than that required by subjects with normal language processing. It was suggested that this deficient sensory processing causes the defect in phonological processing, and later in reading (Studdert-Kennedy & Mody, 1995).

Computer-based training exercises (i.e., Fast ForWord) were devised to drive processing of rapidly successive acoustic stimuli to faster rates and to temporarily extend acoustic speech stimuli to improve speech perception. Fast ForWord is such a program by Scientific Learning Inc. created by Paula

Talal, a neuroscientist at Rutgers University, and Mike Merzenich, a neuroscientist at the university of California medical school.

STUDIES OF THE EFFECTIVENESS OF PHONOLOGICALLY BASED APPROACHES

Phonologically based instruction significantly improved the reading performance of poor readers in first grade. Instruction programs differ in the way in which phonology and other language structures are systematically taught, in the amount of practice given, the mode of delivery (small group or one-on-one) and the use of multisensory enhancing techniques. In general, reading accuracy can be significantly improved in younger and older poor readers using phonologically based methods.

Single-unit recording studies in nonhuman primates after perceptual training, and functional brain imaging studies in children undergoing this type of training, have demonstrated physiological changes (Temple), but a direct comparison between an approach using structured, multisensory language lessons (Orton-Gillingham) and an approach using this structured language teaching plus Fast ForWord showed improved phonological processing in both groups but no long-term reading or language advantage to the group treated with Fast ForWord (Hook).

An issue for the treatment of many developmental abnormalities is whether children with disabilities can generalize from one task or category to another. A study that examined the feasibility of teaching phonological manipulation skills to 4- to 6-year-old children with disabilities enrolled in a special education preschool, compared training in one of three categories of phonological tasks (rhyming, blending, and segmenting) to a control group. Results indicated that children were able to make significant progress in each experimental category, but that they demonstrated little or no generalization either within a category (e.g., from one type of blending task to another) or between categories (e.g., from blending to segmenting), which speaks in favor of comprehensive training programs that use all types of phonological processing.

A study examined whether behavioral remediation ameliorates these dysfunctional neural mechanisms in children with dyslexia (Temple et al., 2003), employed functional MRI in 20 8- to 12-year-old children with dyslexia during phonological processing before and after a remediation program focused on auditory processing and oral language training. Before treatment, the dyslexic group had a mean scaled score on the Woodcock Johnson reading mastery test-revised, word attack, or word identification subtest of less than 85.

Remediation was done using the Fast ForWord language computer intervention program, which includes exercises using nonlinguistic and acoustically modified linguistic speech, so that rapid frequency transitions in speech are slowed and amplified. The patients were taught discrimination between sequences of two brief successive acoustic frequency sweeps, distinguishing between sound changes of individual phonemes, identification of specific phonemes, matching consonant–vowel pairs within simple word structure, distinguishing between words that differed only by their initial or final consonant, following instructions of increasing length or grammatical complexity, and distinguishing grammatical structures. The exercises were done 100 minutes per day, 5 days per week, for an average of 27.9 training days.

Brain imaging was performed before and after training and included paradigms of phonological and nonphonological tests. Areas of interest included the left temporal-parietal region.

Behavioral results varied, but demonstrated that training improved oral language and reading performance, including word identification, pseudoword reading, and passage comprehension, which raised the group's score to the normal range (>85) and improved oral language ability and rapid naming.

Functional magnetic resonance imaging (fMRI) results for the children with dyslexia demonstrated brain activity getting closer to what is seen in normal reading children. There was increased activity in multiple brain areas, including the left temporal-parietal cortex and the left inferior frontal gyrus. There was a correlation between the magnitude of increased activation in the left temporal-parietal cortex and improvement in oral language ability. Increased activity was also seen in areas that were not active in normal reading children performing this task, including the right hemisphere frontal and middle temporal regions and the bilateral cingulate gyri, left hippocampus, inferior temporal gyrus, right parieto occipital, and bilateral thalami regions.

In summary, the study demonstrated a partial remediation of disrupted function in brain regions associated with phonological processing, resulting in improved reading and additional compensatory activation in other brain regions.

In the future, functional brain imaging studies will continue to be used to better understand the neural mechanisms of normal reading development (Schlaggar et al., 2002), but also to further evaluate the efficiency of instructional programs (Simos et al., 2002).

Beyond the type and content of the remediation programs, which are designed to target the intrinsic biological deficiency, other factors are important in the acquisition of knowledge, including the way the person is taught, the intensity of treatment, and the way the information is delivered. Improvement of any kind of reading disorder may depend, to some degree, on these and on the training and skills of the teacher.

USING COMMERCIAL PROGRAMS TO DETECT AND TREAT DYSLEXIA

Several validated tests are now available to identify children with mostly phonological and perhaps orthographic processing weaknesses. These are the children who are likely to experience reading failure. If at-risk children receive remedial teaching in kindergarten and first grade, outcomes are significantly better than if treatment is withheld until later (Eden & Moats, 2002).

In addition, there are many commercial programs for dyslexic students. Examples of commercial programs include the Orton-Gillingham Approach, Alphabetic Phonics, the Slingerland Approach, and many others. These are systematic, sequential approaches that allow professionals to teach language structure at many levels (sounds, syllables, meaningful parts of words, sentence structure, and paragraph and discourse organization). All emphasize the importance of multisensory approach and teach the phonological features of spoken language and word recognition. These programs were shown to bring about significant progress in reading if implemented by a skilled teacher. Earobics and Fast ForWord are examples of software programs directed to phonological and auditory processing skills through interactive computer games.

TREATMENT OF DYSCALCULIA

Treatment of specific math disorder depends on the specific deficit underlying this disability (i.e., whether the main deficit is in spatial reasoning or executive functions). If the main deficit is in executive functions, the child probably experiences the greatest difficulty in complex mathematical word problems and multistep calculations (e.g., long division). Such children can benefit from explicit written, step-by-stem "recipes" or algorithms to guide them through multistep problems. Most of the validated approaches to improving computational skills depend on systematic teaching and supervised drill and practice, but basic approaches to teaching arithmetic to all children are changing. Newer teaching approaches emphasize concept development and understanding the processes of arithmetic, rather than computation. In addition, there is a new emphasis on problem solving and representing quantitative information graphically and through figures (Fleischner, 1995; Thornton et al., 1997).

THERAPY FOR NONVERBAL LEARNING DISABILITIES

Children and adolescents with nonverbal Learning Disabilities (NVLD) have a variety of difficulties with learning, particularly arithmetic, and with visuospatial functions, motor coordination, and social learning. It is recommended that children with these problems get help in school for organizational skills. We also suggest that they have more time to complete assignments and unlimited time for tests.

Occupational therapy may be helpful, especially for younger children. Social training programs may help. Psychological counseling is important to help these children adapt to their difficulties, so their self-esteem will not suffer. Adaptive physical education instead of regular physical education is suggested when children are clumsy.

ORGANIZATIONAL SKILLS

Students with SLDs often require detailed instruction in how to study. This includes teaching the student effective cognitive strategies for comprehension, as well as strategies for organizing and managing study time. An example of a strategy of learning is the following: if one was asked to recall a string of digits (e.g., 2378751314), one might first chunk the digits (237 875 1314) and then rehearse them by saying, "two thirty-seven, eight seventy-five, thirteen, fourteen." By employing these strategies, one has taken a string of numbers that is too long and not easily remembered and converted it to a string that can be practiced until it is remembered. Instructional programs have been developed to teach students with learning disabilities such strategies and to help them select which strategy is most beneficial in particular instances (Fleischner, 1995).

COMMUNICATION STRATEGIES

During the past decade, there has been a growing awareness that social skills are among the brain functions that may be impaired in some types of SLD (i.e., nonverbal learning disabilities [NVLDs]). Delinquency, depression, and substance abuse, problems that have been found to be prevalent in youth and young adults with SLDs, may be helped if children learn social skills that enable them to engage with others.

Programs designed to improve social competence include teaching coping strategies in response to emotional upsets, the ability to adapt to situations that are new or unexpected, the ability to communicate effectively with others, and the ability to make and maintain friends (Fleischner, 1995).

THERAPY FOR MOTOR COORDINATION DIFFICULTIES

Although learning disabled children often have fine motor coordination difficulties, the relationship between this maladroitness and academic underachievement is not clear. If the child's visuospatial and fine motor skills are especially deficient, occupational therapy should be considered, especially for younger patients, but treating motor coordination problems will probably not improve reading or mathematical difficulties.

THE ROLE OF PARENTS

It is important that parents recognize, understand, and accept the diagnosis of SLD. Parents have a significant role in the treatment of their child with SLD from the early stage of recognition of the problem and the facilitation of testing, to the later stage of assuring and participation in the intervention. Currently our educational system does not always provide for the early screening and intervention that are essential for an optimal outcome of learning disabilities. Parents have an important role in advocacy for the appropriate testing and school help for their child. One of the most important roles of parents is preserving their child's self-esteem, through encouragement and looking for extracurricular activities in which the child can succeed. Many parents of children with disabilities, including learning disabilities, may not be ready for those tasks. Frequently, they pass through phases similar to those experienced in the grief process: denial, anger, guilt, blame, and finally acceptance. Parents need guidance and support from the professionals involved in diagnosis and treatment, the school, and their extended family. The physician can educate the parents, empowering them to work both inside and outside the educational system, as well as to join appropriate parent organizations, so that they can become effective educational advocates for their child (Linday, 1995). A very sensitive question is whether the parents should be tutors for their learning disabled children. Parents have a role as organizers and providers of the appropriate learning environment for their child. They should observe and report when the child's workload is too heavy, maintain necessary contact with the teacher, and answer their child's questions. However, there are a number of reasons why they should not act as tutors. They are not special education teachers and may not be acquainted with the appropriate academic approach needed for their child. More important, they are not independent professionals. They may bring into the tutorial sessions their own frustration and anger. Children may not cooperate with their parents because they don't wish to display weakness to the people who they sometimes see as their main critics. The result may be increased frustration on the parents' side, and decreased self-esteem and an increased feeling of isolation and despair on the child's side. Tutoring, when recommended, should not be administered by a family member, and preferably by a person who has special education knowledge.

THE ROLE OF THE PHYSICIAN

The physician has an important role in the early detection of SLD. This role is accomplished through knowledge of normal developmental milestones, performing periodic developmental and educational screenings, and following the child's school progress. Once a problem is identified, the physician has a role ascertaining that the child goes through the diagnostic process, and later, interprets and explains the diagnosis to the parents and child. The physician's role does not end when the diagnostic process is finished. Longitudinal monitoring should continue with support and intervention when needed to ensure that treatment and outcome are optimal (Shapiro & Gallico, 1993).

THE LEGAL BASIS FOR HELP FOR CHILDREN WITH SPECIFIC LEARNING DISABILITIES

Two different federal laws might be used to obtain assistance for children with learning disabilities, the Individuals with Disabilities Education Act (IDEA) and the Rehabilitation Act. The Rehabilitation Act defines physical or mental impairment as (a) any physiological disorder or condition affecting one or more body systems (including neurological, musculoskeletal, cardiovascular, respiratory, and special senses organs), and (b) any mental or psychological disorder. Examples of impairments include chronic asthma, allergies, spina bifida, and diabetes as well as mental retardation, organic brain syndrome, emotional or mental illness, and SLD. SLD is included in the Rehabilitation Act because it constitutes an impairment that substantially limits a major life activity for school-aged students. The affected children are, therefore, entitled to help under this act.

The cornerstone treatment offered to children and youth with SLD is special education. Resources are available in most school districts for these needs, and parents should be informed about this law. Section 504 of the Civil Rights Act (1973) also assures appropriate educational accommodations throughout one's life for those who do not qualify under PL 94-142.

Another law, the Individuals with Disabilities Education Act (IDEA), guarantees a free, appropriate public education to students with disabilities (Cavanaugh, Tervo, & Fogas, 1997), and IDEA recognizes SLD as such a disability. As previously noted, a common interpretation of the legal criteria for determining eligibility for a student with SLD under the IDEA are whether (a) the child shows a severe discrepancy between intellectual potential ("intelligence") and actual achievement in any one of several academic areas; (b) the discrepancy is not primarily due to other factors; and (c) the child needs special education because of the learning disability. It is, therefore, not enough to demonstrate that a child has a learning disability. It is also necessary to demonstrate that he or she is disabled and needs special education because of the learning disability. Children with high IQs often struggle for years before getting special education help. Their academic achievements may not be low enough for an achievement/intelligence discrepancy to occur, or even when they qualify for the discrepancy criteria, it may be argued that they do not need special education because they do not fail. This may also occur when the method assessing disability is by the number of years or months a child's academic performance is lagging behind grade level. Such children have difficulty obtaining special education services, and sometimes legal help needs to be obtained.

The broader definition of disability under the Rehabilitation Act and the fact that it does not require that the student needs special education results in more students being protected by the Rehabilitation Act than by the IDEA. For school-aged students all that is required for Rehabilitation Act eligibility is a mental or physical impairment that substantially limits a major life activity. For example, children who have mental retardation have obvious learning difficulties. However, they are not included in the category of SLD, and may not comply with the legal definition of learning disability. They may not be eligible for special education help because of their learning disabilities but qualify under the Rehabilitation Act. Another example are students diagnosed with attention deficit hyperactivity disorder (ADHD) who qualify under the Rehabilitation Act, even though they may need only minor academic modification and no special education. Attention deficit hyperactivity disorder is a common comorbidity for SLD. A child diagnosed with both ADHD and a learning disability can qualify for special education either as having SLD under the IDEA, or as "Other Health Impaired" if they fulfill the criteria for ADHD. Many have criteria for both (Bateman, 1995).

Either the parents or the school can seek a medical diagnosis relevant to the question of whether a student fits the eligibility criteria of either the IDEA or the Rehabilitation Act. Many parents are not aware that there are two different federal laws and definitions of disabilities that might provide roads to the needed special education assistance for their children. The diagnostic process is carried out by a multidisciplinary team that determines whether an LD exists.

All evaluations (including medical evaluation) that may have educational programs implications must be provided at no cost to the parents (Fennell, 1995). The law also provides that if the parents disagree with the assessment of the child provided by the school district, they are entitled to an independent evaluation by a person at no expense to them.

Special education is defined by law as specially designed instruction to meet the student's unique needs. It includes transportation and such developmental, corrective, and other supportive services that are required to assist a child with a disability so that he or she can benefit from special education, including speech pathology and audiology, psychological services, physical and occupational therapy, and recreation. The services must be spelled out in a written document called an Individualized Educational Plan. Knowing what is available in local schools can be of assistance in helping children with various types of SLDs (Berkovitz, 1995).

Federal law does not always require a neurological or neurodevelopmental examination for eligibility. A medical examination is usually required, however, for a diagnosis of "other health impaired"—the classification designated for ADHD. I believe that every child with school-related problems should have a medical examination by a developmental pediatrician or pediatric neurologist.

Lack of uniformity exists in the classification of SLDs by different school systems. Discussion of the ways by which different countries as well as states within the United States provide help for children with SLDs is beyond the scope of this book. Studies examining school classification of SLDs find both under- and over-classification, by inclusion of children with mental retardation (MacMillan et al., 1996).

Children with SLDs are entitled, through federal and state law, to free appropriate public education and other services, including reasonable accommodation. The services are spelled out in a written document called an Individual Education Plan (IEP), formulated in writing by the student's educators and parents in association with other professionals, which specifies the programs and services to be provided to the student and the goals and objectives of the student's instructional program. The IEP must be implemented, monitored, and reassessed at appropriate intervals. Parents have final say and ultimate responsibility in determining content of the IEP. The mandated IEP can also include modifications of the student's grading, exemptions from state educational tests that limit one's opportunities for further education, and untimed standardized tests (Levy, Harper, & Weinberg, 1992). Other services given to the students may include speech pathology and audiology, psychological services, physical and occupational therapy, counseling, medical services for diagnostic or evaluation purposes, and transportation.

THE ENVIRONMENT

An important part of the educational treatment of SLD is creating instructional environments that encourage students' active involvement in the learning process. The learning method includes student engagement in the design of solutions to problems and the evaluation of the products of their work. These goals are especially important for students with disabilities, many of whom may be passive learners who experience difficulty with flexible use of knowledge and skills. Therefore, the use of collaborative project-based instructional environments, especially multimedia design projects, should be encouraged.

When Should Treatment Start?

Interventions are most likely to be successful if applied early. Therefore, we should focus on early identification and early intervention programs. Unfortunately, the majority of children with SLD are not identified until the third grade. The longer children with disabilities, at any level of severity, go without identification and intervention, the more difficult the task of reme-diation and the lower the rate of success.

It is commonly assumed that children "outgrow" learning disabilities and by adolescence require fewer services. In fact, adolescence may well be a time when increased services are needed because there is increased need for time management, long-term projects, organization of materials, and completion of the multiple assignments and long-term projects that are required in high school (Shapiro & Gallico, 1986).

Psychological Therapy

Introduction

Psychological consequences of learning disorders stem from constant class-room failure frequently accompanied by social difficulties, and include reduced self-esteem, anxiety, anger, and features of depression, which may continue in varied forms into adult life. These children are faced with daily academic and social demands that they cannot fulfill. Ongoing academic failure reduces their motivation to learn, and some students may refuse to go to school. They may try to defend themselves by lying or blaming others, and project blame and anger toward parents and teachers. Reduced self-esteem may also lead to provocative behaviors in the classroom. Studies show that learning disabled people are over-represented in the juvenile delinquency population.

Psychotherapy, which is essential for many children with SLD, often is not offered, and when offered is sometimes not accepted because children usually do not ask for help, and parents do not initially realize the emotional compo-nents of SLD. It may become obvious later in the high school years when it is often too late. In addition, it is still the belief of some that SLD are temporary problems that disappear later in life.

Although psychological problems in SLD are usually explained as stem-ming from low self-esteem secondary to continued academic failure, it is pos-sible that psychological–emotional difficulties are related to the biological abnormalities underlying SLD, as is the case in NVLDs. Once it is understood that SLD syndromes are the result of a basic neurobiological central nervous system dysfunction, one can postulate that this dysfunction may manifest in more ways than simply academic problems (Pennington, 1991).

Therapy: Methods and Forms

The goals of psychological therapy are the maintenance of self-esteem, the development of coping and social skills, and the reduction of anxiety and anger.

Is a psychological evaluation needed for every child with SLD?

The developmental pediatrician or pediatric neurologist who follows children with SLD should be aware of the frequent presence of psychological problems in this group of children. Information regarding the child's self-esteem, social success, life interests, and happiness, as well as information regarding abnormal and delinquent behaviors, should be obtained as part of the clinical history in each case. Behavioral forms (such as the Achenbach Child Behavior Checklist and Teacher Response forms) can be used and completed by parents as well as teachers. A child psychiatry/psychology consultation and intervention should follow when behavioral problems are detected.

Guidelines for therapy include the following. (a) Therapy should be goal directed. The therapist as well as the parents should be clear as to the goals of therapy, and should be able to monitor its success. (b) The therapist should be thoroughly acquainted with the child's cognitive profile, strengths, and weaknesses. For instance, therapy with a child who has a language-based SLD may have to rely on plain and clear conversation and possibly on other, nonverbal modalities. Children with "NVLD" frequently have social communications difficulties as part of their biological deficits. The therapist has to be aware of these deficits. (c) The therapist needs to know when behavioral comorbidities, including ADHD or anxiety, are present. The therapist should also monitor the child for the possible emergence of depression, and together with the physician for the effects and side effects of medications, when given. It is important to note that any psychological approach will not work when intervention for cognitive and learning problems is not available.

The psychologist/therapist should also work with the parents. Much parent understanding is needed regarding the child's abilities and disabilities, and their feelings about the learning disability and their responsibilities (genetic or otherwise). The question, "Where did we go wrong?" needs to be addressed. Family-centered therapy is needed sometimes, and should focus on relieving guilt, diffusing blame, and delivering basic information about the nature of the disability (Shapiro & Gallico, 1993). Parents frequently need adjustment of expectations, patience with immature and difficult behaviors, including the child's defiance and anger, and with the need to work again and again on chores that are considered routine (Silver, 1995). Behavior management programs are a useful technique to facilitate the recognition of desired behaviors and establishment of a positive parent–child relationship.

The task of the psychologist is also to work with the school to get the appropriate classroom placement, help the teacher deal with behavioral problems, and serve as a coordinator of the different interventions (Hagin & Silver, 1990).

Form of Therapy

Therapy may be individual, group, or family therapy. Behavior management techniques and social skills training are also used. Therapy sessions should be highly structured and concrete, because many children are anxious or have attentional deficits (Silver, 1995). Anxiety should be minimized. If a child has language or auditory perceptual problems (which frequently underlies cognitive deficits in children with SLD), therapy should be much less verbal and more in the written and play modes, using tools in the visual mode, including drawing or writing on a blackboard as a preferred mode of communication. Verbal communications should be direct, in short sentences. If a child has a visual perceptual or motor difficulty, therapy can be more verbal.

Anxiety is a frequent behavioral problem in children with SLD. Relaxation techniques can be helpful and may reduce the need for symptomatic psychopharmacological therapy. Similarly, aggression is related to SLDs in some students, and can be treated by providing functional communication training and individual behavioral modification. Providing the appropriate academic help by the school is essential.

Another type of therapy that can be very helpful to some children with SLD is organizational therapy. Learning how to learn and strategize is affected in learning disabilities, and abnormalities of executive functions are common in those students who have comorbid ADHD. Organizational therapy techniques can help develop these skills.

School Role in Psychological Intervention

It was noted that one of the main goals of behavioral interventions is reducing aggression and behavioral problems, which can be present in students with SLD. School work is an imposition for these students, who lack the positive learning experiences of unaffected students and have no success. Finding ways to increase motivation to attend school, find personal identity-building learning projects, reduce the dichotomy between schoolwork and personal projects, articulate how they view the purpose of schooling, and critique what they do not like about it, might change their views of school. Efforts to build self-esteem may include special jobs within the classroom, sports, scouts, music, drama, arts and crafts, and other nonacademic activities in which students with SLD may excel and not differ from their peers (O'Donnell et al., 1995).

School-based prevention programs, which modified classroom teacher practices, offered parent training, and provided child social skills training, were found to be helpful in preventing school failure, drug abuse, and delinquency among low-income urban children (Allen et al., 1994). Schools that promoted student autonomy and relatedness with school personnel and peers and gave them real choices achieved significantly greater levels of success in reducing problem behaviors.

Other Therapies Suggested for SLD

Introduction

Specific learning disabilities are chronic conditions, with continued difficulties encountered by students and their families throughout the student's academic life. Even though students learn and build up knowledge, it frequently seems to parents that they are treading uphill. Parents are, therefore, vulnerable to those who report having a quick remedy and possibly a cure to the problem.

In the past, some suggested "cures" involved nutritional modifications or the treatment of allergies. There are many connections between nutrition and brain function. Severe malnutrition can cause learning abnormalities, as can congenital thyroid deficiency and certain metabolic abnormalities, known as inborn errors of metabolism such as phenylketonuria. Some of these conditions are screened at birth, and children with SLD should be tested for other ones when suspected. For the overwhelming majority of children with SLD who are otherwise healthy and do not have a nutritional deficiency or metabolic disease, changing their diet will not cure their learning disabilities. At the present time, there are no known treatments based on dietary manipulations that have been shown to be clinically successful. Similarly, we do not know of allergies that cause SLD as an exclusive manifestation.

It is important that professionals be informed of controversial therapies so they can educate parents on what is known about these treatments. I usually tell parents that SLD, as well as ADHD, are very common conditions. There are established ways to study the efficacy of new therapies. For any proposed therapy we need to find evidence of efficacy and check for potential harmful side effects. Books, the Internet, magazine articles published by the person proposing the treatment, television interviews, and letters on the Web do not constitute proof of efficacy (Silver, 1995).

"Peripheral" Ocular Abnormalities and Specific Learning Disabilities

It has been suggested that "peripheral" ocular abnormalities, including abnormalities of eye movements or convergence, can cause SLD, particularly reading disabilities. A statement by the American Academy of Optometry and the American Optometric Association suggests that optometric interventions have a role in improving visual function in children with learning disabilities, as part of a multidisciplinary management approach (American Optometric Association, 1997). The definition of SLD states that this diagnosis is made in children who do not have a significant sensory problem (e.g., blindness or deafness) that prevents them from learning normally. Therefore, it is recognized that any visual problem that significantly interfere with visual acuity can cause a disturbance of academic learning. Most learning disabled students discussed in this book do not have such a disturbance. There has not been sufficient evidence that any other optometric problem can cause SLD. A Swedish study found that dyslexic students did not differ significantly from control children in terms of strabismus, accommodation, stereo acuity, vergence function, or ocular dominance (Ygge et al., 1993). Therefore, most learning disabled children will not benefit from optometric therapy (Evans, Drasdo, & Richards, 1996).

- The left angular gyrus and left prefrontal regions are mainly implicated in exact, verbal, memory-based, language-dependent calculation, and in retrieval of learned arithmetic facts, such as multiplication tables.
- Areas of precentral and inferior prefrontal cortex are also activated when subjects are engaged in mental calculation. The dorsolateral prefrontal cortex has a more supporting role, including sequential ordering of operations, control over their execution, and inhibiting verbal response. Neurons in the lateral prefrontal cortex of the monkey are selectively responsive to numerical rank and quantity but typically later than IPS neurons.
- The posterior superior parietal lobe is activated in tasks requiring number manipulation but is not specific to number domain.
- Neurons in the posterior parietal and prefrontal cortices are linked to form a functional network for the representation of numerical information.
- The left angular gyrus and left prefrontal regions are mainly implicated in exact, verbal, memory-based, language-dependent calculation, and in retrieval of learned arithmetic facts, such as multiplication tables.
- Areas of precentral and inferior prefrontal cortex are also activated when subjects are engaged in mental calculation. The dorsolateral prefrontal cortex has a more supporting role, including sequential ordering of operations, control over their execution, and inhibiting verbal response. Neurons in the lateral prefrontal cortex of the monkey are selectively responsive to numerical rank and quantity but typically later than IPS neurons.
- The posterior superior parietal lobe is activated in tasks requiring number manipulation but is not specific to number domain.
- Neurons in the posterior parietal and prefrontal cortices are linked to form a functional network for the representation of numerical information.

A theory for dyslexia suggests an abnormality in the magnocellular visual pathway, the visual pathway in the brain that specializes in the conduction of faster, lower contrast visual stimuli. Dyslexic children were reported to have lower contrast sensitivity at least with some spatial frequencies (Ygge et al., 1993), and differed from normal children in the effect that different color filters had on letter naming accuracy and visual-spatial location (Solman, Dain, Lim, & May, 1995). A condition called scotopic sensitivity syndrome (SSS) that is associated with reading problems was proposed with a suggestion for treatment by the use of colored filters. There is disagreement about the existence of SSS and the efficacy of colored filter therapy, because of lack of scientific evidence, although it has found some support within the medical community (Coyle, 1995). A study of reading disabled children and controls found no significant relationships between academic classification and degree of SSS (Lopez et al., 1994). Another study to determine if tinted lenses cause a measurable improvement in the reading performance of dyslexic children showed neither improvement nor deterioration attributable to lens color or density. In addition, the lens condition that was subjectively preferred by each child did not correlate with actual reading performance. In summary, it is not yet established that magnocellular visual pathway abnormality causes dyslexia, and no evidence that colored filters are helpful.

Other Suggested Treatments

The effects of hemispheric stimulation on the reading performance of individuals with dyslexia performed by presenting words to the left or right visual field were investigated with some evidence of benefit, although there has not been a large study to support such treatment.

Sensory integration (SI) therapy is a controversial, though popular, treatment for the remediation of developmental problems. It has been applied to children with SLD under the assumption that sensory integration abnormalities cause their learning difficulties. There is no valid theory underlying the concept of sensory integration, and no proof that it is a separate entity of disability. There is also no proof of the validity or utility of SI therapy for learning disabled people (Hoehn & Baumeister, 1994).

Pharmacological Therapy

Introduction

Learning is a complex task that involves a number of cognitive processes. Research on the effects of drugs on learning will undoubtedly be enhanced as the different cognitive processes involved with learning become better delineated. Experimentally there are pharmacological agents that influence various cognitive processes. In animal studies, L-dopa has been shown to facilitate episodic memory, but not automatic or semantic memory. Methamphetamine significantly enhanced performance on a visual search task, but not on a time production task. Diphenhydramine accelerated time production but had no effect on visual search.

At the present time there is no pharmacological therapy that ameliorates SLD through a direct effect on the learning process. Therefore, unless a concurrent disorder is present, the use of medication for the treatment of SLD should be considered experimental (Beitchman & Young, 1997). Classroom and test performance are affected, though, by processes other than learning and memory, including attention, motor performance, motor speed, or mood. Drugs that increase alertness, attention, and motivation can be expected to enhance cognitive performance, and such effects may influence learning and subsequent retention.

Medications may also improve academic performance through an effect on behavior or comorbid conditions. The decision of giving a medication depends therefore on identifying comorbid conditions and specific symptoms amenable to drug treatment, and determining how much those interfere with the child's functioning. Such symptoms include mostly disruptive behavior, abnormal movements and attention deficits, spasticity, seizures, anxiety, depression, or self-injurious behavior. Types of medications used in learning disabled children for these purposes include stimulants (i.e., methylphenidate and d-amphetamine) for attentional deficits, hyperactivity, and impulsivity, clonidine or other available medications for tics in Tourette syndrome, and serotonin reuptake blockers for anxiety, obsessive compulsive symptoms, and depression. Many of these medications act by enhancing or inhibiting the effects of various neurotransmitters. For example, stimulants facilitate the action of dopamine and norepinephrine, whereas certain antipsychotics antagonize catecholamines. Drugs that alleviate anxiety, such as benzodiazepines, augment the action of gamma-aminobutyric acid (GABA), an important inhibitory transmitter. Antidepressants such as Prozac enhance the action of serotonin and indoleamine with a wide variety of functions.

Drugs with Possible Effects on the Process of Learning and Memory: Theoretical Considerations

Drugs with possible effects on learning and memory include cholinergic agents, the nootropic medications, stimulants, catecholamines, adrenocorticotropic hormone, opioids, and pituitary-adrenal hormones. There has also been a body of research on the possible effect of the peptide vasopressin on memory (DeWied & Versteeg, 1979).

Cholinergic Agents

Pharmacological attempts to improve memory and learning functions in patients with primary degenerative dementia (mostly Alzheimer disease) frequently involve enhancing cholinergic functions, because the cholinergic system of basal diencephalic origin may be impaired in these disorders. Such attempts have included (a) increasing acetylcholine production by increasing the availability of acetylcholine precursors (i.e., lecithin, choline); (b) inhibiting acetylcholine degradation by inhibiting acetylcholine esterase (mostly physostigmine); and (c) directly stimulating cholinergic receptors by using cholinomimetic agents (i.e., arecoline). Certain cholinesterase inhibitors such as physostigmine have been noted to improve memory in older people and patients with Alzheimer disease. Limitations to the use of these compounds include a short half-life, poor penetration of the blood–brain barrier, and high incidence of side effects (Fuster, 1995). Other compounds have been suggested to restore the ability to learn and remember. Patients treated with phosphatidylserine for age-associated memory impairment improved performance on tasks of daily life relative to those treated with placebo (Crook et al., 1991). There is no knowledge of an abnormality of the cholinergic system in the brains of children with SLDs. Consequently, there is no body of research on the effect of cholinergic agents on learning ability in these children.

Catecholamines

Catecholamines effect different types of learning in animals. Reserpine, which depletes both catecholamines and indolamines, led to impaired performance of rats on both active and passive avoidance learning tasks. When added to reserpine, dihydroxyphenylalanine (DOPA), which raises catecholamine levels, normalized retention of active avoidance learning, but that of passive avoidance remained impaired. Conversely, 5-hydroxytryptamine (5-HTP), which raises indoleamine levels, restored passive but not active avoidance learning to normal.

There is evidence that memory storage may be activated by the adrenergic system through an effect on the amygdaloid complex. Memory is impaired by treatments that reduce norepinephrine release or block norepinephrine receptors in the amygdala. These noradrenergic influences on memory are thought to be mediated by activation of cholinergic neurons within the amygdala. Activation of the amygdala enhanced a caudate-dependent learning task as well as a hippocampal-dependent task, suggesting that the amygdala influences neural activity (McGaugh & Cahill, 1997).

Vasopressin Another compound with a possible effect on enhancing memory is the hypothalamic hormone vasopressin. Vasopressin has an effect on memory, delaying extinction of an active avoidance response in intact rats and restoring the ability of hypophysectomized rats to acquire such a response. A tendency toward improvement of memory functions was found in a group of chronic schizophrenics given vasopressin.

Nootropic Agents Piracetam and oxiracetam are nootropic compounds structurally related to the neurotransmitter GABA. These compounds, which were originally introduced for aging-related memory disturbance in Europe, have been reported to have a positive impact on verbal learning, and possibly enhance long-term potentiation. The pharmacological mechanism of action of piracetam-like nootropics is still unclear. Research work suggests that the memory-enhancing action of these pharmacological agents depends on the presence of the adrenals and the integrity of steroid metabolism, suggesting that their central effects might be mediated by peripheral mechanisms. Although some studies found oxiracetam to be effective in improving simple reaction time and cognitive function in a group of patients with primary degenerative dementia (Rozzine, Zanetti, & Bianchetti, 1993) and improving the amplitude and latency of P300, a brain potential related to the cerebral pathways of attention and memory, other studies did not find this effect.

Dyslexic boys treated with 3.3 grams daily of piracetam or placebo under double-blind conditions showed a positive effect of the drug on verbal conceptualization (similarities) but not on the ability to give verbal definitions (vocabulary). A multisite, 12-week, double-blind, placebo-controlled study of piracetam in dyslexic boys showed improved reading speed but no significant effects for either reading accuracy or reading comprehension measures. A longer (36-week) multisite evaluation reported small improvements in oral passage reading but no improvement on the reading speed measure. Most other measures of information processing, language, and memory were not significantly improved with piracetam treatment. Another more recent study using piracetam in dyslexic subjects did not find an improvement in any aspect of reading (Tallal et al., 1986).

In summary, although the discussed substances may have effects on learning and memory processes, none was proven to have an effect in dyslexia or other SLD.

Medications for Treatment of Behavioral Comorbidities of Specific Learning Disabilities

Children with SLD may receive medications for the treatment of comorbid conditions, including ADHD, anxiety, and depression.

Stimulants

Attention deficit hyperactivity disorder is frequently treated with stimulant medications. Amphetamines have direct effects on the tonic midbrain activating system, similar to that of epinephrine. Methylphenidate has a similar effect to amphetamine but may act more as a diencephalic or thalamic phasic stimulant. It causes cortical activation in cats that is not abolished by lesions of the reticular formation at the level of the red nucleus but is abolished by lesions of the diffuse thalamic projection. Studies have found that the photo metrazol threshold, which is lower in children with hyperkinetic syndrome, rose to normal levels after administration of amphetamines, leading to a theory that amphetamines raise the level of synaptic resistance in the diencephalon (Laufer, Denhoff, & Solomons, 1957).

Clinically, stimulant medications improve classroom behavior and attention in children with ADHD. In the child with coexisting ADHD and LD, stimulant pharmacotherapy can reduce impulsivity and improve attention, organization, goal-directed behavior, and motivation, and thus improve classroom performance. Children are better able to function in their environment, thus improving classroom learning.

Stimulant medications include methylphenidate (Ritalin), dextroamphetamine (Dexedrine), and Adderall. These are short acting and are effective for 4 to 6 hours; therefore, more than one daily dose is usually needed. Longer-acting (sustained release) forms of methylphenidate and Dexedrine are available. Similarly, atomoxetine may have an effect on academic performance either by treating coexisting attentional disorder or, perhaps, having a direct effect on enhancing learning and memory. Stimulants may have side effects, including reduced appetite and growth, and tics, and can enhance symptoms of anxiety and depression in some children.

Recent findings indicate that between 1990 and 1995 there was a significant increase in the prevalence of methylphenidate treatment of children and adolescents, with approximately 2.8% (or 1.5 million) of US youths age 5 to 18 receiving this medication by the mid-1995. This trend has continued in the last years and may be related to a number of factors, including an increased duration of treatment, increased number of girls treated, and pharmacological treatment of inattentive children and adolescents with ADHD-inattentive type (Safer, Zito, & Fine, 1996). These findings sharpen the question of whether stimulant medication actually enhances cognitive performance and whether it is given to children with SLD and adolescents in the hope of improving academic achievements, even without a clear comorbidity of ADHD.

The effects of stimulant drug treatment of children were noted by Bradley and his coworkers in a series of early studies carried out on institutionalized emotionally disturbed children (Bradley, 1950). These behaviorally disturbed children became calmer, more organized, less aggressive, and less disruptive, and their schoolwork improved (Rappoport & Inoff-Germain, 2002). It was believed that these effects were secondary to an improvement of the "emotional attitude" or mood, and improved motivation. More recent studies have revealed similar results. Some effects of Ritalin and Dexedrine were found on Porteus Maze Performance, a test that showed a significant decline in scores after prefrontal lobotomy, suggesting that stimulants may have an effect on planning ability. Similarly, dopaminergic therapy produced improvement on a task dependent on working memory and cognitive sequencing in patients with Parkinson disease. There is no clear evidence that stimulants have a direct effect on the process of learning or long-term academic achievements in children with SLD. Earlier studies suggested benefits when children with "pure" reading disorders were treated with methylphenidate. Significant improvement relative to a placebo control subjects was found on some cognitive measures, although this improvement was not necessarily correlated with improvement in academic performance. Cognitive studies suggest that visual processing mechanisms are the most sensitive to stimulants in learning disabled children. Methylphenidate seems to have a specific effect on visuomotor processes, which in turn positively affect performance but not verbal tasks (Gittelman-Klein & Klein, 1976). Complex intellectual performance may not be affected by amphetamines. A possible direct effect of stimulants on learning could have been masked by the dose given for behavioral control, which may be higher than the optimal dose for a learning effect. It has been shown that with increased doses of methylphenidate, behavior and attention span may improve, but the learning effect has a ceiling (Frank, 2000). A larger dose may not help and may actually interfere with learning ability. In effect, a decrement in learning was shown in children given larger doses (1.0 mg/kg) of methylphenidate (Sprague & Sleator, 1977).

Beta Blockers

The alpha-adrenergic blocker clonidine is used for symptoms of ADHD, usually when there are disturbing side effects from stimulants. It can be used as the first medication when tics or Tourette symptoms are present. It may be more effective in reducing hyperactivity and hyperarousal, whereas stimulants have a more direct effect on distractibility and attention deficit. It may take a long time to effect, may have to be given three to four times per day, and may have disturbing side effects, including sedation, hypotension, bradycardia, cardiac arrhythmia, and dermatitis (when a patch is used). A starting dose may be 0.05 mg at bedtime, but the dose may need to be gradually increased and given four times per day, although a long-acting formula (Intuniv) can be given once a day.

Other Medications

Antidepressants (including selective serotonin reuptake inhibitors, imipramine, and desipramine) can improve overall learning and classroom behavior in children with the comorbidity of SLD and depressive symptoms through an effect on the depression symptomatology. These antidepressant medications usually work by blocking the reuptake of serotonin or norepinephrine or both. Specific serotonin reuptake inhibitors can be quite effective in reducing anxiety and obsessive compulsive symptomatology, and elevating mood.

Other medications given for behavioral modulation, including risperidone, and haloperidol, may have a positive effect on behavioral symptomatology, but a deleterious effect on learning. It is not clear whether anticonvulsants such as carbamazepine or valproic acid have an independent effect on learning disorders in children with epilepsy. Anticonvulsants may improve auditory comprehension in cases of verbal auditory agnosia, a specific disorder with loss of the ability to understand speech. Affected individuals have abnormal electroencephalograms, revealing spike and wave activity.

Patients on any type of medication should be followed regularly by the physician who prescribed the medication, and have telephone contact with their physician between visits to adjust dosages and report possible side effects. Medical monitoring at regular intervals includes blood pressure and pulse measurements, and can include blood tests, electrocardiogram, and cardiac function monitoring, depending on the type of medication.

Other Compounds

There has not been any proof that megavitamin therapy, special diets, or treatment for vestibular dysfunction have any effect on SLD. Similarly, there is no evidence that learning disabilities are caused by allergies or asthma. When treating for these conditions, the physician should try to minimize drowsiness, which may interfere with learning.

The Future of Biological and Pharmacological Therapy for Specific Learning Disabilities

The future of specific psychopharmacological treatment for SLDs may be tied to the identification of genes for specific types of learning disabilities. Animal studies investigate the possible effects of growth factors and tissue implants. Therapy may take the form of specific growth factors or neuronal grafting.

Researchers tested the potential effect of insulin-like growth factor I (IGF-I) on functional recovery in an animal model of cerebellar ataxia. When treated with IGF-I, inferior olive neurons, the targets of a neurotoxin, were rescued to various degrees depending on the time that treatment with IGF-I was initiated (Fernandez, De La Vega, & Torres-Aleman, 1998). There have been animal as well as human studies examining the potential effects of grafting of

DA-producing neurons into the striatum, in Parkinson disease, with promising results. In addition to the enormous difficulties of studies involving cell implantation or growth factors in children, one needs to remember that the nature of brain abnormalities in SLD is different. It is not a degenerative disease and we do not have to restore lost brain tissue, but probably treat an aberrant developmental pattern. This may limit the future usefulness of such treatments for children with SLDs.

SUMMARY

Specific learning disabilities result from abnormal cognitive processing. A most important therapeutic goal for SLD is to treat the learning "academic" deficit. At the present time there is no definitive physiological cure for the learning problem in SLDs. Remedial learning venues include retraining brain systems, helping to store and use information, or developing "bypass" learning techniques. Training the peripheral organs like "eye training" does not cure learning disabilities.

Another important goal is that students with SLDs emerge from school emotionally intact, with positive self-esteem and minimal behavioral and emotional comorbidities, and understanding ways to cope with their difficulties. Therapies aimed toward these goals include emotional support and treatment of comorbid behavioral and emotional conditions.

We need to look upon a specific learning disability as a chronic disorder—a type of static encephalopathy, which can be successfully treated but not completely eliminated. As in the case of many similar developmental disabilities, there may not be fast "cure" at the present time, but there is usually steady progress and improvement. With timely remediation, the prognosis is certainly good. Children with SLD improve, learn, and can live a normal life.

OUTCOME

Introduction

Specific learning disabilities are a lifelong condition. This means that a degree of abnormalities related to SLD may remain. Children and adolescents with a reading disability, given the appropriate intervention, will improve and advance, but may continue to have some deficits. For instance, reading may stay slow, and errors and spelling abnormalities may persist into adulthood.

The goals of therapy for children and adolescents with these conditions is that they can learn and acquire knowledge, keep up with their peers academically, compete in the employment market, and achieve social and economic success.

Children with Specific Learning Disabilities
Lag Academically

Almost all children (95% or more) achieve significant literary skills by the spring of third grade. They can identify common sight words, words in context in reading, and recognize word sequence. In mathematics, they can add and subtract. By the end of third grade many of these students have also acquired more complex skills, such as making interpretations beyond text. In math, they are able to multiply and divide, and solve mathematical word problems (US Government Printing Office, 2005). The percentage of these children who had mastered more complex literary skills by the spring of third grade vary according to the number of family risk factors identified in kindergarten, and include living in poverty, non-English primary home language, mother's education less than high school/GED, and single parent household. Dyslexic peers of these children, are already at a significant literary handicap by the third grade. These risk factors that determine the academic success in non disabled children translate into more handicaps in children with SLD.

Functional Outcome of Specific Learning Disabilities

To what degree do appropriate diagnosis and treatment ameliorate the learning disability handicap? Shaywitz et al. (1999) reported that more than 70% of poor readers in third grade read poorly in 12th grade in spite of the fact that many of these children received special education services. This means that some parts of the literary handicap remains by the end of high school, although other parts may gradually improve. Studies of older, dyslexic college students found that they had superior passage comprehension and rapid naming performance compared with younger dyslexic children, and demonstrated significant progress over time. It is possible that passage comprehension and rapid naming differences disappear with age as dyslexic children learn to compensate for their reading problems (Leonard et al., 2001; Brambati et al., 2004).

How do these data translate into academic and professional success or failure? The degree and functional importance of SLD depends on many factors previously outlined—the degree of learning disability, the strengths of the subjects' cognitive structure, behavioral comorbidities, self-esteem and other emotional factors, family and school support structures, and the effectiveness of therapy.

Dropping Out of School

One of the possible unwanted outcomes of SLD is dropping out of school. Students who drop out of school have decreased opportunities in the competitive employment market, earn less than their peers, and are more likely to be involved in sociopathic activity. Dropouts make up near half of the prison population. There are certain groups of young people who are more likely than others to leave school before graduating, and some of the determining factors relate to ethnic and social background. Nevertheless, SLD are one of the important causes of school dropout, subjecting people with these disabilities to the disadvantages and risks of this group.

The Early Childhood Longitudinal Study, kindergarten class of 1998–1999 collected information on a cohort of children who began kindergarten in fall 1998, followed them, and assessed their achievements in reading, math, and general knowledge through spring 2004, when most had completed the fifth grade. A number of family risk factors—household below poverty level, non-English primary home language, mother's highest education less than a high school diploma/GED, and single parent household—were found to be negatively associated with children's achievement gains in reading and mathematics.

Although some students who drop out of school may come back to supplement their education, a significant number do not. More than 40% of school dropouts later received a high school diploma or an alternative high school credentials, whereas 37% did not earn a high school diploma or alternative credentials. These findings demonstrate that many students who drop out of high school at least once go on to earn a high school diploma or alternative credentials within few years or enroll in a postsecondary institution. Almost half of those who did not complete high school belonged to the bottom 25% socioeconomic group.

SUMMARY

As a group—SLD subjects are at a higher risk for academic, occupational, and social failures. The goals of early identification and therapy are to decrease these risks and improve outcome.

The degree of achievement of these goals depends on several issues: early identification, an accurate diagnosis of SLDs, the type and severity of the disability, and the temperament and intelligence of the child, as well as the presence of other factors, including ADHD and comorbid emotional disturbance, coping mechanisms of the child, and response of the school and parents (Silver, 1989). Early recognition and diagnosis and effective treatment can reduce these risks. It should be remembered, though, that effective treatment also includes attention to the psychological effects of SLDs.

Familial and social factors are more difficult to tackle, but better understanding of these conditions and their potential effects on the child will assist these factors.

CHAPTER 17

Conclusions

INTRODUCTION

Although Specific Learning Disability (SLD) are defined in terms of academic failure, children with SLD differ from unaffected children on a variety of dimensions. In addition to academic difficulties, they may have problems with motor coordination, attentional deficits, and behavioral difficulties. These additional problems are not the reason for the learning difficulties (e.g., dyslexia), but may be related to the underlying brain differences.

SLD have been recognized in different forms and described for more than a century. The etiologies for these brain differences, including genetic, neurological, social, and educational are better recognized. Advanced neuroimaging techniques demonstrate brain abnormalities that may explain the nature of SLD and may allow us to arrive at more specific diagnoses. Although genetics factors seem to be important etiological factors, the pathophysiology by which genetic abnormality brings about a specific learning disability Is not yet known.

PATHOPHYSIOLOGY OF SPECIFIC LEARNING DISABILITY

The pathophysiology underlying SLD syndromes occurs very early in a child's life, much before the start of academic learning, and is most likely congenital. The factors that cause SLD occur either in utero and/or early in the child's life and affect brain development. There have been many theories attempting to explain the pathogenesis of SLD in general, and specific reading disability (dyslexia) in particular. Some are reviewed in this book: The visual system has a role in reading. Written words are perceived visually and the neural network involved in reading includes processing of graphophonemic features through the occipital-temporal region. The visual theory of dyslexia describes abnormalities in the magnocellular visual system (Eden et al., 1995) but it is not clear how the magnocellular system can be involved in single word recognition. It is more likely that the role of visual processing is only as an initial part of a broader neural network responsible for dyslexia.

The proponents of an auditory deficit theory suggested that the problem with dyslexia is in auditory perception. There is evidence that dyslexics have difficulty processing rapidly changing auditory stimuli and do not discriminate between speech and nonspeech stimuli as well as good readers (Farmer & Klein, 1995). Abnormal processing was correlated with reading ability. This theory places the deficit responsible for reading impairment in "lower order" brain processing, rather than the phonological or higher level language processing. Some of the studies leading to this theory could not be replicated, and other experiments in which discrimination of auditory stimuli was examined did not reveal significant differences between good and poor readers (Mody et al., 1997).

A theory of cerebellar abnormality underlying SLD argues that the cause for the cognitive abnormality in SLD is the inability of to perform automatic tasks including reading and especially rapid naming (Nicholson, Fawcett, & Dean, 2001), and to estimate time, suggesting a cerebellar abnormality (Nicholson, 1995, 1999; Fawcett & Nicholson, 1999; Rae, 1998). Functional neuroimaging studies of dyslexics gave some support to this theory, revealing abnormalities in the right cerebellum. It is hard to explain, though, why most people with cerebellar pathology do not have dyslexia or an other SLD. Also, there has not been good evidence that dyslexic children have "classical" cerebellar deficits including abnormalities of balance, gait and other motor skills (Wimmer et al., 1999).

How does the brain process lexical (reading) information? The visual input of reading can be processed in different ways. One major way is through phonological processing.

The current theory for specific reading disability (dyslexia) is that it is the result of abnormality of phonological processing (difficulty to process language sounds) (Bradely & Bryant, 1983; Stanovich, 1988). Phonological processing includes speech sound awareness and sound–symbol association. Phonological awareness (PA) -is the ability to identify and mentally manipulate the constituent speech sounds, and has been found to predict much of the variance in reading skills.

The current understanding of a core phonological deficit causing dyslexia is consistent with the results of recent anatomical neuroimaging studies. These studies, especially functional brain imaging studies, demonstrate that phonological processing is executed through a network across the brain, and that dyslexic brains have abberent left hemisphere activation during the performance of tasks involving phonological processing including reading, in particular in the brain regions normally associated with the processing of phonological information (Hulme & Snowling, 1997; Fiez & Petersen, 1998).

The exact mechanism by which the brain recovers phonemes and associates them with visually presented orthography is still unknown. The phonological deficits of dyslexia may still be related to a more basic auditory processing deficit or a sensory perception deficit, although there has not been conclusive proof for such abnormality. It is more likely that the brain changes in dyslexia involve faulty network transmission within the phonological brain network centers (Boets et al., 2013).

The current theory on the pathophysiology of dyscalculia suggests that the fundamental abnormality is a deficit in the representation of numerosities— a specific deficit in core numerical abilities (e.g. the number of objects in a set). According to this theory there is no language processing deficits at the core of dyscalculia. There are, though, other cognitive factors that effect mathematical abilities, including attention and working memory. The brain area involved is located in the intraparietal sulcus.

BIOLOGICAL ABNORMALITIES

The evidence for biological brain abnormalities in SLD, especially dyslexia, is strong. Historically there have been interesting findings, in imaging as well as postmortem studies, on the present of neocortical malformations and aberrant left-right brain asymmetries, especially in temporal speech regions, and differences in cell size in thalamic sensory nuclei (the magnocellular divisions of the thalamus). The association of these findings with dyslexia has not been adequately validated.

Functional Anatomy Studies in Dyslexia

The advance in our understanding of the biological changes in SLD has come, in recent years, from functional neuroimaging. Brain areas that are activated during reading include areas in the left temporal lobe and left frontal lobe. The functional anatomical abnormalities of dyslexia include abnormalities in multiple brain regions involved in reading, as well as finding of disconnection of these regions (Eden & Zeffiro, 1998). Diffusion tensor MRI studies found that white matter diffusion anisotropy in the temporal-parietal region of the left hemisphere was significantly correlated with reading scores for reading-impaired and control readers, demonstrating the importance of the connections between the cortical centers involved in reading (Kingberg et al., 2000).

The anomalous brain activity seen in dyslexics is quite consistent across different cultures (Paulesco et al., 2000).

An instructional reading program improves phonological processing, and increases metabolic activation in deficient brain areas (Aylward et al., 2003). This corresponds to evidence from electrophysiological studies of sensory fields in the cortex of primates showing that the underlying neural circuitry is altered after specific, temporally cohesive training regimens leading to "remapping," demonstrating the plasticity of the brain.

In dyscalculia, the intraparietal sulcus IPS is activated in most neuroimaging studies of number processing and may constitute a central amodal representation of quantity (Dehaene et al., 2003). Other brain areas that participate in the brain networks involved with calculation are the left angular gyrus and left prefrontal regions.

Genetics of Reading

The cause of SLD is in many cases genetic, but the genetics of SLD is complex. We have known all along that certain genetic, chromosomal conditions can cause learning abnormalities. Those have usually been more global (e.g., Down syndrome), although more detailed neuropsychological studies show a preponderance of one type of academic learning (e.g., Williams syndrome). The search has been for genetic abnormalities in individuals and families in which the main or only abnormality is SLD (e.g., dyslexia, dyscalculia). There are a number of chromosomal linkages which have been replicated at independent laboratories across the world. Linkage analyses in families with dyslexia have reported nine chromosomal regions in which the presence of susceptibility genes is suspected. These are dyslexia susceptibility 1 (DYX1) to dyslexia susceptibility 9 (DYX9), on chromosomes 1, 2, 3, 6, 15, and 18. Candidate genes include *DCDC2* and *K1AA0319*, both identified within DYX2 on chromosome 6p22, *ROBO1* (roundabout Drosophila homolog 1) and *DYX1C1*. The multigenetic nature of dyslexia is likely to be one explanation for its observed heterogeneity and its coexistence with disorders of attention. Also- specific regions of the genome have been identified as being involved with a number of different reading related processes. (Grigorenko, 2001) and separate genes are probably involved in a number of reading-related processes. For example - orthographic coding and phoneme awareness have unique genetic foundations (Gayan & Olson, 2001).

Although genetic studies have shown that much of one's PA skills can be accounted for by hereditary factors, significant variance also stems from one's environment (Grigorenco, 2001). Reading and attention deficit hyperactivity disorder (ADHD) may have different genetic origin but reading (decoding) problems and ADHD have shared genetic risk factors that influence the development of both disorders.

NEUROPSYCHOLOGY

There is no one typical neuropsychological abnormality for dyslexia, dyscalculia or other SLD, although there are some neuropsychological findings commonly found in SLD. An example is a variability of the scores of the Wechsler Intelligence Scale for Children subtests. A significant discrepancy between verbal and performance IQ scores means that the different measures of intelligence do not correlate, possibly because brain functions are not well integrated. Although this discrepancy is common in SLD students, there is no correlation with the degree of SLD. Another example is reduced verbal scores, which may be a result of language processing deficits that sometimes underlie reading disability. More significantly abnormalities of language processing tests, in particular phonological processing tests or rapid naming tests, are suggestive of dyslexia. Reduced scores on visuospatial tests may underlie mathematical difficulties, and Non Verbal Learning Disabilities, while executive functions abnormalities are compatible with Attention Deficit Hyperactivity Disorder, and with some cases of dyscalculia.

A BIOLOGICAL MODEL OF SPECIFIC LEARNING DISABILITY

We can attempt to draw a biological model of SLD. Some parts of this model have experimental proof, whereas some parts are still hypothesized. The model for SLD has a number of layers. The first, most evident, level is a classification of academic skills deficit (e.g., reading or calculation). The second level will identify the core cognitive deficits that determine the academic skills deficits (e.g., in dyslexia - phonological awareness and rapid letter naming). Adding to these deficits are other metacognitive characteristics that influence academic strengths and weaknesses, including psychosocial and emotional factors (e.g., attention, motivation, social skills, behavioral problems including anxiety and depression), as well as environmental factors (e.g., socioeconomic, schooling, intervention). The third level is the neurological, brain, abnormalities (e.g., functional and/or structural brain abnormalities). The fourth and most basic layer is the congenital/genetic layer. There is an interaction between different factors on the same level and on different levels.

Abnormal genes cause the neurological abnormalities in one or more of the brain circuits. These, in turn, causes the cognitive abnormality that causes the specific learning disability.

How does a genetic abnormality cause changes in brain development and how does a brain abnormality manifest itself as a learning disability? There are partial answers to these questions, some involving multiple variables with multiple possible outcomes. Gene abnormality can causes aberrant brain development (for instance – through interference with neural migration, lack of appropriate axonal arborization, synaptogenesis or myelination or appropriate cortical organization), causing abnormal connectivity. Abnormal connectivity results in abnormal brain circuits, which interferes with learning of complex subjects like reading and mathematics.

We need to know more about the mechanisms of normal learning, the interaction of neurobiological factors and environmental factors, and the mechanisms of action of intervention (Rayner et al., 2001; Vellutino et al., 2004; Plomin & Kovas, 2005).

There is a learning plasticity in the brain, and a brain area or network can anatomically or functionally change with learning, training, and experience. The brain networks involved in different types of learning may use different basic mechanisms and neurotransmitters. The basic networks of learning are also influenced through other synaptic connections by other factors including emotional factors, motivation, and reward. A network of neurons can change its pattern of connectivity. Thus, networks that support cognitive skills, such as pattern recognition and language acquisition, can be modified. Early in the development of networks, basic patterns of connectivity are formed by the interaction of genetic determinants and unsupervised forms of learning. Neurons involved in classical conditioning are found in the brainstem, cerebellum and, cortex (Knuden, 1994). Later during life, plasticity may be determined more by experience and training.

Because the abnormalities that cause SLD have to affect brain development, and occur either in utero or early in the child's life, it is more likely that SLD children have, in addition to the impairment of academic learning, fine motor difficulties as well as frequent behavioral abnormalities. This comorbidity of developmental dyslexia with both internalizing and externalizing behavioral disturbances and with other learning disabilities suggests that developmental dyslexia may be one of the manifestations of a larger underlying syndrome— the result of an early developmental aberration.

There are many questions that need to be answered. Scientists have to answer the question of the mode of transmission of SLD, how it is inherited, and how genes affect learning. Physicians and psychologists have to find better tests for SLD—possibly biological tests—which will enable them to diagnose it earlier and with better precision. Educators have to find better teaching methods and appropriate school environment for SLD children. And society needs to recognize that SLD is a very significant problem and allocate the resources needed to effectively treat it.

Who should be involved in the diagnosis and treatment of SLD?

It is interesting to note that although neurology is the medical profession responsible for diagnosing and treating brain disorders, the diagnosis and treatment of children with SLD has not been, for many years, a traditional role of the neurologist. Rather it has been an important domain of psychologists, special education teachers, and other disciplines, with "peripheral" involvement of pediatricians. This is gradually changing. Dyslexics have brain abnormalities involving brain areas in the left (and to a lesser degree, bilateral) temporal and frontal lobes. They may have characteristic genetic abnormalities. In the future, brain imaging, especially functional imaging, and genetic testing, will be used to diagnose dyslexia. The need to analyze brain functions, with neuro imaging, genetics, neurophysiology, and neuropsychological tools has put the neurologist and neuropsychologist in the forefront of understanding and studying learning disorders.

DIAGNOSIS OF SPECIFIC LEARNING DISABILITY

Diagnosis and early identification are the essential first steps in the process of treatment. A delay in diagnosis until the third grade (which sometimes may be the result of using the discrepancy method for diagnosis), delays remediation and causes secondary emotional problems.

The deficit in the phonological component of language that many dyslexic people have is present early in life. By testing Kindergarten children for deficits in phonological and orthographic weaknesses, we can identify those children who are at risk of having a reading disability, earlier in life, and give them the appropriate instruction (Wagner et al., 1997). Children can put a name to a picture before they learn to read. Checking picture naming skills in preschool children may give us an early measure of a child's semantic and phonological knowledge, and therefore provide information on later reading performance (Jansky & de Hirsch, 1972; Wolf & Goodglass, 1986).

TREATMENT

Reading can be improved by the early initiation of treatment programs that include the teaching of phonetic awareness (orally identifying and manipulating syllables and speech sounds), phonics (making associations between sounds and letters), fluency, and vocabulary. Phonological awareness-based instruction significantly improves reading performance of poor readers in the first grade (National Reading Panel, 2000). It has been demonstrated that remediation can normalize the brain pathways that are deviant in people with dyslexia. Future measures of improvement of dyslexia and dyscalculia may include e functional brain imaging to evaluate the results of remediation.

Most intensive instructional approaches for students with dyslexia include the same strategies as recommended for the general classroom (National Reading Panel, 2000), but differ in treatment intensity, the mode of delivery (taking into consideration that the students may have language processing difficulties), and using multisensory enhancing techniques (Swanson, 1999, 2003; Torgesen et al., 2001). Starting treatment for a reading disability earlier or in first grade improves outcome, and prevents secondary emotional abnormalities. Improving reading speed and reading comprehension are more difficult to achieve.

Dyslexics may have abnormal rapid temporal processing. They may require longer time intervals between successive auditory stimuli in order to discriminate between them or sequence them (Tallal, 1996). This may interfere with the ability to segment speech into phonemes. Although there has been no clear proof that there is a link between sensory processing in the form of poor temporal processing and poor reading, computer-based programs were devised to improve the analysis of rapid successive acoustic stimuli and also extend acoustic speech stimuli (i.e., Fast ForWord). Single unit recording studies in nonhuman primates after such training and functional brain imaging in children show physiological improvement (Temple, 2000).

LIMITATIONS OF BIOLOGICAL FINDINGS

Although the biological studies have been very effective in revealing the brain abnormalities seen in SLD, especially in dyslexia; the cognitive differences of SLD children; and the genetic deviations that may lead to reading and other learning abnormalities, there are a number of limitations to these studies.

Some of the studies involve a relatively small number of subjects, and some are adults or college students, of different populations, with different cognitive deficits, and may not represent the majority of SLD children and adolescents. Many of the studies of the neurological bases of dyslexia and other types of SLD reflect statistical tendencies and do not represent systematic rule, so cannot yet be used for diagnosis.

FUTURE DIRECTIONS

Future work needs to continue to identify the brain structures and connections in dyslexia and dyscalculia. For instance, do areas including area V5/MT and the fusiform gyrus, which have a role in dyslexia (Eden et al., 1996; Demb et al., 1997, 1998; Brunswick et al., 1999; Shaywitz et al., 2002), constitute a separate structural network that accounts for the orthographic deficits in dyslexia

Future research needs also to continue to consider the various hypotheses, which may be complementary rather than mutually exclusive.

There is also a need to understand how genes affect learning, to continue identifying the different genes responsible for different aspects of reading and calculating, and identify genetic markers for risk of dyslexia. Better under-standing of the genetics of dyslexia may help diagnose and treat susceptible children more effectively, in ways that account for their individual disabilities (Francks & MacPhie, 2002). In addition, attempts need to be made to explore the complex genotype/phenotype relations.

There is a need to find better tests for SLD—possibly biological tests—that will enable us to diagnose SLD earlier and with better precision.

There is only little research on the cognitive and neural effects of therapy and compensatory mechanisms occurring spontaneously. Further, functional brain imaging studies are needed to better understand the neural mechanisms of normal reading development (Schlaggar et al., 2002) and reading remedia-tion (Simos et al., 2002), and evaluate the efficiency of instructional programs.

Educators have to find better teaching methods for SLD. Better therapeutic technology can be developed based on information acquired from neurosci-ence and from long-term educational and clinical studies.

Most biological research in dyslexia has involved single word reading. There is need for more research on sentence and text processing.

There is also a need for larger behavioral and neuroimaging studies in dys-lexia in different linguistic communities.

It is extremely important to develop an appropriate school environment for SLD children, to minimize social and psychological effects of these condi-tions and prevent the development of low self-esteem and long-term psycho-logical damage (Goodley & Rapley, 2001).

BIBLIOGRAPHY

A

Aaron PG. The impending demise of the discrepancy formula. *Rev Educ Res.* 1997; 67: 461–502.

Ackerman PT, Dykman RA. Phonological processes, confrontational naming and immediate memory in dyslexia. *J Learn Disabil.* 1993; 26: 597–609.

Ackerman PT, Dykman RA, Oglesby DM, Newton JE. EEG power spectra in children with dyslexia, slow learners and normally reading children and ADD during verbal processing. *J Learn Disabil.* 1994; 27: 619–630.

Ackermann H, Riecker A, Mathiak K, et al. Rate-dependent activation of a prefrontal-insular-cerebellar network during passive listening to trains of click stimuli: an fMRI study. *Neuroreport.* 2006; 12: 4087–4092.

Adair JC, Schwartz RL, Williamson DJ, Raymer AM, Heilman KM. Articulatory processes and phonologic dyslexia. *Neuropsychiatry Neuropsychol Behav Neurol.* 1999; 12: 121–127.

Adams JW, Hitch GJ. Working memory and children's mental addition. *J Exp Child Psychol.* 1997; 67: 21–38.

Adlard A, Hazan V. Speech perception in children with specific reading difficulties (dyslexia). *Q J Exp Psychol.* 1998; 51A: 153–177.

Ahissar M, Protopapas A, Reid M, Merzenich MM. Auditory processing parallels reading abilities in adults. *Proc Natl Acad Sci USA.* 2000; 97: 6832–6837.

Akshoomoff NA, Courchesne E, Press GA, Iragui V. Contribution of the cerebellum to neuropsychological functioning: evidence from a case of cerebellar degenerative disorder. *Neuropsychologia.* 1992; 30: 315–328.

Alarcon M, DeFries JC. Reading performance and general cognitive ability in twins with reading difficulty and control pairs. Personality and individual differences. *J Person Soc Psychol.* 1997; 22: 793–803.

Allen JP, Kuperminc G, Philliber S, Herr K, et al. Programatic prevention of adolescent problem behaviors: the role of autonomy, relatedness, and volunteer service in the teen outreach program. *Am J Commun Psychol.* 1994; 22: 617–638.

Allen LS, Richey MF, Chai YM, Gorsky RA. Sex differences in the corpus callosum of the living human being. *J Neuro Sci.* 1991; 11: 933–942.

Alster EH. The effects of extended time on algebra test scores for college students with and without learning disabilities. *J Learn Disabil.* 1997; 30: 222–227.

American Psychiatric Association. *Diagnostic and Statistical Manual of Mental Disorders.* 3rd ed. Washington, DC: American Psychiatric Association; 1987.

American Psychiatric Association. *Diagnostic and Statistical Manual of Mental Disorders.* 4th ed. Washington, DC: American Psychiatric Association; 1994.

Anderson A, Gore J. The physical basis of neuroimaging techniques. In: Lewis M, Peterson B, eds. *Child and Adolescent Psychiatric Clinics of North America.* Philadelphia, PA: Saunders; 1997:213–264.

Anderson JR, Betts S, Ferris JL, Fincham JM. Cognitive and metacognitive activity in mathematical problem solving: prefrontal and parietal patterns. *Cog Affect Behav Neurosci.* 2011; 11(1): 52–67.

Ansari D. Effect of development and enculturation on number representation in the brain. *Nat Rev Neurosci.* 2008; 9: 278–291.

Ansari D, Garcia N, Lucas E, et al. Neural correlates of symbolic number processing in children and adults. *Neuroreport.* 2005; 16: 1769–1773.

Ansari D, Karmiloff-Smith A. Atypical trajectories of number development: a neuro-constructive perspective. *Trends Cog Sci.* 2002; 6(12): 511–516.

Ardila A, Rosselli M. Acalculia and dyscalculia. *Neuropsychol Rev.* 2002; 12: 179–231.

Ashburner J, Friston KJ. Voxel-based morphometry—the methods. *Neuroimage.* 2000; 11: 805–821.

Ashkenazy S, Rubinsten O, Henik A. Attention, automaticity and developmental dyscalculia. *Neuropsychology.* 2009; 23: 535–540.

Aylward E, Richards T, Berninger V, Nagy W, Field K, Grimme A, et al. Instructional treatment associated with changes in brain activation in children with dyslexia. *Neurology.* 2003; 61: 212–219.

B

Badian NA. Dyscalculia and nonverbal disorders of learning. In: Mykelbust HR, ed. *Progress in Learning Disabilities.* New York: Grune and Stratton, 1983:235–264.

Badian NA, MaAnulty GB, Duffy FH, et al. Prediction of dyslexia in kindergarten boys. *Ann Dyslexia.* 1990; 40: 152–169.

Baharloo S, Johnston PA, Service SK, et al. Absolute pitch: an approach for identification of genetic and nongenetic components. *Am J Hum Genet.* 1998; 62: 224–231.

Bakwin H. Reading disability in twins. *Dev Med Child Neurol.* 1973; 15: 184–187.

Baldweg T, Richardson A, Watkins S, et al. Impaired auditory frequency discrimination in dyslexia, detected with mismatch evoked potentials. *Ann Neurol.* 1999; 45: 495–503.

Barnea A, Lamm O, Epstein R, et al. Brain potentials from dyslexic children recorded during short term memory tasks. *Int J Neurosci.* 1994; 74: 227–237.

Bashir AS, Scavuzzo A. Children with language disorders: natural history and academic success. *J Learn Disabil.* 1992; 25: 53–65.

Bateman B. The physician and the world of special education. *J Child Neurol.* 1995; (suppl 1): S114–120.

Baum DD, Duffelmeyer F, Geelan M. Resource teacher perceptions of the prevalence of social dysfunction among students with learning disabilities. *J Learn Disabil.* 1988; 21: 380–381.

Beauliew C, Plewes C, Paulson LA, et al. Imaging brain connectivity in children with severe reading disability. *Neuroimage.* 2005; 25: 1266–1271.

Beauregard M, Chertkow H, Bub D, et al. The neural substrate for concrete, abstract, and emotional word lexica: a positron emission tomography study. *J Cogn Neurosci.* 1997; 9: 441–461.

Beitchman JH, Young AR. Learning disorders with a special emphasis on reading disorders: a review of the past 10 years. *J Am Acad Child Adolesc Psychiatry.* 1997; 36(8): 1020–1033.

Bell JM, McCallum RS, Cox EA. Towards a research based assessment of dyslexia: using cognitive measures to identify reading disabilities. *J Learn Disabil.* 2003; 36: 505–516.

Benaish AA, Tallal P. Infant discrimination of rapid auditory cues predict later language impairment. *Behav Brain Res.* 2002; 136: 31–49.

Bender BG, Linden MG, Robinson A, et al. Neuropsychological impairment in 42 adolescents with sex chromosome abnormalities. *Am J Med Genet.* 1993; 48: 169–173.

Benton A, Hannay HJ, Varney NR. Visual perception of line direction in patients with unilateral brain disease. *Neurology.* 1975; 25: 907–910.

Berkovitz IH. The adolescent in the school. A therapeutic guide. *Adol Psychiatry.* 1995; 20: 343–363.

Berninger V, Abbot R, Thomson J, Raskin W. Language phenotype for reading and writing disability: a family approach. *Scient Stud Read.* 2001; 15: 59–106.

Best M, Demb JB. Normal planum temporale asymmetry in dyslexics with a magnocellular pathway deficit. *Neuroreport.* 1999; 10: 607–612.

Biederman J, Milberger S, Paraone SV. Impact of adversity on functioning and comorbidity in children with attention deficit hyperactivity disorder. *J Am Child Adolesc Psychiatry.* 1995; 34: 1495–1503.

Binder M, Urbanik AS. Materia ldependent activation in prefrontal cortex: working memory for letters and texture patterns: initial observations. *Radiology.* 2006; 238: 256–263.

Bishop DV. Commentary: cerebellar abnormalities in developmental dyslexia: cause, correlate or consequence? *Cortex.* 2002; 38: 491–498.

Bishop DV, Bishop SJ, Bright P, James C, Delaney T, Tallal P. Different origin of auditory and phonological processing problems in children with language impairment: evidence from a twin study. *J Speech Language Hear Res.* 1999; 42: 155–168.

Bishop DV, Clarkson B. Written language as a window into residual language deficits. A study of children with persistent and residual speech and language impairments. *Cortex.* 2003; 39: 215–237.

Blachman BA, ed. *Foundations of Reading Acquisition and Dyslexia.* Mahwah, NJ: Erlbaum; 1997.

Blachman BA, Ball EW, Black RS, Tangel DM. Kindergarten teachers develop phoneme awareness in low-income, inner-city classrooms. *Read Write: Interdisc J.* 1994; 6: 1–18.

Bliss TV, Collingridge GL. A synaptic model of memory: long term potentiation in the hippocampus. *Nature.* 1993; 361: 31–39.

Bloom SW. Institutional tendencies in medical sociology. *J health Soc Behav.* 1986; 27: 265–276.

Blumsack J, Lewanowski L, Waterman B. Neurodevelopmental precursors to learning disabilities: a preliminary reportfrom a parent survey. *J Learn Disabil.* 1997; 30: 226–237.

Booth JR, Burman DD, Meyer JR, Gitelman DR, Parrish TB, Mesulam M. Relation between brain activation and lexical performance. *Hum Brain Map.* 2003; 19: 155–169.

Booth JR, Burman DD, Meyer JR, et al. Development of brain mechanisms for processing orthographic and phonologic representations. *J Cogn Neurosci.* 2004; 16: 1234–1249.

Bradley C. Benzadrine and Dexedrine in the treatment of children's behavior disorders. *Pediatrics.* 1950; 57: 24–28.

Bradley L, Bryant PE. Difficulties in auditory organization as a possible cause of reading backwardness. *Nature.* 1978; 271: 746–747.

Bradley L, Bryant PE. Categorizing sounds and learning to read: a causal connection. *Nature.* 1983; 301: 419–421.

Brady S, Shankweiler D, Mann V. Speech perception and memory coding in relation to reading ability. *J Exp Child Psychol.* 1983; 35: 345–367.

Brambati SM, Termine CM, Ruffino MG, et al. Regional reductions of gray matter volume in familial dyslexia. *Neurology.* 2004; 63: 742–745.

Branch WB, Cohen MJ, Hynd GW. Academic achievement and attention deficit hyperactivity disorder in children in children with left or right hemisphere dysfunction. *J Learn Disabil.* 1995; 28: 35–43.

Brewer VR, Moore BD, Hiscock M, et al. Learning disability subtypes in children with neurofibromatosis. *J Learn Disabil.* 1997; 30: 521–533.

Brookeshire BL, Butler IJ, Ewing-Cobbs L, Fletcher EM. Neuropsychological characteristics of children with Tourette syndrome: evidence for a Nnonverbal learning disability? *J Clin Exp Neuropsychol.* 1994; 16: 289–302.

Brown WE, Eliez S, Menon V, Rumsey JM, et al. Preliminary evidence of widespread morphological variations of the brain in dyslexia. *Neurology.* 2001; 56: 781–783.

Bruck M. Persistence of dyslexics' phonological awareness deficits. *Dev Psychol.* 1992; 28: 874–886.

Brumback RA, Stanton RD. An hypothesis regarding the commonality of right-hemisphere involvement in learning disability, attentional disorder, and childhood major depressive disorder. *Percept Motor Skills.* 1982; 55: 1091–1097.

Brunswick N, McCrory E, Price CJ, Frith CD, Frith U. Explicit and implicit processing of words and pseudowords by adult developmental dyslexics: a search for Wernicke's Wortschatz? *Brain.* 1999; 122: 1901–1917.

Bull R, Johnston RS. Children's arithmetical difficulties: contribution from processing speed, item identification and short term memory. *J Exp Child Psychol.* 1997; 65: 1–24.

Bryan T, Smiley A. Learning disabled boys' performance and self-assessments on physical fitness tests. *Percep Mot Skills.* 1983; 56: 443–450.

Bryan T, Sullivan-Burstein K, Mathur S. The influence of affect on social information processing. *J Learn Disabil.* 1998; 31: 418–426.

Butterworth B. The development of arithmetic abilities. *J Child Psychol Psychiatr.* 2005; 46: 3.

Butterworth B. Foundational numerical capacities and the origins of dyscalculia. *Trends Cogn Sci.* 2010; 14: 534–541.

Butterworth B, Cipolotti L, Warrington EK. Short-term memory impairment and arithmetical ability. *Q J Exp Psychol.* 1996; 49a: 251–262.

Butterworth B, Varma S, Laurilland D. Dyscalculia: from brain to education. *Science.* 2011; 332: 1049–1053.

C

Cahill L, McGaugh JL. Modulation of memory storage. *Curr Opin Neurobiol.* 1996; 6: 237–242.

Cantlon JF, Platt ML, Brannon EM. Beyond the number domain. *Trends Cogn Sci.* 2009; 13: 83–91.

Cantwell DP, Baker L. Association between attention deficit hyperactivity disorder and learning disorders. *J Learn Disabil.* 1991; 24: 88–95.

Cao F, Bitan T, Chou TL, et al. Deficient orthographic and phonologic representations in children with dyslexia revealed by brain activation patterns. *J Child Psychol Psychiatry*. 2006; 47(10): 1041–1050.

Cardon LR, Smith SD, Fulker DW, et al. Quantitative trait locus for reading disability on chromosome 6. *Science*. 1994; 266: 276–279.

Carrol J, Maughan B, Goodman R, Meltzer H. Literary difficulties and psychiatric disorders: evidence for comorbidity. *J Child Psychol Psychiatr*. 2005; 46: 524–532.

Castles A, Datta H, Gayan J, Olson RK. Varieties of developmental reading disorder: genetic and environmental influences. *J Exp Child Psychol*. 1999; 72: 73–94.

Castro-Caldes A, Cavaleiro MP, et al. Influence of learning to read and write on the morphology of the corpus callosum. *Eur J Neurol*. 1999; 6: 23–28.

Castro-Caldes A, Peterson KM, Reis A, et al. The illiterate brain: learning to read and write during childhood influences the functional organization of the adult brain. *Brain*. 1990; 121: 1053–1063.

Catalino SM, Shatz CZ. Activity dependent cortical target selection by thalamic axons. *Science*. 1998; 281: 559–562.

Catani M, Allin MP, Husain M, Puglese L, Mesulam MM, et al. Symmetries in human brain language pathwas correlate with verbal recall. *Proc Natl Acad Sci USA*. 2007; 104: 1716–1718.

Catani M, Ffytche DH. The rises and falls of disconnection syndromes. *Brain*. 2005; 128: 2224–2239.

Cavanaugh S, Tervo RC, Fogas R. The child with attention deficit hyperactivity disorder and learning disability. *SDJ Med*. 1997; 50: 193–197.

Cestnick L. Cross-modality temporal processing deficits in developmental phonological dyslexics. *Brain Cogn*. 2001; 46: 319–325.

Chabot RJ, Merkin H, Wood LM, et al. Sensitivity and specificity of QEEG in children with attention deficit or specific developmental learning disorders. *Clin Electroencephalogr*. 1996; 27: 26–34.

Chao LL, Weisberg J, Martin A. Experience-dependent modulation of category-related cortical activity. *Cereb Cortex*. 2002; 12: 545–551.

Chapman CA, Waber DP, Bassett N, et al. Neurobehavioral profiles of children with neurofibromatosis 1 referred for learning disabilities, are sex specific. *Am J Med Genet*. 1996; 67: 127–132.

Chi JG, Dooling EC, Gilles FH. Left-right asymmetries of the temporal speech areas of the human fetus. *Arch Neurol*. 1977; 34: 346–348.

Cipolotti L, van Harskamp N. Disturbances of number processing and calculation. In: Bernt RS, ed. *Handbook of Neuropsychology*. vol 3, 2nd ed. St. Louis, MO: Elsvier Science; 2001:305–334.

Cirino PT, Israelian MK, Morris MK, et al. Evaluation of the double deficit hypothesis in college students referred for learning difficulties. *J Learn Disabil*. 2005; 38: 29–43.

Clarkson ED, Rosa FG, Edwards Prasad J, Weiland DA, et al. Improvement of neurological deficits in 6-hydroxydopamine-lesioned rats after transplantation with allogenetic simian virus 40 large tumor antigen iduced immortalized dopamine. *Proc Natl Acad Sci USA*. 1998; 95: 1265–1270.

Cohen JD, Servan-Schreiber D. A theory of dopamine function and its role in cognitive deficits in schizophrenia. *Schizophrenia Bull*. 1993; 19: 85–104.

Cohen L. Abstract representations of numbers in the animal and human brain. *Trends Neurosci*. 1998; 21(8): 355–361S.

Cohen L, Dehaene S. Calculating without reading: unsuspected residual abilities in pure alexia. *Cogn Neuropsychol*. 2000; 17: 563–583.

Cohen L, Dehaene F, Chochon F, et al. Language and calculation within the parietal lobe. *Neuropsychologia*. 2000; 38: 1426–1440.

Cohen L, Dehaene S, Naccache L, et al. The visual word form area: spatial and temporal characterization of an initial stage of reading in normal subjects and posterior split-brain patients. *Brain*. 2000; 123: 291–307.

Cohen L, Lehéricy S, Chochon F, et al. Language-specific tuning of visual cortex? Functional properties of the visual word form area. *Brain*. 2002; 125: 1054–1069.

Cohen M, Campbell R, Yaghmai F. Neuropathological abnormalities in developmental dysphasia. *Ann Neurol*. 1989; 25: 567–570.

Coltheart M, Rastle K, Perry C, et al. DRC: a dual route cascaded model of visual word recognition and reading aloud. *Psychol Rev*. 2001; 108: 204–256.

Cooper H, Nye B. Homework for students with learning disabilities: the implications of research for policy and practice. *J Learn Disabil*. 1994; 27: 470–479.

Corina DP, Richards TL, Serafini S, et al. fMRI auditory language differences between dyslexic and able reading children. *Neuroreport*. 2001; 12: 1195–1201.

Corrigan N, Steward M, Scott M, et al. Predictive value of preschool surveilliance in detecting learning difficulties. *Arch Dis Child*. 1996; 74: 517–521.

Corrigan N, Stewart M, Scott M, Fee F. Fragile X, Iron and neurodevelopmental screening in 8 year old children with mild to moderate learning difficulties. *Arch Dis Child*. 1997; 76: 264–267.

Costa LD, Scarola LM, Rapin I. Purdue pegboard scores for normal grammer school children. *Percept Mot Skills*. 1964; 18: 748.

Cowell PE, Allen LS, Zalatimo NS, Denenberg VH. A developmental study of sex and age interactions in the human corpus callosum. *Dev Brain Res*. 1992; 66: 187–192.

Coyle B. Use of filters to treat visual perceptual problem creats adherence and sceptics. *CMAJ*. 1995; 152: 749–750.

Crawford SG, Kaplan BJ, Kinsbourne M. Are families of children with reading difficulties at risk for immune disorders and nonrighthandedness. *Cortex*. 1994; 30: 281–292.

Critchley M. *The Dyslexic Child*. London, UK: Heinemann Medical, 1970.

Critchley M, Critchley EA. *Dyslexia Defined*. London, UK: Heinemann Medical Books, 1978.

Crook TH, Tinkleberg J, Yesavage J, Petrie, et al. Effects of phosphatidylserine in age associated memory impairment. *Neurology*. 1991; 41: 644–649.

D

Damasio H, Grabowski T, Frank R, Galaburda AM, Damasio AE. The return of Phineas Gage. Clues about the brain from the skull of a famous patient. *Science*. 1994; 264: 1102–1105.

Deb S, Prassad KB. The prevalence of autistic disorder among children with a learning disability. *Br J Psychiatr*. 1994; 165: 395–399.

Decker MW, McGaugh JL. The role of interaction between the cholinergic system and other neuromodulatory systems in learning and memory. *Synapse*. 1991; 7: 151–168.

DeFries JC, Alarcon M, Oison RK. Genetics and dyslexia: developmental differences in the etiologies of reading and spelling deficits. In: Hulme C, Snowling M, eds. *Dyslexia: Biological Bases Identification and Intervention*. London, UK: Whurr, 1997:20–37.

DeFries JC, Alercon M. Genetics of specific reading disability. *Ment Retard Dev Disabil Res Rev*. 1996; 2: 39–47.

DeFries JC, Fulker DW. Multiple regression analysis of twin data. *Behav Genet*. 1985; 15: 467–473.

DeFries JC, Singer SM, Foch TT, Lewitter FI. Familial nature of reading disability. *Br J Psychiatry*. 1978; 132: 361–367.

Dehaene S. *The Number Sense*. New York, NY: Oxford University Press; 1997.

Dehaene S, Cohen L. cerebral pathways to calculation: double dissociation between rote verbal and quantitative knowledge of arithmetic. *Cortex*. 1997; 33: 219–250.

Dehaene S, Dehaene-Lambertz G, Cohen L. Abstract representations of numbers in the animal and human brain. *Trends Neurosci*. 1998; 21: 355–361.

Dehaene S, Molko N, Cohen L, Wilson A. Arithmatic and the brain. *Curr Opin Neurobiol*. 2004; 14: 218–224.

Dehaene S, Piazza M, Pinel P, Cohen L. Three parietal circuits for number processing. *Cogn Neuropsychol*. 2003; 20: 487–506.

Dehaene S, Piazza M, Pinel P, et al. Three parietal circuits for number processing. *Cogn Neuropsychol*. 2003; 20: 487–506.

Dehaene S, Spelke E, Pinek P, et al. Sources of mathematical thinking. Behavioral and brain imaging evidence. *Science*. 1999; 284: 970–974.

Dehaene S, Tzourio N, Frak V, et al. Central activation during number multiplication and comparison: a PET study. *Neuropsychologia*. 1996; 34: 1097–1106.

Dejerine J. *Sur un cas de cécité verbale avec agraphie, suivi d'autopsie*. C. R. Société du Biologie 1891; 43: 197–201.

Delazar M, Domahs F, Bertha C, et al. Learning complex arithmetic: an fMRI study. *Cogn Brain Res*. 2003; 18: 76–88.

Demb JB, Boynton GM, Best M, Heeger DJ. Psychophysical evidence for a magnocellular pathway deficit in dyslexia. *Vision Res*. 1998; 38: 1555.

Demb JB, Boynton GM, Heeger DJ. Brain activity in visual cortex predicts individual differences in reading performance. *Proc Natl Acad Sci USA*. 1997; 94: 13363–13366.

Demonet JF, Taylor MJ, Chaix Y. Developmental dyslexia. *Lancet*. 2004; 363(9419): 1451–1460.

Demonet JF, Thierry G, Cardebat D. Renewal of the neurophysiology of language. *Funct Neuroimag Physiol Rev*. 2005; 85(1): 49–95.

Denckla MB. Development of speed in repetitive and successive finger movements in normal children. *Dev Med Child Neurol*. 1973; 15: 635–645.

Denckla MB. A theory and model of executive function. In: Lyon GR, Krasnegor NA, eds. *Attention, Memory and Executive Function*. Baltimore, MD: Paul H. Brookes; 1996:263–278.

Denckla MB. Academic and extracurricular aspects of nonverbal learning disabilities. *Psychiatr Ann*. 1991; 21: 717–724.

Denckla MB. The child with developmental disabilities grown up: adult residua of childhood disorders. *Behav Neurol*. 1993; 11(1): 105–125.

Denckla MB, Rudel RG. Rapid 'automatized' naming (R.A.N.): dyslexia differentiated from other learning disabilities. *Neuropsychologia*. 1976; 14: 471–479.

Denckla MB, Rudel RG, Chapman C, Krieger J. Motor proficiency in dyslexic children with and without attentional disorders. *Arch Neurol*. 1985; 42: 228–231.

Denhoff E, Laufer MW, Solomons G. Hyperkinetic disorder in children's behavior problems. *Psychosom Med*. 1957; 19: 38–49.

Desimone R, Duncan J. Neural mechanisms of selective visual attention. *Annu Rev Neurosci*. 1995; 18: 193–222.

Desmond JE, Gabrieli JD, Glover GH. Dissociation of frontal and cerebellar activity in a cognitive task: evidence for a distinction between selection and search. *Neuroimage*. 1998; 7: 368–376.

Deutsch GK, Dougherty RF, Bammer R, et al. Children's reading performance is correlated with white matter structure measured by diffusion tensor imaging. *Cortex*. 2005; 41: 354–363.

DeWied D, Versteeg DH. Neurohypophyseal principles and memory. *Fed Proc*. 1979; 38: 2348–2354.

Dmonet JF, Taylor MJ, Chaix Y. Developmental dyslexia. *Lancet*. 2004; 363: 1451–1452.

Dobrunz LE. Long term potentiation and the computational synapse. *Proc Natl Acad Sci USA*. 1998; 95: 4086–4088.

Donchi E, Miller GA, Farwell LA. The endogenous components of the event related potentials—a diagnostis tool? *Prog Brain Res*. 1986; 70: 87–102.

Dorsaint-Pierre R, Penhune VB, Watkins KE, Neelin P, et al. Asymmetries of the planum temporale and Heschl's gyrus: relationship to language lateralization. *Brain*. 2006; 12: 1164–1176.

Duane DD. Alertness, vigilance, and waskefulness in developmental disorders of reading and attention. *Ann NY Acad Sci*. 1993; 682: 333–334.

Duara R, Kushch A, Gross-Glen K, et al. Neuroanatomic differences between dyslexic and normal readers on magnetic resonance imaging scans. *Arch Neurol*. 1991; 48: 410–416.

Dubeau F, Tampieri D, Lee N, et al. Periventricular and subcortical nodular heterotropia. A study of 33 patients. *Brain*. 1995; 118: 1273–1287.

Duffy FH, Denckla MB, Bartels PH, et al. Dyslexia: automated diagnosis by computerized classification of brain electrical activity. *Ann Neurol*. 1980; 7: 421–428.

E

Eckert M. Neuroanatomical markers for dyslexia: a review of dyslexia structural imaging studies. *Neuroscientist*. 2003; 10(4): 362–371.

Eckert MA, Leonard CM, Richards TL, Aylwards EH, et al. Anatomical correlations of dyslexia: frontal and cerebellar findings. *Brain*. 2003; 126(2): 482–494.

Eden GF, Jones KM, Cappell K, et al. Neural changes following remediation in adult developmental dyslexia. *Neuron*. 2004; 44: 411–422.

Eden GF, Moats L. The role of neuroscience in the remediation of students with dyslexia. *Nat Neurosci*. 2002; 5: 1080–1084.

Eden GF, Stein JF, Wood HM, Wood FB. Temporal and spatial processing in disabled and normal children. *Cortex*. 1995; 31(3): 451–468.

Eden GF, Stein JF, Wood HM, Wood FB. Differences in eye movements and reading problems in dyslexic and normal children. *Vision Res*. 1994; 34: 1345–1358.

Eden GF, VanMeter JW, Rumsey JM, et al. Abnormal processing of visual motion in dyslexia revealed by functional brain imaging. *Nature*. 1996; 382: 66–69.

Eden GF, Zeffiro TA. Neural systems affected in developmental dyslexia revealed by functional neuroimaging. *Neuron*. 1998; 21: 279–282.

Eger P, Sterzer P, Russ MO, et al. A supramodal number representation in human intraparietal cortex. *Neuron*. 2003; 37: 719–725.

Ehri L, Nunes SR, Willow DM, et al. Phonemic awareness instruction helps children to learn to read: Evidence from the National Reading Panel's meta analysis. *Read Res Quart*. 2001; 36: 250–287.

Eichenbaum H. To cortex: thanks for the memories. *Neurology*. 1997; 19: 481–484.

Eidelberh D, Galaburda AR. Symmetry and asymmetry in the human posterior thalamus. 1. Cytoarchitectonic analysisin normal persons. *Arch Neurol*. 1982; 39: 325–332; 333–336.

Elbert T, Pantev C, Wienbruch C, Rockstroh B, Taub W. Increased representation of the fingers of the left hand in string players. *Science*. 1995; 270: 305–307.

Eliez S, Rumsey JM, Geidd JN, et al. Morphological alteration of temporal lobe gray matter in dyslexia: an MRI study. *J Child Psychol Psychiatry*. 2000; 41: 637–644.

Evans BJ, Drasdo N, Richards IL. Dyslexia: the link with visual deficits. *Ophthalmic Physiol Opt*. 1996; 161: 3–10.

F

Fagerheim T, Raeymaekers P, Tonnessen FE, et al. A new gene (DYX3) for dyslexia is located on chromosome 2. *J Med Genet*. 1999; 36: 664–669.

Faraone SV, Biederman J, Lehman BK, et al. evidence for independent familial transmission of attention deficit hyperactivity disorder and learning disabilities: results from a family genetic study. *Am J Psychiatry*. 1993; 150: 891–895.

Farmer ME, Klein RM. The evidence for a temporal processing deficit linked to dyslexia: a review. *Psychonom Bull Rev*. 1995; 2: 460–493.

Fawcett AJ, Nicholson RI. Automatization deficits in balance for dyslexic children. *Percep Motor Skills*. 1992; 75: 507–529.

Fawcett AJ, Nicholson RI. Performance of dyslexic children on cerebellar and cognitive tests. *J Mot Behave*. 1999; 31: 68–78.

Fawcett AJ, Nicolson RI. Dyslexia: the role of the cerebellum. In: Fawcett AJ, ed. *Dyslexia: Theory and Good Practice*. London, UK: Whurr; 2001:89–105.

Fawcett AJ, Nicolson RI, Dean P. Impaired performance of children with dyslexia on a range of cerebellar tasks. *Ann Dyslexia*. 1996; 46: 259–283.

Feldman H, Yeatmen J, Lee E. Diffusion tensor imaging: a review for pediatric reaserchers and clinicians. *J Dev Behav Pediatr*. 2010; 31: 346–356.

Feller MB, Wellis DP, Stellwagen D, et al. Requirement for cholinergic synaptic transmission in the propagation of spontaneous retinal waves. *Science*. 1996; 272: 1182–1187.

Fennell EB. The role of neuropsychological assessment in learning disabilities. *J Child Neurol*. 1995; 10(suppl 1): S36–S41.

Fie JA, Petersen SE. Neuroimaging studies of word reading. *Proc Natl Acad Sci USA*. 1998; 95(3): 914–921.

Fiebach CJ, Frederici AD, Muller K, von Cramon DY. fMRI evidence for duel routes to the mental lexicon in visual word recognition. *J Cogn Neurosci*. 2002; 14: 11–23.

Fiez JA, Petersen SE. Neuroimaging studies of word reading. *Proc Natl Acad Sci USA*. 1998; 95: 914–921.

Fiez JA, Tallal P, Miezin FM, et al. Studies of auditory processing. Passive presentation and detection. *Neurosci Abst*. 1992; 18: 932.

Filipek P. Structural variations in measures in the developmental disorders. In: Thatcher R, Lyon G, Rumsey J, Krasnegor N, eds. *Developmental Neuroimaging: Mapping the Development of Brain and Behavior*. San Diego, CA: Academic; 1996:169–186.

Finch AJ, Nicholson RI, Fawcett AJ. Evidence for neuroanatomical differences within the olivo cerebellar pathway of adults with dyslexia. *Cortex*. 2002; 38: 529–539.

Finucci JM, Guthric JT, Childs AL, et al. The genetics of specific reading disability. *Ann Hum Genet*. 1976; 40: 1–23.

Fisher BL, Allen R, Kose G. The relationship between anxiety and problem solving skills in children with and without learning disabilities. *J Learn Disabil*. 1996; 29: 439–446.

Fisher SE, DeFrics JC. Developmental dyslexia: genetic dissection of a complex cognitive trait. *Nat Neurosci*. 2002; 3: 767–780.

Fisher SE, Francks C, Marlow AJ, et al. Independent genome-wide scans identify a chromosome 18 quantitative-trait locus influencing dyslexia. *Nat Genet*. 2002; 30: 86–91.

Fisher SE, Marlow AJ, Lamb J, et al. A quantitative-trait locus on chromosome 6p influences different aspects of developmental dyslexia. *Am J Hum Genet*. 1999; 64: 146–156.

Fleischner JE. Educational management of students with learning disabilities. *J Child Neurol*. 1995; Suppl 1: S81–5.

Fletcher-Flinn C, Elmes H, Strugnell D. Visual perceptual and phonological factors in the acquisition of literacy among children with congenital developmental coordination disorder. *Dev Med Child Neuro*. 1997; 39: 158–166.

Fletcher J, Lyon G, Fuchs L, Barnes M. *Learning Disabilities: From Identification to Intervention*. New York, NY: Guilford Press; 2007.

Fletcher JM, Denton C, Francis DJ. Validity of alternative approach for the identification of learning disabilities: operationalizing unexpected underachievement. *J Learn Disabil*. 2005; 38: 345–352.

Fletcher JM, Shaywitz SE, Shankweiler DP, et al. Cognitive profiles of reading disability: comparisons of discrepancy and low achievement definitions. *J Educ Psychol*. 1994; 86: 6–23.

Flowers DL, Wood FB, Naylor CE. Regional cerebral blood flow correlates of language processes in reading disability. *Arch Neurol*. 1991; 48: 631–643.

Fogerheim T, Raeymaekers P, Tonnessen FE, et al. A new gene (DYX3) for dyslexia is located on chromosome 2. *J Med Genet*. 1999; 36: 144–147.

Frackowiak RS. Brain activity during reading. The effects of exposure duration and task. *Brain*. 1994; 117: 1255–1269.

Francis DJ, Shaywitz SE, Steubing KK, et al. Measurements of change: assessing behavior over time and within a developmental context. In: Lyon GR, ed. *Frames of Reference for the Assessment of Learning Disabilities: New View on Measurement Issues*. Baltimore, MD: Paul H. Brookes; 1994.

Francks C, MacPhie IL, Monaco AP. The genetic basis of dyslexia. *Lancet Neurol*. 2002; 1(8): 483–490.

Frank Y. Learning Disabilities. In: Palmar KJ, ed. *Topics in Pediatric Psychiatry*. Auckland, New Zeland: Adis International; 2000.

Frank Y, Pavlakis SG. Brain imaging in neurobehavioral disorders. *Pediatr Neurol*. 2001; 25: 278–287.

Frank Y, Seiden J, Napolitano B. Visual event related potentials and reaction time in normal adults, normal children and children with attention deficit hyperactivity disorder: differences in short term memory processing. *Int J Neurosci*. 1996; 88: 109–124.

Frith U, Frith C. Modularity of mind and phonological deficit. In: von Euler C, Lundberg I, Linas R, eds. *Basic Mechanisms in Cognitive and Language with Special Reference to Phonological Problems in Dyslexia*. Amsterdam, The Netherlands: Elsevier; 1998: 3–17.

Frnandez AM, de la Vega AG, Torres-Aleman I. Insulin like growth factor 1 restores motor coordination in a rat model of cerebellar ataxia. *Proc Natl Acad Sci USA*. 1998; 95: 1253–1258.

Fuchs LS, Fuchs D. Treatment validity: a simplifying concept for reconceptualizing the identification of learning disabilities. *Learn Disabil Res and Prac*. 1998; 4: 204–219.

Fulbright RK, Jenner AR, Mencl WE, et al. The cerebellum's role in reading: a functional MR imaging study. *AJNR.* 1999; 20: 1925–1930.

Fuster JM. Temporal processing. *Ann NY Acad Sci.* 1995; 769: 173–181.

G

Gabel LA, Gibson CJ, Gruen JR, LoTurco JJ. Progress towards a cellular neurobiology of reading disability. *Neurobiol Dis.* 2010; 38(2): 173–180.

Gaillard WD, Sachs BC, Whitnah JR, Ahmad Z, et al. Developmental aspects of language processing: fMRI of verbal fluency in children and adults. *Hum Brain Mapp.* 2003; 18: 176–185.

Galaburda AM, Kemper TL. Cytoarchitectonic abnormalities in developmental dyslexia: a case study. *Ann Neurol.* 1979; 6: 94–100.

Galaburda AM, LeMay M, Kemper TL, et al. Right-left asymmetries in the brain. *Science.* 1978; 199: 852–856.

Galaburda AM, Menard M, Rosen GD. Evidence for aberrant auditory anatomy in developmental dyslexia. *Proc Natl Acad Sci USA.* 1994; 91: 8010–8013.

Galaburda AM, Sanides F, Geschwind N. Human brain: cytoarchitectonic left-right asymmetries in the temporal speech region. *Arch Neurol.* 1978; 35: 812–817.

Galaburda AM, Sherman GF, Rosen GD, et al. Developmental dyslexia: four consecutive patients with cortical anomalies. *Ann Neurol.* 1985; 18: 222–233.

Gale SD, Perkel DJ. Anatomy of a songbird basal ganglia circuit essential for vocal learning and plasticity. *J Chem Neuroanat.* 2010; 39: 124–131.

Gan WB, Lichtman JW. Synaptic segregation of the developing neuromuscular junction. *Science.* 1998; 282: 1508–1511.

Garcia-Molina A. Phineas Gage and the enigma of the prefrontal cortex. *Neurology.* 2012; 27: 370–375.

Gardner H. *Frames of Mind.* New York, NY: Basic Books; 1983.

Garrett AS, Flowers DL, Absher JR, et al. Cortical activity related to accuracy of letter recognition. *Neuroimage.* 2000; 11: 111–123.

Gauger LM, Lombardino LJ, Leonard CM. Brain morphology in children with specific language impairment. *J Speech Lang Hear Res.* 1997; 40: 1272–1284.

Gauthier I, Tarr M, Moylan J, et al. The fusiform "face area" is part of a network that processes faces at the individual level. *J Cogn Neurosci.* 2000; 123: 495–504.

Gayan J, Olson RK. Genetic and environmental influences on orthographic and phonological skills in children with reading disabilities. *Dev Neuropsychol.* 2001; 20: 483–507.

Gayan J, Smith SD, Cherny SS, et al. Quantitative-trait locus for specific language and reading deficits on chromosome 6p. *Am J Hum Genet.* 1999; 64: 157–164.

Geary DC. Basic number, counting and arithmetic skills in infancy and preschool reflect a biologically inherent arithmetic system. *Eur J Child Adol Psychiatr.* 2000; 9: II/11–II/16.

Geary DC. Mathematical disabilities: cognitive, neuropsychological, and genetic components. *Psychol Bull.* 1993; 114: 345–362.

Georgiewa P, Rzanny R, Gazer L, et al. Phonological processing in dyslexic children: a study combining functional imaging and event related potentials. *Neurosci Lett.* 2002; 318: 5–8.

Georgiewa P, Rzanny R, Hopf JM, et al. fMRI during word processing in dyslexic and normal reading children. *Neuroreport.* 1999; 10: 3459–3465.

Gerstmann J. Fingeragnosie: eine unschriebene storuny der orientierung am eigenen. *Korper, Wiener Klinishe Wochenschrift* 1924; 37: 1010–1012.

Geschwind N. Disconnection syndrome in animals and man. *Brain.* 1965; 88: 237–294, 585–644.

Geschwind N, Galaburda AM. Cerebral lateralization: biological mechanisms, associations, and pathology. I. Hypothesis and a program for research. *Arch Neurol.* 1985; 42: 428–458.

Geschwind N, Levitsky W. Human brain: left-right asymmetries in temporal speech region. *Science.* 1968; 161: 186–187.

Gillon G, Dodd B. Enhancing the phonological processing skills of children with specific reading disability. *Eur J Disord Commun.* 1997; 32: 67–90.

Gittelman-Klein R, Klein DF. Methylphenidate effects in learning disabilities: psychometric changes. *Arch Gen Psychiatry.* 1976; 33: 655–664.

Glaser WR. Picture naming. *Cognition.* 1992; 42: 61–105.

Goda Y, Stevens CF. Long term depression properties in a simple system. *Neuron.* 1996; 16: 103–111.

Goda Y, Stevens CF. Synaptic plasticity: the basis of particular types of learning. *Curr Biol.* 1996; 6: 375–378.

Goldberg E. *The Executive Brain: Frontal Lobes and the Civilized Mind.* New York, NY: Oxford University Press; 2001.

Goldman-Rakic PS. Topography of cognition: parallel distributed networks in primate association cortex. *Ann Rev Neurosci.* 1988; 11: 137–156.

Goodley D, Rapley M. How do you understand "learning difficulties"? Towards a social theory of impairment. *Mental Retardation.* 2001; 39: 229–232.

Goswami U, Thomson J, Richardson U, et al. Amplitude envelope onsets and developmental dyslexia: a new hypothesis. *Proc Natl Acad Sci USA.* 2002; 99: 10911–10916.

Grabner RH, Ansari D, Koschutnig K, et al. To retrieve or to calculate left angular gyrus mediates the retrieval of arithmetic facts during problem solving. *Neuropsychologia.* 2009; 47: 604–608.

Grabner RH, Ansari D, Reishofer G, et al. Individual differences in mathematical competence predict parietal lobe activation during mental calculation. *Neuroimage.* 2007; 38: 346–356.

Grabner RH, Ischebeck A, Reishofer G, et al. Fact learning in complex arithmetic and figural-spatial tasks. The role of the angular gyrus and its relation to mathematical competence. *Hum Brain Mapp.* 2009; 30: 2936–2952.

Grabner RH, Reishofer G, Koschutnig K, Ebner F. Competence in processing mathematical representations. *Frontiers Hum Neurosci.* 2011; 5: 1–11.

Greatrex JC, Drasdo N. The magnocellular deficit hypothesis in dyslexia: a review of reported evidence. *Ophthalmic Physiolog Opt.* 1995; 15: 501–506.

Gresham FM. Response to treatment. In: Bradely R, Danielson L, Hallihan D, eds. *Identification of Learning Disabilities: Research to Practice.* Mahwah, NJ: Erlbaum; 2002:467–517.

Grigorenko EL, Wood FB, Meyer MS, Pauls DL. Chromosome 6p influences on different dyslexia-related cognitive processes: further confirmation. *Am J Hum Genet.* 2000; 66: 715–723.

Grigorenko EL, Wood FB, Meyer MS, et al. Linkage studies suggest a possible locus for developmental dyslexia on chromosome 1p. *Am J Med Genet.* 2001; 105: 120–129.

Grigorenko EL, Wood FB, Meyer MS, et al. Susceptibility loci for distinct components of developmental dyslexia on chromosomes 6 and 15. *Am J Hum Genet.* 1997; 60: 27–39.

Grigorenko E. Developmental dyslexia: an update on genes, brains and environments. *J Child Psychol Psychiatr.* 2001; 42: 91–125.

Grills-Taquechel AE, Fletcher JM, Vaughn SR, Stuebing KK. Anxiety and reading difficulties in early elementary school: evidence for unidirectional or bidirectional relations. *Child Psychiatry Hum Dev*. 2012; 43: 35–47.

Gross-Glenn K, Duara R, Barker WW, Lowenstein D, et al. Positron emission tomographic studies during serial word reading by normal and dyslexic adults. *J Clic Neuropsychol*. 1991; 13: 541–544.

Gross-Tsur V, Manor O, Shalev R. Developmental dyscalculia: prevalence and demographic features. *Dev Med Child Neurol*. 1996; 38: 25–33.

Gross-Tsur V, Shalev RS, Manor O, Amir N. Developmental right hemisphere syndrome: clinical spectrum of the nonverbal learning disability. *J Learn Disabil*. 1995; 28: 80–86.

H

Habib M. The neurological basis of developmental dyslexia: an overview and working hypothesis. *Brain*. 2000; 123: 2373–2399.

Hagin R, Silver A. *Learning Disorders in Childhood*. New York, NY: Wiley; 1990.

Hagman JD, Wood F, Buchsbaum MS, et al. Cerebral brain metabolism in adult dyslexic subjects, assessed with positron emission tomography during performance of an auditory task. *Arch Neurol*. 1992; 49: 734–739.

Hallgren B. Specific dyslexia: a clinical and genetic study. *Acta Psychiatr Neurolog Scand*. 1950; 65(suppl): 1–287.

Halperin JM, Wolf LE, Pascualvaca DM, et al. Differential assessment of attention and impulsivity in children. *J Amer Acad Chil Adolesc Psychiatry*. 1988; 27: 326–329.

Hammill DD. On defining learning disabilities: an emerging consensus. *J Learn Disabil*. 1990; 23: 74–84.

Hammill DD. A brief look at the learning disabilities movement in the United States. *J Learn Disabil*. 1993; 26: 295–310.

Hammill DD, Leigh J, McNutt G, et al. A new definition of learning disabilities. *J Learn Disabil*. 1987; 20: 109–113.

Hannula-Jouppi K, Kaminen-Ahola N, Taipale M, et al. The axon guidance receptor gene ROBO1 is a candidate gene for developmental dyslexia. *PLoS Genet*. 2005; 1: e50.

Hari R, Kiesila P. Deficit of temporal auditory processing in dyslexic adults. *Neurosci Lett*. 1996; 205: 138–140.

Hari R, Renvall H. Impaired processing of rapid stimulus sequences in dyslexia. *Trends Cogn Sci*. 2001; 5: 525–532.

Hari R, Renvall H, Tanskanen T. Left minineglect in dyslexic adults. *Brain*. 2001; 124: 1373–1380.

Harmony T, Marosi E, Becker J, et al. Longitudinal quantitative EEG study of children with different performances on a reading-writing test. *Electroencephalogr Clin Neurophysiol*. 1995; 95: 426–433.

Hastings RP, Sonuga-Barke EJ, Remington B. An analysis of labels for people with learning disabilities. *Br J Clin Psychol*. 1993; 32: 463–465.

Heilman KM, Voeller K, Alexander AW, et al. Developmental dyslexia: a motor-articulatory feedback hypothesis. *Ann Neurol*. 1996; 39: 407–412.

Helenius P, Tarkiainen A, Cornelissen P, et al. Dissociation of normal feature analysis and deficient processing of letter-strings in dyslexic adults. *Cerebral Cortex*. 1999; 4: 476–483.

Henik A, Rubinstein O, Ashkenazy S. The "where" and "what" in developmental dyslexia. *Clin Neuropsychol*. 2011; 25: 989–1008.

Henry M, Ganschow L, Miles TR. The issue of definition. Some problems and perspectives. *Int Dyalexia Assoc*. 2000; 26(4): 38–43.

Hermann K, Norrie E. Is congenital word blindness a hereditary type of Gerstmann's syndrome. *Psychiatria Neurologia*. 1958; 136: 59–73.

Hier DB, LeMay M, Rosenberger PB, Perlo V. Developmental dyslexia: evidence for a subgroup with reversed cerebral asymmetry. *Arch Neurol*. 1978; 35: 90.

Hillier LW, Fulton RS, Fulton LA, Graves TA, et al. The DNA sequence of chromosome 7. *Nature*. 2003; 424: 157–164.

Hinshelwood J. *Congenital Word-Blindness*. London, UK: H.K. Lewis; 1917.

Ho CS, Chan DW, Lee SH, Tsang SM, Luan VH. Cognitive profiling and preliminary subtyping in Chinese developmental dyslexia. *Cognition*. 2004; 91: 43–75.

Hoeft F, Meyler A, Hernandez C, et al. Functional and morphometric brain dissociation between dyslexia and reading ability. *Proc Natl Acad Sci*. 2007; 104(10): 4234–4239.

Hoehn TP, Baumeister AA. A critique of the application of sensory integration therapy to children with learning disabilities. *J Learn Disabil*. 1994; 27: 338–350.

Hofman KJ, Harris EL, Bryan RN, Denckla MB. Neurofibromatosis type I: the cognitive phenotype. *J Pediatr*. 1994; 124: S1–8.

Holoway ID, Ansari ID. Developmental specialization in the right intraparietal sulcus for the abstract representation of numerical magnitude. *J Cogn Neurosci*. 2010; 22: 2627–2637.

Horne MK, Butler EG. The role of the cerebello-thalamo-cortical pathway in skilled movement. *Prog Neurobiol*. 1995; 46: 199–213.

Horwitz B, Rumsey JM, Donohue BC. Functional connectivity of the angular gyrus in normal reading and dyslexia. *Proc Natl Acad Sci USA*. 1998; 95: 8939–8944.

Hubel DH, Wiesel TN. Receptive fields and functional architecture of monkey striate cortex. *J Physiol*. 1968; 195: 215–243.

Hugdahl K, Thornsen T, Ersland L, et al. The effects of attention on speech perception: an MRI study. *Brain Language*. 2003; 85: 37–48.

Hulme C, Roodenruy S. Practitioner review: verbal working memory development and its disorders. *J Child Psychol Psychiatry*. 1995; 36: 373–398.

Hulme C, Snowling M. *Dyslexia: Biology, Cognition, and Intervention*. San Diego, CA: Singular Publishing; 1997.

Humphreys P, Kaufmann WE, Galaburda AM. Developmental dyslexia in women: neuropathological findings in three patients. *Ann Neurol*. 1990; 28: 727–738.

Hynd GW, Hall J, Novey ES, et al. Dyslexia and corpus callosum morphology. *Arch Neurol*. 1995; 36: 373–398.

Hynd GW, Semrud-Cliceman M, Lorys AR, et al. Brain morphology in developmental dyslexia and attention deficit disorder/hyperactivity. *Arch Neurol*. 1990; 47: 919.

I

Indefrey P, Levelt WJM. The neural correlates of language production. In Gazzaniga MS, ed. *The New Cognitive Neuroscience*. Cambridge, MA: MIT Press; 2000: 845–865.

Ingram TT, Mason AW, Blackburn I. A retrospective study of 82 children with reading disability. *Dev Med Child Neurol*. 1970; 12: 271–281.

Isaacs EB, Edmonds CJ, Lucas A, Gadian DG. Calculation difficulties in children of very low birthwight: a neural correlate. *Brain.* 2001; 124: 1701–1707.

Ivry RB, Keele SW. Timing functions of the cerebellum. *J Cogn Neurosci.* 1989; 1: 136–152.

Ivry RB, Justus TC. A neural instantiation of the motor theory of speech perception [review]. *Trends Neurosci.* 2001; 24: 513–515.

J

Jansky J, de Hirsch K. *Preventing Reading Failure: Prediction, Diagnosis and Intervention.* New York, NY: Harper & Row; 1972.

Jenson WR, Sheridan SM, Olympia D, Andrews D. Homework and students with learning disabilitirs and behavioral disorders: a practical, parent-based approach. *J Learn Disabil.* 1994; 27: 538–548.

Jernigan TL, Hesselink JR, Sowekk E, Tallal PA. Cerebral structure of magnetic cerebral imaging in language and learning impaired children. *Arch Neurol.* 1991; 48: 539–545.

Jezzard P, Matthews P, Smith S. *Functional MRI: An Introduction to Methods.* Oxford, UK: Oxford University Press; 2001.

Jobard G, Crivello F, Tzourio-Mazoyer N. Evaluation of the dual route theory of reading: a metanalysis of 35 neuroimaging studies. *Neuroimage.* 2003; 20: 693–712.

Johannes S, Kussmaul CL, Munte TF, Mangun GR. Developmental dyslexia: passive visual stimulation provides no evidence for a magnocellular processing defect. *Neuropsychologia.* 1996; 34: 1123–1127.

Johnson DJ. An overview of learning disabilities: psychoeducational perspectives. *J Child Neurol.* 1995; Suppl 1: S2–5.

Johnson DJ, Myklebust HR. *Learning disabilities. Educational principles and practice.* New York: Grune and Straton; 1967.

Jusczyk PW, Hohne EH. Infant's memory for spoken words. *Science.* 1997; 277: 1984–1986.

K

Karni A, Meyer G, Rey-Hipolito C, Jezzard P, et al. The acquisition of skilled motor performance: fast and slow experience driven changes in primary motor cortex. *Proc Natl Acad Sci USA.* 1998; 95: 861–868.

Katzir T, Wolf M, O'Brien B, et al. reading fluency—whole is more than the parts. *Ann Dyslexia.* 2006; 56: 51–82.

Kawai N, Matsuzawa T. Numerical memory span in a chimpsnze. *Nature.* 2000; 403: 39–40.

Keenan JM, Betjemann RS, Wadsworth SJ, et al. Genetic and environmental influences on reading and listening comprehension. *J Res Read.* 2006; 29: 75–91.

Keller TA, Carpenter PA, Just MA. Brain imaging of tongue-twister sentence comprehension: twisting the tongue and the brain. *Brain Language.* 2003; 84: 189–203.

Kentros C, Hargreaves E, Hawkins RD, et al. Abolition of long term stability of new hippocampal place cell maps by NMDA receptor blockade. *Science.* 1998; 280: 2121–2126.

Kim SG, Ugurbil K, Strick PL. Activation of a cerebellar output nucleus during cognitive processing. *Science.* 1994; 265: 949–951.

Kinsbourne M, Warrington EK. The developmental Gerstmann syndrome. *Arch Neurol.* 1963; 8: 490–501.

Kirk SA. *Educating Exceptional Children.* Boston, MA: Houghton Mifflin; 1978.

Kirstein CL, Philpot RM, Dark T. Fetal alcohol syndrome: early olfactory learning as a model system to study neurobehavioral deficit. *Int J Neurosci.* 1997; 89: 119–132.

Kleinschmidt A, Rusconi E. Gerstmann meets Gescwind: a crossing (or kissing) variant of a subcortical disconnection syndrome? *Neuroscientist.* 2011; 17: 633–644.

Klingberg T, Hedehus M, Temple E, et al. Microstructure of temporo parietal white matter as a basis for reading. Evidence from diffusion tensor magnetic imaging. *Neuron.* 2000; 25: 493–500.

Klingberg T, Hedehus M, Temple E, et al. Microstructure of temporo-parietal white matter as a basis for reading ability: evidence from diffusion tensor magnetic resonance imaging. *Neuron.* 2000; 25: 493–500.

Klingberg T, Vaidya CJ, Gabrieli JD, Moseley ME, Hedehus ME. Myelination and organization of the frontal white matter in children: a diffuse tensor MRI study. *Neuroreport.* 1999; 10: 2817–2821.

Knudsen EL. Supervised learning in the brain. *J Neurosci.* 1994; 14: 3985–3997.

Koepp MJ, Gunn RN Lawrence AD, et al. Evidence for striatal dopamine release during a video game. *Nature.* 1998; 393: 266–268.

Kolb B, Wilson B, Taylor L. Developmental changes in the recognition and comprehension of facial expression: implicatins for frontal lobe functions. *Brain Cogn.* 1992; 20: 74–84.

Koumoula A, Tsironi V, et al. An epidemiological study of number processing and mental calculation in Greek schoolchildren. *J Learn Disabil.* 2004; 37: 377–388.

Kramer AF, Donchin E. Brain potentials as indices of orthographic and phonological interaction during word matching. *J Exp Psych Learn Memory Cog.* 1987; 13: 76–86.

Kraus N, McGee TJ, Carrell TD, Zecker SG, et al. Auditory neurophysiologic responses and discrimination deficits in children with learning problems. *Science.* 1996; 273: 971–973.

Kronbichler M, Hutzler F, Wimmer H. Dyslexia: verbal impairments in the absence of magnocellular impairments. *Neuroreport.* 2002; 13: 617–620.

Kubova Z, Kuba M, Peregrin J, Novakova V. Visual evoked potential evidence for magnocellular system deficit in dyslexia. 1996; 45: 87–89.

Kucian K, Loenneker T, Dietrich T, et al. Impaired neural networks for approximate calculations in dyscalculic children. A functional MRI study. *Behav Brain Funct.* 2006; 2: 31.

Kucian K, Loenneker T, Martin E, Von Aster M. Non symbolic numerical distance effect in children with and without developmental dyscalculia. *Dev Neuropsychol.* 2011; 36: 741–762.

Kucian K, Von Aster M, Loenneker T, et al. Development of neural networks for exact and approximate calculation: an FMRI study. *Dev Neuropsychol.* 2008; 33: 447–473.

Kujala T, Myllyviita K, Tervaniemi M, Alho K, Kallio J, Näätänen R. Basic auditory dysfunction in dyslexia as demonstrated by brain activity measurements. *Psychophysiology.* 2000; 37: 262–266.

Kuriki S, Takeuchi F, Hirata Y. Neural processing of words in the human extrastriate visual cortex. *Brain Res Cogn Brain Res.* 1998; 6: 193–203.

Kushch A, Gross-Glen K, Jallad B, Lubs H, et al. Temporal lobe surface areameasurment on MRI in normal and dyslexic readers. *Neuropsychologia.* 1993; 31: 811–821.

L

Landrel K, Bevan A, Butterworth B. developmental dyscalculia and basic numerical capacities: a study of 8-9 year old students. *Cognition.* 2004; 93: 99–125.

Larsen JP, Hoien T, Lundberg I. MRI evaluation of the size and symmetry of the planum temporale in adolescents with developmental dyslexia. *Brain Lang.* 1990; 39: 289–301.

Latvala ML, Korhonen TT, Penttinen M, Laippala P. Ophthalmic findings in dyslexic schoolchildren. *Br J Ophthalmol.* 1994; 78: 339–343.

Lee SK, Kim DI, Kim J, et al. Diffusion-tensor MR imaging and fiber tractography: a new method of describing aberrant fiber connections in developmental CNS anomalies. *Radiographics.* 2005; 25: 53–65.

Lehmkuhle S, Garzia R, Turner L, et al.A defective visual pathway in children with reading disability. *N Engl J Med.* 1993; 328: 989–996.

Leonard CM, Eckert MA, Lombardino LJ, et al. Anatomical risk factors for phonological dyslexia. *Cereb Cortex.* 2001; 11: 148–157.

Leonard CM, Voeller KK, Lombardino LJ, et al. Anomalous cerebral structures in dyslexia revealed with magnetic resonance imaging. *Arch Neurol.* 1993; 50: 461–469.

Leppanen PH, Lyytinen H. Auditory event related potentials in the study of developmental language related disorders. *Audiol Neurootol.* 1997; 2: 308–340.

Levin BE. Organizational deficits in dyslexia: possible frontal lobe dysfunction. *Dev Neuropsychol.* 1990; 6: 95–110.

Levin PM. The efferent fibers of the frontal lobe of the monkey, Macaca mulatta. *J Comp Neurol.* 1936; 63: 369–419.

Levin HS, Scheller J, Rickard T, et al. Dyscalculia and dyslexia after right hemisphere injury in infancy. *Arch Neurol.* 1996; 53: 88–96.

Levy HB, Harper CR, Weinberg WA. A practical approach to children failing in school. *Pediatr Clin North Am* 1992; 39: 895–924.

Lewis C, Hitch GJ, Walker P. The prevalence of specific arithmetic difficulties and specific reading difficulties in 9 to 10 year old boys and girls. *J Child Psychol Psychiatry.* 1994; 35: 283–292.

Li Y, Field PM, Raisman G. Repair of adult rat corticospinal tract by transplant of olfactory ensheathing cells. *Science.* 1997; 277: 2000–2002.

Liberman IY, Shankweiler D. Phonology and beginning reading: a tutorial. In: Reiben L, Perfetti CA, eds. *Learning to Read: Basic Research and Its Implications.* Hillsdale, NJ: Erlbaum; 1991:3–17.

Lieberman IY, Shankwiler D. Phonology and the problems of learning to read and write. *Remed Spec Educ.* 1985; 6: 8–17.

Liberman IY, Shankweiler D, Orlando C, et al. Letter confusions and reversals of sequence in the beginning reader: implications for Orton's theory of developmental dyslexia. *Cortex.* 1971; 7: 127–142.

Light JG, DeFries JC, Olson RK. Multivariate behavioral genetic analysis of achievement and cognitive measures in reading disabled and control twin pairs. *Hum Biol.* 1998; 70: 215–237.

Linday LA. Dyslexia: empowering parents to become their child's educational advocate. *J Dev Behav Pediatr.* 1995; 15: 353–360.

Linkersdorfer J, Lonnemann J, Lindberg S, et al. Grey matter alterations co-localize with functional abnormalities in developmental dyslexia: an ALE meta-analysis. *PLOS One.* 2012; 7: e43122: 1–10.

Lisberger SG. The neural basis for learning of simple motor skills. *Science.* 1988; 242: 728–735.

Liston C, Watts R, Tottenham N, et al. Frontostriatal microstructure modulates efficient recruitment of cognitive control. *Cereb Cortex.* 2006; 16: 553–560.

Livingstone MS, Rosen GD, Drislane FW, Galaburda AM. Physiological and anatomical evidence for a magnocellular defect in developmental dyslexia. *Proc Natl Acad Sci USA.* 1991; 88: 7943–7947.

Llinas R. Is dyslexia a dyschronia? *Ann NY Acad Sci.* 1993; 682: 48–56.

LoCasto, PC, Krebs-Noble D, Gullapalli RP, Burton MW. An fMRI investigation of speech and tone segmentation. *J Cogn Neurosci.* 2004; 16: 1612–1624.

Logan G. Toward an instance theory of automatization. *Psychol Rev.* 1988; 95: 492–527.

Loppez R, Yolton RL, Kohl P, Smith DL, Saxerud MH. Comparison of Itlen scotopic sensitivity syndrome test results to academic and visual performance data. *J Am Optom Assoc.* 1994; 65: 705–714.

Lovegrove W, Slaghuis W, Bowling A, et al. Spatial frequency processing and the prediction of reading ability: a preliminary investigation. *Percept Psychophysiol.* 1986; 40: 440–444.

Lovegrove WJ, Bowling A, Badcock B, Blackwood M. Specific reading disability: differences in contrast sensitivity as a function of spatial frequency. *Science.* 1980; 210: 439–440.

Loveless N, Koivikko H. Sluggish auditory processing in dyslexics is not due to persistence in sensory memory. *Neuroreport.* 2000; 11: 1903–1906.

Lovett MW, Barron RW, Forbes JE, et al. Computer speech based training and literacy skills in neurologically impaired children: a controlled evaluation. *Brain Language.* 1994; 47: 117–154.

Lovett MW, Borden SL, Deluca T, et al. Treating the core deficits of developmental dyslexia: evidence of transfer of learning after phonologically and strategy based reading programs. *Dev Psychol.* 1994; 30: 805–822.

Lovett MW, Steinbach KA, Frijters J. Remediating the core deficits of developmental reading disability: a double-deficit perspective. *J Learn Disabil.* 2000; 33: 334–358.

Lundberg I, Frost J, Petersen OP. Effects of an extensive program for stimulating phonological awareness in preschool children. *Read Res Quart.* 1988; 23: 263–284.

Luria AR. *The Higher Cortical Functions in Man.* New York, NY: Basic Books; 1966.

Lyons GR. Learning disabilities. *Fut Child.* 1996; 6: 54–76.

Lyons GR. Research initiatives in learning disabilities: contributions from scientists supported by the National Institute of Child Health and Human Development. *J Child Neurol.* 1995; 10(suppl 1): 120–126.

Lyons GR. Towards a definition of dyslexia. *Ann Dyslexia.* 1995; 45: 3–27.

M

Macmillan M. Inhibition and the control of behavior. From Gall to Freud via Phineas Gage and the frontal lobes. *Brain Cogn.* 1992; 19: 72–104.

MacMillan DL, Gresham FM, Siperstein GN, Bocian KIN. The labyrinth of IDEA: school decisions on referred students with subaverage intelligence. *Am J Ment Retard.* 1996; 20: 161–170.

Magistretti PJ, Pellerin L. Cellular bases of brain energy metabolism and their relevance to functional brain imaging: evidence for. *Mapp.* 2000; 10: 120–131.

Manis FR, Mcbride-Chang C, Seidenberg MS, et al. Are speech perception deficits associated with developmental dyslexia? *J Exp Child Psychol.* 1997; 66: 211–235.

Manis FR, Seidenberg MS, Doi LM. See Dick RAN: rapid naming and the longitudinal prediction of reading subskills in first and second graders. *Sci Stud Reading.* 1999; 3: 129–157.

Margalit M. Loneliness and coherence among preschool children with learning disabilities. *J Learn Disabil.* 1998; 31: 173–180.

Martin A, Haxby JV, Lalonde FM, et al. Discrete cortical regions associated with knowledge of color and knowledge of action. *Science.* 1995; 270: 102–103.

Martin F, Lovegrove W. Flicker contrast sensitivity in normal and specifically disabled readers. *Perception.* 1987; 16: 215–221.

Mataro M, Garcia-Sanchez C, Junque C,et al. Magnetic resonance imaging measurement of the cadate nucleus in adolescents with attention deficit hyperactivity disorder andits relationship with neuropsychological and behavioral measures. *Arch Neurol.* 1997; 54: 963–968.

Mathews PJ, Ober LK, Albert ML. Wernicke and Alzheimer on the language disturbances of dementia and aphasi. *Brain Language.* 1994; 46: 439–462.

Mattis S, French J, Rapin I. Dyslexia in children and young adults: three independent neuropsychological syndromes. *Dev Med Child Neurol.* 1975; 17: 150–163.

Maughan B, Pickles A, Hagell A, et al. Reading problems and antisocial behavior: developmental trends in comorbidity. *J Child Psychol Psychiatr.* 1996; 37: 405–418.

Maurer U, Brem S, Bucher Ke, Brandeis D. Emerging neurophysiological specialization for letter strings. *J Cogn Neurosci.* 2005; 17: 1532–1552.

Mazzocco MM. Defining and differentiating mathematical learning disabilities and difficulties. In: Berch DB, Mazzocco MM, eds. *Why Is Math So Hard for Some Children? The Nature and Origins of Mathematical Learning Difficulties and Disabilities.* Baltimore, MD: Paul H. Brookes; 2011:29–47.

McAnally KI, Stein JF. Auditory temporal coding in dyslexia. *Proc Natl Acad Sci USA.* 1996; 263: 961–965.

McCandliss BD, Cohen L, Dehane S. The visual word form area: expertise for reading in the fusiform gyrus. *Trends Cogn Sci.* 2003; 7: 293–299.

McCloskey M, Caramazza A, Basili A. Cognitive mechanisms in number processing and calculation: evidence from dyscalculia. *Brain Cog.* 1985; 4: 171–196.

McCrory E. *A Neurocognitive Investigation of Phonological Processing in Dyslexia.* London, UK: University College London; 2000.

McCrory E, Frith U, Brunswick N, Price C. Abnormal functional activation during a simple word repetition task: a PET study of adult dyslexics. *J Cogn Neurosci.* 2000; 12: 753–762.

McCrory EJ, Mechelli A, Frith U, Price CJ. More than words: a common neural basis for reading and naming deficits in developmental dyslexia. *Brain.* 2004; 128: 261–267.

McDermott S. Explanatory model to describe school district prevalence rated for mental retardation and learning disabilities. *Am J Ment Retard.* 1994; 99: 175–195.

McGarth LM, Smith SD, Penington BF. Breakthroughs in the search for dyslexia genes. *Trends Mol Med.* 2006; 12: 333–341.

McGaugh JL, Cahill L. Interaction of neuromodulatory systems in modulating memory storage. *Behav Brain Res.* 1997; 83: 31–38.

McKelvey JR, Lambert R, Molton R, Shevell MI. Right hemisphere dysfunction in Asperger syndrome. *J Child Neurol.* 1995; 10: 310–314.

McPherson WB, Ackerman PT, Oglesby DM, et al. Event related brain potentials elicited by rhyming and nonrhymng differentiate subgroups of reading disabled adolescents. *Integ Physiol Behav Science.* 1996; 31: 3–17.

Meng H, Smith SD, Hager K, et al. DCDC2 is associated with reading disability and modulates neuronal development in the brain. *Proc Natl Acad Sci USA.* 2005; 102: 17053–17058.

Meyer-Lindenberg A, Mervis CB, Berman KF. Neural mechanisms in Williams syndrome: a unique window to genetic influences on cognition and behavior. *Nat Rev Neurosci.* 2006; 7: 380–393.

Middleton FA, Strick PL. Anatomical evidence for cerebellar and basal ganglia involvement in higher cognitive function. *Science.* 1994; 266: 458–461.

Middleton FA, Strick PL. Cerebellar output channels. *Int Rev Neurobiol.* 1997; 41: 61–82.

Miller CJ, Hynd GW, et al. What ever happened to developmental Gerstmann's syndrome? Link to other pediatric, genetic and neurodevelopmental syndromes. *J Child Neurol.* 2004; 19: 282–290.

Mitchell KG. Curiouse and curiouser: genetic disorders of cortical specialization. *Curr Opin Genet Dev.* 2011; 21: 271–277.

Mody M, Studdert-Kennedy M, Brady S. Speech perception deficits in poor readers: auditory processing or phonological coding? *J Exp Child Psychol.* 1997; 64: 199–231.

Molko N, Cachia A, Riviera D, et al. Brain anatomy in Turner syndrome. Evidence for impaired social and spatial numerical networks. *Cerebral Cortex.* 2004; 14: 840–850.

Molko N, Cachia A, Riviere D, et al. Functional and structural alterations of the intraparietal sulcus in a developmental dyscalculia of genetic origin. *Neuron.* 2003; 40: 847–858.

Mooney R, Spiro JE. Bird song: of tone and tempo in the telencephalon. *Curr Biol.* 1997; 7: 289–291.

Moore CJ, Price CJ. Three distinct ventral occipitotemporal regions for reading and object naming. *Neuroimage.* 1999; 10: 181–192.

Moore LH, Brown WS, Markee TE, Theberge DC, Zvi JL. Bimanual coordination in dyslexic adults. *Neuropsychologia.* 1995; 33: 781–793.

Moore LH, Brown WS, Markee TE, Theberge DC, Zvi JC. Callosal transfer of finger localization information in phonologically dyslexic adults. *Cortex (Italy)* 1996; 32(2): 311–322.

Morgan WP. A case of congenital word-blindness. *Br Med J.* 1896; 2(378): 1896.

Morris DW, Robinson L, Turic D, et al. Family-based association mapping provides evidence for a gene for reading disability on chromosome 15q. *Hum Mol Genet.* 2000; 9: 843–848.

Moruzzi G, Magoun HW. Brain stem reticular formation and activation of the EEG. *Electroencephalog Clin Neurophysiol.* 1949; 4: 455–473.

Murphy LA, Pollatsek A, Well AD. Developmental dyslexia and word retrieval deficits. *Brain Language.* 1988; 35: 1–23.

Murphy MM, Mazzocco MM, Hanich LB. Cognitive characteristics of childrenwith mathematics learning disability (MLD) as a function of the cutoff criterion used to define MLD. *J Learn Disabil.* 2007; 40: 458–478.

Mussolin C, De Volder A, Grandin C, et al. Neural correlates of symbolic number comparison in developmental dyscalculia. *J Cogn Neurosci.* 2010; 22: 860–874.

Myklebust HR. Nonverbal learning disabilities: assessment and intervention. In: Myklebust HR, ed. *Progress in Learning Disabilities.* vol. 3. New York, NY: Grune & Stratton; 1975: 85–121.

Myklebust HR, Johnson DJ. Dyslexia in children. *Exceptional Children.* 1962; 29: 14–25.

N

Naccache L, Dehaene S. The priming method: imaging unconscious repetition priming reveals an abstract representation of number in the parietal lobes. *Cereb Cortex.* 2001; 11: 966–974.

Nader K, Bechara A, Kooy Van Der D. Neurological constraints on behavioral models of activation. *Ann Rev Psychol.* 1997; 48: 85–114.

Naglieri JA, Reardon SM. Traditional IQ is irrelevant to learning disabilities—intelligence is not. *J Learn Disabil.* 1993; 26: 127–133.

Natin K, Snowling MJ. Individual differences in contextual facilitation: evidence from dyslexia and poor reading comprehension. *Child Dev.* 1998; 69: 996–1011.

Nation K, Snowling M. Assessing reading difficulties: the validity and utility of current measures of reading skill. *Br J Educ Psychol.* 1997; 67: 359–370.

National Reading Panel. *Teaching Children to Read: An Evidence-Based Assessment of the Scientific Research Literature on Reading and Its Implications for Reading Instruction.* Washington, DC: National Institute of Child Health and Human Development; 2000.

Neville HJ, Bavelier D. Neural organization of plasticity of language. *Curr Opin Neurobiol.* 1998; 8: 254–258.

Neville HJ, Holcomb PJ, Tallal P. The neurobiology of sensory and language processing in language impaired children. *J Cogn Neurosci.* 1993; 5: 235–253.

Newman SD, Twieg D. Differences in auditory processing of words and pseudowords: an fMRI study. *Hum Brain Mapp.* 2001; 14: 39–47.

Nicoll RA, Malenka RC. A tale of two transmitters. *Science.* 1998; 281: 360–361.

Nicolson R, Fawcett AJ, Dean P. Dyslexia, development and the cerebellum. *Trends Neurosci.* 2001; 24: 515–516.

Nicolson RI, Fawcett AJ, Berry EL, Jenkins IH, Dean P, Brooks DJ. Association of abnormal cerebellar activation with motor learning difficulties in dyslexic adults. *Lancet.* 1999; 353: 1662–1667.

Nicolson RI, Fawcett AJ, Dean P. Developmental dyslexia: the cerebellar deficit hypothesis [review]. *Trends Neurosci.* 2001; 24: 508–511.

Nicolson RI, Fawcett AJ, Dean P. Time estimation deficits in developmental dyslexia: evidence of cerebellar involvement. *Proc R Soc Lond B Biol Sci.* 1995; 259: 43–47.

Nicolson RI, Fawcett AJ. Automaticity: a new framework for dyslexia research? *Cognition.* 1990; 35: 159–182.

Nieder A, Diester I, Tudusciuc D. Temporal and spatial enumeration process in the primate parietal cortex. *Science.* 2006; 313: 1431–1435.

Nieder A, Freedman DJ, Miller EK. Representation of the quantity of visual items in the primate prefrontal cortex. *Science.* 2002; 297: 1708–1711.

Nieder A, Miller EK. A parieto-frontal network for visual numerical information in the monkey *Proc Natl Acad Sci USA.* 2004; 101: 7457–7462.

NJCLD Interagency Committee on Learning Disabilities. *Learning Disabilities: a Report to the US Congress.* Bethesda MD: National Institutes of Health; 1987.

Nopola-Hemmi J, Myllyluoma B, Haltia T, et al. A dominant gene for developmental dyslexia on chromosome 3. *J Med Genet.* 2001; 38: 658–664.

Nopola-Hemmi J, Taipale M, Haltia T, Lehesjoki AE, Voutilainen A, Kere J. Two translocations of chromosome 15q associated with dyslexia. *J Med Genet.* 2000; 37: 771–775.

North K, Joy P, Yuille D, et al. Specific learning disability in children with Neurofibromatosis type I: significance of MRI abnormalities. *Neurology.* 1994; 44: 878–883.

Nothen MM, Schulte-Korne G, Grimm T, et al. Genetic linkage analysis with dyslexia: evidence for linkage of spelling disability to chromosome 15. *Eur Child Adolesc Psychiatry.* 1999; 8(suppl 3): 56–59.

O

O'Donnell J, Hawkins JD, Catalano RF, Abbott RD, Day LE. Preventing school failure, drug use, and delinquency among low income children: long term intervention in elementary schools. *Am J Orthopsychiatry*. 1995; 65: 87–100.

Ogawa S, Lee TM. Magnetic resonance imaging of blood vessels at high fields: in vivo and in vitro measurements and image simulation. *Magn Resort Med*. 1990; 16: 9–18.

Olson RK. Dyslexia nature and nurture. *Dyslexia*. 2002; 8143–8159.

Orton ST. *Reading, Writing and Speech Problems in Children: A Presentation of Certain Types of Disorders in the Development of the Language Faculty*. New York, NY: W.W. Norton; 1937.

Orton ST. Word blindness in school children. *Arch Neurol Psychiatr*. 1925; 14: 581–615.

Ostrosky-Solis F, Canseco E, Meneses LS, et al. Neuroelectric correlates of a neuropsychological model of word decoding and semantic processing in reading disabled children. *Int J Neurosci*. 1987; 35: 1–20.

Ouvrier RA, Goldsmith RF Ouvrier S, Williams IC. The value of the mini-mental state examination in childhood: a preliminary study. *J Child Neurol*. 1993; 8: 145–148.

P

Padget SY, Knight DF, Sawyer DJ. Tennessee meets the challenge of dyslexia. *Ann Dyslexia*. 1996; 46: 49–72.

Paller KA, Kutas M, Mayes AR. Neural correlates of encoding in an incidental learning paradigm. *Electroencephalogr Clin Neurophysiol*. 1987; 67: 360–371.

Parent A, Hazrati LN. Functional anatomy of the basal ganglia. The cortico-basal ganglia-thalamo-cortical loop. *Brain Res Rev*. 1995; 20: 91–127.

Paulesu E, Démonet J-F, Fazio F, et al. Dyslexia: cultural diversity and biological unity. *Science*. 2001; 291: 2165–2167.

Paulesu E, Frith U, Snowling M, et al. Is developmental dyslexia a disconnection syndrome? Evidence from PET scanning. *Brain*. 1996; 119: 143–157.

Paulesu E, et al. A cultural effect on brain function. *Nat Neurosci*. 2000; 3: 91–96.

Pauls DL, Leckman JF, Cohen DJ. Familial relationship betweek Gilles de la Tourette's syndrome, attention deficit disorder, learning disabilities, speech disorder and stuttering. *J Am Acad Child Adolesc Psychiatr*. 1993; 32: 1044–1050.

Pelletier PM, Ahmed SA, Rourke BP. Classification rules for basic phonological processing disabilities and nonverbal learning disabilities: formulation and external validity. *Child Neuropsychol*. 2001; 7: 84–98.

Pennington BF. The genetics of dyslexia. *J Child Psychol Psychiatr*. 1990; 31: 193–201.

Pennington BF. *Diagnosing Learning Disorders: A Neuropsychological Framework*. New York, NY: Guilford Press; 1991.

Pennington BF, Filipek PA, Lefly D, et al. Brain morphometry in reading-disabled twins. *Neurology*. 1999; 53: 723–729.

Pennington BF, Gilger JW, Olson RK, DeFries JC. The external validity of age- versus I.Q.-discrepancy definitions of reading disability: Lessons from a twin study. *J Learn Disabil*. 1992; 25: 562–573.

Pennington BF, Gilger JW, Pauls D, et al. Evidence for major gene transmission of developmental dyslexia. *JAMA*. 1991; 266: 1527–1534.

Perviainen T, Helenius P, Poskiparta E, et al. Cortical sequence of word perception in beginning readers. *J Neurosci*. 2006; 26: 6052–6061.

Peterson KM, Reis A, Ingvar M. Cognitive processing in literate and illiterate subjects: a review of some recent behavioral and functional neuroimaging data. *Scand J Psychol*. 2001; 42: 251–267.

Petryshen TL, Kaplan BJ, Fu Liu M, et al. Evidence for a susceptibility locus on chromosome 6q influencing phonological coding dyslexia. *Am J Med Genet*. 2001; 105: 507–517.

Petryshen TL, Kaplan BJ, Hughes ML, Tzenova J, Field LL. Supportive evidence for the DYX3 dyslexia susceptibility gene in Canadian families. *J Med Genet*. 2002; 39: 125–126.

Piazza M. Pinel P, LeBihan D, Dehaene S. A magnitude code common to neumerosities and number symbols in human intraparietal cortex. *Neuron*. 2007; 53: 293–305.

Plaut DC, McClelland JL, Seidenberg MS, Patterson K. Understanding normal and impaired word reading: computational principles in quasi-regular domains. *Psychol Rev*. 1996; 103: 56–115.

Plomin R, Kovas Y. Generalist genes and learning disabilities. *Psychol Bull*. 2005; 131: 592–617.

Poblano A, Cordoba de Caballero B, Castillo I, Cortes V. Electro oculographic recordings reveal readin deficiencies in learning disabled children. *Act Med Res*. 1996; 27: 509–512.

Poeppel D. A critical review of PET studies of phonological processing. *Brain Language*. 1006; 55: 317–351.

Poldrack RA, Wagner AD, Prull MW, Desmond JE, Glover GH, Gabrieli JD. Functional specialization for semantic and phonological processing in the left inferior prefrontal cortex. *Neuroimage*. 1999; 10: 15–35.

Polk TA, Farah MJ. The neural development and organization of letter recognition: evidence from functional neuroimaging, computational modeling and behavioral studies. *Proc Natl Acad Sci USA*. 1998; 95: 847–852.

Price CJ, Devlin JT. The myth of the visual word form area [review]. *Neuroimage*. 2003; 19: 473–481.

Price CJ, Friston KJ. Cognitive conjunction: a new approach to brain activation experiments. *Neuroimage*. 1997; 5: 261–270.

Price GR, Holloway I, Rasanen P, Vesterinen M, Ansari D. Impaired parietal magnitude processing in developmental dyscalculia. *Curr Biol*. 2007; 17: R1042–1043.

Price C, Moore C, Frackowiak RSJ. The effect of varying stimulus rate and duration brain activity during reading. *Neuroimage*. 1996; 3: 40–52.

Pringle Morgan W. A case of congenital word blindness. *Br Med J*. 1896; 2: 1378.

Public Law 94-142 (1975). The Education for all Handicapped Children Act, and the subsequent Individuals with Disabilities Education Act (1992).

Public Law 94-142: Education for All Handicapped Children Act of 1975. (August 23, 1977). 20 USC 1401 et seq. *Fed Reg*. 42 (163), 42474–42518.

Pugh KR, Mencl WE, Shaywitz BA, et al. The angular gyrus in developmental dyslexia: task-specific differences in functional connectivity within posterior cortex. *Psychol Sci*. 2000; 11: 51–56.

Pugh KR, Shaywitz BA, Shaywitz SE, et al. Cerebral organization of component processes in reading. *Brain*. 1996; 119: 1221–1238.

Pugh KR, Shaywitz BA, Shaywitz SE, et al. Predicting reading performance from neuroimaging profiles: a relation between phonological effects in printed word identification and cerebral organization of language processes. *J Exper Psychol*. 1997; 23: 299–318.

Pujol J, Vendrell P, Junque C, et al. When does human brain development end? Evidence of corpus callosum growth up to adulthood. *Ann Neurol*. 1993; 34: 71–75.
Purvis KL, Tannock B. Language abilities in children with attention deficit hyperactivity disorder, reading disabilities and normal controls. *J Abnorm Child Psychol*. 1997; 25: 133–144.

Q

Quine L, Rutter DR. First diagnosis of severe mental and physical disability: a study of doctor-patient communication. *J Child Psychol Psychiatry*. 1994; 35: 1273–1287.

R

Rae C, Harasty JA, Dzendrowskyj TE, et al. Cerebellar morphology in developmental dyslexia. *Neuropsychologia*. 2002; 40: 1285–1292.
Rae C, Lee MA, Dixon RM, et al. Metabolic abnormalities in developmental dyslexia detected by 1H magnetic resonance spectroscopy. *Lancet*. 1998; 351: 1849–1852.
Raichle ME. Imaging the mind. Semin Nucl Med 1998; 28: 278–289.
Raichle ME, Fiez JA, Videen TO, et al. Practice-related changes in human brain functional anatomy during nonmotor learning. *Cereb Cortex*. 1994; 4: 342–353.
Ramus F. Neurobiology of dyslexia: a reinterpretation of the data. *Trends Neurosci*. 2004; 27: 720–726.
Ramus F, Pidgeon E, Frith U. The relationship between motor control and phonology in dyslexic children. *J Child Psychol Psychiatry*. 2003; 44: 712–722.
Ramus F, Rosen S, Dakin SC, et al. Theories of developmental dyslexia: insights from a multiple case study of dyslexic adults. *Brain*. 2003; 126: 841–865.
Rappoport JL, Inoff-Germain G. Responses to methylphenidate in Attention-Deficit/Hyperactivity Disorder and normal children: update 2002. *J Atten Disord*. 2002; Suppl 1: S57–60.
Rauscheker AM, Deutc GK, Ben-Shachar M, Schwartzman A, Perry LM, Dougherty RF. Reading impairment in a patient with missing arcuate fasciculus. *Neuropsychologia*. 2009; 47: 180–194.
Raymond JL, Lisberger SG, Mauk MO. The cerebellum: a neuronal learning. *Science*. 1996; 272: 1126–1131.
Rayner K, Foorman BR, Perfetti CA, et al. How psychological science informs the teaching of reading. *Psychol Sci*. 2001; 2: 31–74.
Reschly DJ, Tilly WD. Reform trend and system design alternatives. In: Reschly, D, Tilly W., Grimes, J, eds. *Special Education in Transition*. Longmont CO: Sopris West; 1999:19–48.
Renvall H, Hari R. Auditory cortical responses to speech-like stimuli in dyslexic adults. *J Cogn Neurosci*. 2002; 14: 757–768.
Renvall H, Hari R. Diminished auditory mismatch fields in dyslexic adults. *Ann Neurol*. 2003; 53: 551–557.
Reynolds CA, Hewitt JK, Erikson MT, et al. The genetics of children's oral reading performance. *J Child Psychol Psychiatry*. 1996; 37: 425–434.
Rezaie R, Simos PG, Fletcher JM, et al. Engagement of temporal lobe regions predicts response to educational interventions in adolescent struggling readers. *Dev Neuropsychol*. 2011; 36: 869–888.
Rezaie R, Simos PG, Fletcher JM, et al. The timing and strength of regional brain activation associated with word recognition in children with reading difficulties. *Front Hum Neurosci*. 2011; 5: 45.

Richards T, Corina D, Serafini S, et al. Effects of a phonologicallydriven treatment for dyslexia on lactate levels measured by proton MRI spectroscopic imaging. *Am J Neuroradiol.* 2000; 21: 916–922.

Richardson U, Leppänen PHT, Leiwo M, Lyytinen H. Speech perception differs in infants at familial risk for dyslexia as early as six months of age. *Dev Neuropsychol.* 2003.

Richlan F, Kronbichler M, Wimmer H. Functional abnormalities in the dyslexic brain: a quantitative meta-analysis of neuroimaging studies. *Hum Brain Mapp.* 2009; 30: 3299–3308.

Rimrod SL, Peterson DJ, Denckla MB, et al. White matter microstructural differences linked the left perisylvian language network in children with dyslexia. *Cortex.* 2010; 46(6): 739–749.

Risold PY, Swanson LW. Structural evidence for functional domains in the rat hippocampus. *Science.* 1996; 272: 1484–1486.

Riva D, Giorgi C. The cerebellum contributes to higher functions during development: evidence from a series of children surgically treated for posterior fossa tumours. *Brain.* 2000; 123: 1051–1061.

Rivera SM, Menon V, White CD, Glaser B, Reiss AL. Functional brain activation during arithmetic processing in females with Fragile X syndrome is related to FMR1 protein expression. *Hum Brain Mapp.* 2002; 16: 206–218.

Rivera SM, Reiss AL, Eckert MA. Menon V. Developmental changes in mental arithmetic: evidence for increased functional specialization in the left inferior parietal cortex. *Cereb Cortex.* 2005; 15: 1779–1790.

Roarke BP. Arithmatic disabilities, specific and otherwise: a neuropsychological perspective. *J Learn Disabil.* 1993; 26: 214–226.

Robichon F, Bouchard P, Demonet J, Habib M. Developmental dyslexia: re-evaluation of the corpus callosum in male adults. *Eur Neurol.* 2000b; 43: 233–237.

Robichon F, Levrier O, Farnarier P, Habib M. Developmental dyslexia: atypical cortical asymmetries and functional significance. *Eur J Neurol.* 2000a; 7: 35–46.

Rosenberger PB. Perceptual-motor and attentional correlates of developmental dyscalculia. *Ann Neurol.* 1989; 26(2): 216–220.

Ross ED. The aprosodias: functional anatomic organization of the affective components of language in the right hemisphere. *Arch Neurol.* 1981; 38: 561–569.

Rosseli M, Matute E, Pinto N, Ardila A. Memory abilities in children with subtypes of dyscalculia. *Dev Neuropsychol.* 2006; 30: 801–818.

Rothenberger A, Moll GH. Standard EEG and dyslexia in children—new evidence for specific correlates? *Acta Paedopsychiatr.* 1994; 56: 209–218.

Rotzer S, Loenneker T, Kucina K, Martin E, et al. Dysfunctional neural network of spatial working memory contributes to developmental dyscalculia. *Neuropsychologia.* 2009; 47: 2859–2865.

Rourke BP. Syndrome of nonverbal learning disabilities: the final common pathway of white-matter disease/dysfunction. *Clin Neuropsychol.* 1987; 1: 209–234.

Rourke BP, Young GC, Leenaars AA. A childhood learning disability that predisposes those afflicted to adolescent and adult depression and suicide risk. *J Learn Disabil.* 1989; 22: 169–175.

Rovet JF. The psychoeducational characteristics of children with Turner syndrome. *J Learn Disabil.* 1993; 26: 333–341.

Rozzini R, Zanetti O, Bianchetti A. Treatment of cognitive impairment secondary to degenerative dementia. Effectiveness of oxiracetam therapy. *Acta Neurol (Napoli).* 1993; 15: 44–52.

Rubinstein O, Henik A. Developmental dyscalculia: heterogeneity might not mean differenct mechanisms. *Trends Cogn Sci.* 2009; 13: 92–99.

Rubishon F, Habib M. Abnormal callosalmorphology in male adult dyslexics: relationship to handedness and phonological abilities. *Brain Lang.* 1998; 62: 127–146.

Rudel RG, Tauber HL, Twitchell TE. Levels of impairment of sensory-motor functions in children with early brain damage. *Neuropsychologia.* 1974; 12: 95–108.

Rugg MD, Walla P, Schioerscheidt AM, et al. Neural correlates of depth of processing effects on recollection: evidence from brain potentials and positron emission tomography. *Exp Brain Res.* 1998; 123: 18–23.

Rumsey JM, Andreason P, Zametkin AJ, et al. Failure to activate the left temporoparietal cortex in dyslexia. *Arch Neurol.* 1992; 49: 527–534.

Rumsey JM, Nace K, Donohue B, Wise D, Maisog JM, Andreason P. A positron emission tomographic study of impaired word recognition and phonological processing in dyslexic men. *Arch Neurol.* 1997; 54: 562–573.

Rusconi E, Pinel P, Eger E, et al. A disconnection account of Gerstmann syndrome. *Ann Neurol.* 2009; 66: 654–662.

S

Safer DJ, Zito JM, Fine EM. Increased methylphenidate usage for attention deficit disorder in the 1990. *Pediatrics.* 1996; 98: 1084–1088.

Sagi D, Tanne D. Learning: Learning to see. *Curr Opin Neurobiol.* 1994; 4: 195–199.

Salmelin R, Service E, Kiesila P, Uutela K, Salonen O. Impaired visual word processing in dyslexia revealed with magnetoencephalography. *Ann Neurol.* 1996; 40: 157–162.

Scarborough HS. Very early language deficits in dyslexic children. *Child Development.* 1990; 61: 1728–1743.

Schacter DL. Memory and awareness. *Science.* 1998; 280: 59–60.

Schatschneider C, Torgesen JK. Using our current understanding of dyslexia to support early identification and intervention. *J Child Neurol.* 2004; 19: 759–765.

Schlaggar BL, Brown TT, Lugar HM, et al. Functional neuroanatomical differences between adults and school-age children in the processing of single words. *Science.* 2002; 296: 1476–1479.

Schmahamann JD. From movement to thought: anatomic substrates of the cerebellar contribution to cognitive processing. *Hum Brain Map.* 1996; 4: 174–198.

Schneider W, Kuspert P, Roth E et al. Short and long term effects of training phonological awareness in kindergarten: evidence for two German studies. *J Exp Child Psychol* 1997; 66: 311–340.

Schonfeld IS, Shaffer D, Barmack JE. Neurological soft signs and school achievement: the mediating effects of sustained attention. *J Abnorm Child Psychol.* 1989; 17: 575–596.

Schulte-Körne G, Deimel W, Bartling J, Remschmidt H. Auditory processing and dyslexia: evidence for a specific speech processing deficit. *Neuroreport.* 1998a; 9: 337–340.

Schulte-Körne G, Deimel W, Bartling J, Remschmidt H. Role of auditory temporal processing for reading and spelling disability. *Percept Motor Skills.* 1998b; 86: 1043–1047.

Schulte-Körne G, Grimm T, Nothen MM, et al. Evidence for linkage of spelling disability to chromosome 15. *Am J Hum Genet.* 1998; 63: 279–282.

Schultz RT, Cho NK, Staib LH, Kiev LE, et al. Brain morphology in normal and dyslexic children: the influence of sex and age. *Ann Neurol.* 1994; 35: 732–742.

Schumacher J, Antoni H, Dahdough F, Konig IR et al. Strong genetic evidence of DCDC2 as a susceptibility gene for dyslexia. *Am J Hum Genet*. 2006; 78: 52–63.

Schumacher J, Hoffman P, Schmal C, et al. Genetic of dyslexia: the evolving landscape. *J Med Genet*. 2007; 44: 289–297.

Scoville WB. Amnesia after bilateral mesial temporal lobe excision. Introduction to case MH. *Neuropsychologia*. 1968; 6: 211–213.

Segui J, Fraisse P. Le temps de réaction verbale. III. Réponses spécifiques et réponses catégorielles à des stimulus objets. *Année Psychol*. 1968; 68: 69–82.

Seki A, Koeda T, Sugihara S, et al. A functional magnetic resonance imaging study during reading in Japanese dyslexic children. *Brain Dev*. 2001; 23: 312–316.

Semrud-Clikeman M, Biederman J, Sprich-Buckminster S, Lehman BK, Faraone SV, Norman D. Comorbidity between ADHD and learning disability: a review and report in a clinically referred sample. *J Am Acad Child Adolesc Psychiatry*. 1992; 31(3): 439–448.

Semrud-Clikeman M, Hynd GW. Right hemispheric dysfunction in nonverbal learning disabilities: social, academic, and adaptive functioning in adults and children. *Psychol Bull*. 1990; 107: 196–209.

Shadmehr R, Holcomb HH. Neural correlates of motor memory consolidation. *Science*. 1997; 277: 821–825.

Shalev RS, Auerbach J, Manor O, Gross-Tsur V. Developmental dyscalculia: prevalence and prognosis. *Eur J Child Adol Psychiatr*. 2000; 9(suppl 2): 1158–1164.

Shalev RS, Gross-tsur V. Developmental dyscalculia. *Pediatr Neurol*. 2001; 24: 337–342.

Shalev RS, Manor O, Auerbach J, Gross-Tsur V. Persistence of developmental dyscalculia: what counts? Results from a 3-year prospective follow-up study. *J Pediatr*. 1998; 133(3): 358–362.

Shalev RS, Manor O, Gross-Tsur V. Developmental dyscalculia: a perspective six year follow up. *Dev Med Child Neurol*. 2005; 47: 1215.

Shapiro BS, Gallico RP. Learning disabilities. *Pediatr Clin North Am*. 1993; 40: 491–505.

Shapiro BS, Gallico RP. Learning disabilities. *Res Q*. 1986; 21: 360–407.

Share DL, Mcbee R, Silva PA. IQ and reading progress: a test of the capacity notion of IQ. *J Am Acad Child Adol Psychiatry*. 1989; 28: 97–100.

Shatz CJ. The developing brain. *Sci Am*. 1992; 9: 61–67.

Shaywitz BA. The role of functional magnetic resonance imaging in understanding reading and dyslexia. *Dev Neuropsychol*. 2006; 30(1): 613–632.

Shaywitz SE. Current concepts: dyslexia. *N Engl J Med*. 1998; 338: 307–312.

Shaywitz SE. *Overcoming Dyslexia: A New and Complete Science-Based Program for Reading Problems at Any Level*. New York, NY: Knopf; 2003.

Shaywitz SE, Shaywitz B. Dyslexia: specific reading disability. *Pediatr* Rev. 2003; 24: 147–153.

Shaywitz SE, Shaywitz BA. Reading disability and the brain. *Educ Leader*. 2004; 61: 6–11.

Shaywitz SE, Shaywitz BA. The science of reading and its implications for overcoming dyslexia. *Educ Canada*. 2004; 44: 20–23.

Shaywitz SE, Shaywitz BA. Dyslexia (specific reading disability). *Biol Psychiatry*. 2005; 57: 1301–1309.

Shaywitz BA, Fletcher JM, Shaywitz SE. Defining and classifying learning disabilities and attention deficit hyperactivity Disorder. *J Child Neurol*. 1995; 10(suppl 1): 550–557.

Shaywitz SE, Morris R, Shaywitz BA. The education of dyslexic children from childhood to young adulthood. *Annu. Rev. Psychol*. 2008; 59: 451–475.

Shaywitz SE, Shaywitz BA, Fletcher JM, Escobar MD. Prevalence of reading disability in boys and girls: results of the Connecticut Longitudinal Study. *JAMA.* 1990; 264: 998–1002.

Shaywitz SE, Escobar MD, Shaywitz BA, et al. Evidence that dyslexia may represnt the lower tail of a normal distribution of reading ability. *N Engl J Med.* 1992; 326: 145–150.

Shaywitz SE, Fletcher JM, Holahan JM, et al. Persistence of dyslexia: the Connecticut Longitudinal Study at adolescence. *Pediatrics.* 1999; 104: 1351–1359.

Shaywitz SE, Shaywitz BA, Fulbright RK, et al. Neural systems for compensation and persistence: young adult outcome of childhood reading disability. *Biol Psychiatry.* 2003; 54: 25–33.

Shaywitz BA, Shaywitz SE, Blachman BA, et al. Development of left occipitotemporal systems for skilled reading in children after a phonologically-based intervention. *Biol Psychiatry.* 2004; 55: 926–933.

Shaywitz SE, Shaywitz BA, Pugh KR, et al. Functional disruption in the organization of the brain for reading in dyslexia. *Proc Natl Acad Sci USA.* 1998; 95: 2636–2641.

Shaywitz BA, Shaywitz SE, Pugh KR, et al. Disruption of posterior brain systems for reading in children with developmental dyslexia. *Biol Psychiatry.* 2002; 52: 101–110.

Sherrington CS. Santiago Ramon J Cajal 1852-1934. *Obit Fell R Soc.* 1935; 1: 424–441.

Silani G, Frith U, Demonet J-F, et al. Brain abnormalities underlying altered activation in dyslexia: a voxel based morphometry study. *Brain.* 2005; 128(10): 2453–2461.

Silva AJ, Paylor R, Wehner JM, Tonegawa J. Impaired spatial learning in alpha calcium calmodulin kinase II mutant mice. *Science.* 1992; 257: 206–211.

Silver L. Psychological and family problems associated with learning disabilities: assessment and intervention. *J Amer Acad Child Adol Psychol.* 1989; 28(3): 319–325.

Silver LB. Controversial therapies. *J Child Neurol.* 1995; (suppl 1): S96–100.

Simos PG, Fletcher JM, Bergman E, et al. Dyslexia specific brain activation profile becomes normal following successful remedial training. *Neurology.* 2002; 58: 1203–1213.

Simos P, Fletcher J, DentonC, et al. Magnetic source imaging studies of dyslexia interventions. *Dev Neuropsychol.* 2006; 30: 591–611.

Simos PG, Breier JI, Bergman E, Papanicolau AC. Cerebral mechanisms involved in word reading in dyslexic children: a magnetic source imaging approach. *Cerebral Cortex.* 2000; 10: 809–816.

Simos PG, Fletcher JM, Bergman E, et al. Dyslexia-specific brain activation profile becomes normal following successful remedial training. *Neurology.* 2002; 58: 1203–1213.

Simos PG, Kanatsouli K, Fletcher JM, Sarkari S, et al. Aberrant spatiotemporal activation profile associated with mat difficulties in children: a magnetic source imaging study. *Neuropsychology.* 2008; 22(5): 571–584.

Simos PG, Rezaie R, Fletcher JM, et al. functional disruption of the brain mechanism for reading: effects of comorbidity and task difficulty among children with developmental learning problems. *Neuropsychology.* 2011; (25)4: 520–534.

Sing WT, Perfetti CA, Jin Z, Tan LH. Biological abnormality of impaired of impaired reading is constrained by culture. *Nature.* 2004; 431: 71–76.

Singer HS, Scheurholz LJ, Denckla MB. Learning difficulties in children with Tourette syndrome. *J Chil Neurol.* 1995; (suppl 7): S58–61.

Sinyor D, Jacques P, Kaloupek DG, Becker R, et al. PostStroke depression and lesion location. An attempted replication. *Brain.* 1986; 109: 537–546.

Skottun BC. The magnocellular deficit theory of dyslexia: the evidence from contrast sensitivity. *Vision Res.* 2000; 40: 111–127.

Slaghuis WL, Ryan JF. Spatio-temporal contrast sensitivity, coherent motion, and visible persistence in developmental dyslexia. *Vision Res.* 1999; 39: 651–668.

Smart D, Sanson A, Prior M. Connections between reading disability and behavioral problems: testing temporal and causal hypotheses. *J Abnorm Child psychol.* 1996; 24: 363–383.

Smith SD, Kimberling WJ, Pennington BF, Lubs HA. Specific reading disability: identification of an inherited form through linkage analysis. *Science.* 1983; 219: 1345–1347.

Snowling M, van Wagtendonk B, Stafford C. Object naming deficits in developmental dyslexia. *J Res Reading.* 1988; 11: 678–685.

Snowling MJ. *Dyslexia.* 2nd ed. Oxford, UK: Blackwell; 2000.

Snowling MJ. Phonemic deficits in developmental dyslexia. *Psychol Res.* 1981; 43: 219–234.

Snowling MJ, Hulme C. Evidence based interventions for reading and language difficulties: creating a virtuous circle. *Br J Educ Psychol.* 2011; 81: 1–23.

Solman RT, Dain SJ, Lim HS, May JG. Reading related wavelength and spatial frequency effects in visual spatial location. *Ophthalmic Physiol Opt.* 1995; 15: 125–132.

Soltesz F, et al. A combined event related potential and neuropsychological investigation of developmental dyscalculia. *Neurosci Lett.* 2007; 417: 181–186.

Soorani-Lunsing RJ, Hadders-Algra M, Olinga AA, et al. Is minor neurological dsfunction at 12 years related to behavior and cognition? *Dev Med Child Neurol.* 1993; 35: 321–330.

Sprague RL, Sleator EK. Methylphenidate in hyperkinetic children: differences in dose effects on learning and social behavior. *Science.* 1977; 198: 1274–1276.

Squire LR, Zola SM. Structure and function of declarative and nondeclerative memory systems. *Proc Natl Acad Sci USA.* 1996; 93: 13515–13522.

Stanescu-Cosson R, Fiez JA, Videen TO, et al. Practice-related changes in human brain functional anatomy during nonmotor learning. *Cereb Cortex.* 1994; 4: 342–353.

Stanescu-Cosson R, Pinel PF, van De Moortele D, et al. Understanding dissociations in dyscalculia: a brain imaging study of the impact of number size on the cerebral networks for exact and approximate calculation. *Brain.* 2000; 123: 2240–2250.

Stanley PD, Dai Y, Nolan RF. Differences in depression and self esteem reported by learning disabled and behavior disordered middle school students. *J Adolesc.* 1997; 20: 219–222.

Stanowich KE. Explaining the difference between the dyslexic and the garden variety poor reader: the phonological—care variable—difference model. *J Learn Disabil.* 1988; 21: 590–604.

Stanovich KE. Explaining the difference between the dyslexic and the gardern variety poor reader: the phonological core variable difference model. *J Learn Disabil.* 1988; 21: 590–604.

Stanovich KE. Discrepancy definitions of reading disability: Has intelligence led us astray? *Read Res Quart.* 1991; 26: 7–29.

Stanovich KE, Siegel LS. Phenotypic performance profile of children with reading disabilities: a regression-based test of the phonological-core variable-difference model. *J Educ Psychol.* 1994; 86: 24–53.

Stanovich KE, Siegel LS, Gottardo A. Converging evidence for phonological and surface subtypes of reading disability. *J Educ Psychol.* 1997; 89: 114–127.

Stein J. The magnocellular theory of developmental dyslexia. *Dyslexia.* 2001; 7: 12–36.

Stein J. Visual motion sensitivity and reading. *Neuropsychologia.* 2003; 41: 1785–1793.

Stein J, Walsh V. To see but not to read: the magnocellular theory of dyslexia. *Trends Neurosci.* 1997; 20: 147–152.

Steinman BA, Steinman SB, Lehmkuhle S. Transient visual attention is dominated by the magnocellular stream. *Vision Res.* 1997; 37: 17–23.

Stelmack RM, Saxe BJ, Noldy-Cullum N, Campbell KB, Armitage R. Recognition memory for words and event related potentials: a comparison of normal and disabled readers. *J Clin Exp Neuropsychol.* 1988; 10: 185–200.

Stoodley CJ. The cerebellum and cognition: evidence fromfunctional imaging studies. *Cerebellum.* 2012; 11: 352–365.

Stothard SE, Hulme C. A comparison of reading comprehension and decoding difficulties in children. In: Cornoldi, C, Oakhill, J, eds. *Reading comprehension difficulties: Processes and intervention.* Mahawah, NJ: Erlbaum; 1996:93–112.

Stough LM, Aguirre-Roy AR. Learning disabilities in Costa Rica: challenges for "an army of teachers". *J Learn Disabil.* 1997; 30: 566–571.

Strauss AA, Lehtinen LE. *Psychopathology and Education of the Brain-Injured Child.* vol. 1. New York, NY: Grune & Stratton; 1947.

Studdert-KennedyM,ModyM.Auditorytemporalperceptiondeficitsinreading-impaired:a critical review of the evidence. *Psychol Bull Rev.* 1995; 2: 508–514.

Sutton JP, Whitten JL, Topa M, et al. Evoked potential maps in learning disabled children. *Electroenceph Clin Neurophysiol.* 1986; 65: 399–404.

Swan D, Goswami U. Picture naming deficits in developmental dyslexia: the phonological representations hypothesis. *Brain Language.* 1997; 56: 334–353.

Swanson HL. Reading research for students with LD: a meta-analysis of intervention outcomes. *J Learn Disabil.* 1999; 32: 504–532.

Swanson HL. Working memory in learning disability subgroups. *J Exp Child Psychol.* 1993; 56(1): 87–114.

Swanson HL, Ashbaker MH, Lee CJ. Working memory in learning disability subgroups. *Exp Child Psychol (US)* 1996; 61(3): 242–275.

Swanson HL, Harris K, Graham S, eds. *Handbook of Learning Disabilities.* New York, NY: Guilford Press; 2003.

T

Taipale M, Kaminen N, Nopola-Hemmi J, et al. A candidate gene for developmental dyslexia encodes a nuclear tetratricopeptide repeat domain protein dynamically regulated in the brain. *Proc Natl Acad Sci USA.* 2003; 100: 11553–11558.

Tallal P. Auditory temporal perception, phonics and reading disabilities in children. *Brain Language.* 1980; 9: 182–198.

Tallal P. The science of literacy: from the laboratory to the classroom. *Proc Natl Acad Sci USA.* 2000; 97: 2402–2404.

Tallal P, Chase C, Russell G, Schmitt RL. Evaluation of the efficacy of piracetam in treating information processing, reading and writing disorders in dyslexic children. *Int J Psychophysiol.* 1986; 4: 41–52.

Tallal P, Miller SL, Bedi G, et al. Language comprehension in language-learning impaired children improved with acoustically modified speech. *Science.* 1996; 271: 81–84.

Tallal P, Miller S, Fitch RH. Neurobiological basis of speech: a case for the preeminence of temporal processing [review]. *Ann NY Acad Sci.* 1993; 682: 27–47.

Tallal P, Piercy M. Defects of non-verbal auditory perception in children with developmental dyslexia. *Nature.* 1973; 241: 468–469.

Tarkiainen A, Helenius P, Salmelin R. Category specific occipitotemporal activation during face perception in dyslexic individuals: an MRG study. *Neuroimage*. 2003; 19: 1194–1204.

Taylor MJ, Keenan NK. Event related potential to visual and language stimuli in normal and dyslexic children. *Psychophysiology*. 1990; 271: 318–327.

Temple CM. Developmental and acquired dyslexia. *Cortex*. 2006; 42: 898–910.

Temple E, Deutsch GK, Poldrack RA. Neural deficits in children with dyslexia ameliorated by behavioral remediation: evidence from functional MRI. *PNAS*. 2003; 100: 2860–2865.

Temple E, Poldrack RA, Protopapas A, et al. Disruption of the neural response to rapid acoustic stimuli in dyslexia: evidence from functional MRI. *Proc Natl Acad Sci USA*. 2000; 97: 13907–13912.

Temple E, Poldrack RA, Salidis J, et al. Disrupted neural responses to phonological and orthographic processing in dyslexic children: an fMRI study. *Neuroreport*. 2001; 12: 299–307.

Thornton CA, Langrall CW, Jones GA. Mathematics instructions for elementary students with learning disabilities. *J Learn Disabil*. 1997; 30: 142–150.

Tonnessen FE, Lokken A, Hoien T, Lundberg L. Dyslexia, left handedness andimmune-disorders. *Arch Neurol*. 1993; 50: 411–416.

Torgesen J, Alexander A, Wagner R, et al. Intensive remedial instruction for children with severe reading disabilities: immediate and long-term outcomes from two instructional approaches. *J Learn Disabil*. 2001; 34: 33–58.

Torgesen JK. Recent discoveries on remedial interventions for children with dyslexia. In: Snowling MJ, Hulme C, eds. *The Science of Reading: A Handbook*. Oxford, UK: Blackwell; 2005:521–537.

Torgesen JK, Wagner RK, Rashotte CA, et al. Preventing reading failure on young children with phonological processing disabilities. Group and individual responses to instruction. *J Educ Psychol*. 1999; 91: 579–593.

Tranel D, Hall LE, Olson S, et al. Evidence for a right-hemisphere developmental learning disability. *Dev Neuropsychol*. 1987; 3: 113–127.

Tsatsanis KD, Fuerst DR, Rourke BP. Psychosocial dimensions of learning disabilities: external validation and relationship with age and academic functioning. *J Learn Disabil*. 1997; 30: 490–502.

Tur-Kaspa H, Bryan T. Teacher's ratings of the social competence and school adjustments of students with LD in elementary and junior high school. *J learn Disabil*. 1995; 28: 44–52.

Turkeltaub PE, Gareau L, Flowers DL, Zeffiro TA, Eden GF. Development of neural mechanisms for reading. *Nat Neurosci*. 2003; 6: 767–767.

U

Uchida I, Kikyo H, Nakujima K, Konishi S, et al. Activation of lateral extrastriate areas during orthographic processing of Japanese characters studied with fMRI. *Neuroimage*. 1999; 9: 208–215.

Ungerleider LG. Functional brain imaging studies of cortical mechanisms for memory. *Science*. 1995; 270: 769–775.

V

Vallance DD, Winter MG. Discourse processes underlying social competence in children with language learning disabilities. *Dev Psychopathol*. 1997; 9: 95–108.

Van Eimeren L, Gruber RH, Koschutnid K, Reishofer G, Ebner F, Ansari D. Structure-function relationship underlying calculations: a combined diffusion tensor imaging and fMRI study. *Neuroimage*. 2010; 52: 358–363.

van Harskamp NJ, Rudge P, Cipolotti L. Are multiplication facts implemented by the left supramarginal and angular gyri. *Neuropsychologia*. 2002; 40: 1786–1793.

van Ingelghem M, van Wieringen A, Wouters J, et al. Psychophysical evidence for a general temporal processing deficit in children with dyslexia. *Neuroreport*. 2001; 12: 3603–3607.

Vellutino FA. An understanding of dyslexia: psychological factors in specific reading disability. In: Benton AL, Pearl D, eds. *Dyslexia: An Appraisal of Current Knowledge*. New York, NY: Oxford University Press; 1978:61–111.

Vellutino FR. *Dyslexia: Research and Theory*. Cambridge, MA: MIT Press; 1979.

Vellutino FR, Fletcher JM, Snowling MJ, Scanlon DM. Specific reading disability (dyslexia): what have we learned in the past four decades? *J Child Psychol Psychiatry*. 2004; 45: 2–40.

Victor JD, Conte MM, Burton L, Nass RD. Visual evoked potentials in dyslexics and normals: failure to find a difference in transient or steady-state responses. *Vis Neurosci*. 1993; 10: 939–946.

Voeller KKS. Right-hemisphere deficit syndrome in children. *Am J Psychiatry*. 1986; 143: 1004–1009.

Voeller KKS. Social-emotional learning disabilities. *Psychiatr Ann*. 1990; 21: 735–741.

Von Aster M. Developmental dyscalculia in children: review of the literature and clinical validation. *Acta Paedopsychiatrica*. 1994; 56: 169–178.

von Plessen K, Lundervold A, Duta N, et al. Less developed corpus callosum in dyslexic subjects—a structural MRI study. *Neuropsychologia*. 2002; 40: 1035–1044.

W

Wagner R, Torgesen JK, Rashotte CA, et al. Changing relations between phonological processing abilities and word-level reading as children develop from beginning to skilled readers: a 5-year longitudinal study. *Dev Psychol*. 1997; 33: 468–479.

Warren C, Morton J. The effects of priming on picture recognition. *Br J Psychol*. 1982; 73: 117–129.

Warrington EK, James M. Tachistoscopic number estimation in patients with unilateral lesions. *J Neurol Neurosurg Psychiatry*. 1967; 30: 468–474.

Webb DW, Fryer AE, Osborne JP. Morbidity associated with tuberous sclerosis: a population study. *Dev Med Child Neurol*. 1996; 38: 146–155.

Weintraub S, Mesulam M-M. Developmental learning disabilities of the right hemisphere: emotional, interpersonal, and cognitive components. *Arch Neurol*. 1983; 40: 463–468.

Wiederholt JL. Historical perspectives on the education of the learned disabled. In Mann L, Sabatino DA, eds. *The Second Review of Special Education*. Austin, TX: PRO-ED; 1974.

Wiesel TN, Hubel DH. Comparison of the effects of unilateral and bilateral eye closure on cortical unit response in kitten. *J Neurophysiol*. 1965; 28: 1029–1040.

Wildgruber D, Ackerman H, Grodd W. Differential contributions of motor cortex, basal ganglia and cerebellum to speech motor control: effects of syllable repetition rate evaluated by fMRI. *Neuroimage*. 2001; 13: 101–109.

Wilkinson GS. *Wide Range Achievement Test 3*. Wilmington, DE: Wide Range; 1993.

Wilson A, Revkin S, Cohen D, et al. *Behavioral Brain Function*. 2006 [software for mathematics].

Wimmer H, Mayringer H, Raberger T. Reading and dual-task balancing: evidence against the automatization deficit explanation of developmental dyslexia. *J Learn Disabil*. 1999; 32: 473–478.

Witelson SF. Sex differences in neuroanatomical changes with aging. *N Engl J Med*. 1991; 325: 211–212.

Witelson SF, Kigar Di, Harvey T. The exceptional brain of Albert Einstein. *Lancet*. 1999; 353: 2149–2153.

Withers GS, Greenough WT. Reach training selectivity alters dendritic branching in subpopulations of layer II-III pyramids in rat motor somatosensory forelimb cortex. *Neuropsychologia*. 1989; 27: 61–69.

Witruk E. Memory deficits of dyslexic children. *Ann NY Acad Sci*. 1993; 682: 43.

Witton C, Talcott JB, Hansen PC, et al. Sensitivity to dynamic auditory and visual stimuli predicts nonword reading ability in both dyslexic and normal readers. *Curr Biol*. 1998; 8: 791–797.

Wolf M. Naming speed and reading: the contribution of the cognitive neurosciences. *Reading Res Q*. 1991; 26: 123–141.

Wolf M, Bowers PG. The double-deficit hypothesis for the developmental dyslexias. *J Educ Psychol*. 1999; 91: 415–438.

Wolf M, Goodglass H. Dyslexia, dysnomia, and lexical retrieval: a longitudinal investigation. *Brain Language*. 1986; 28: 154–168.

Wolf M, Obergon M. Early naming deficits, developmental dyslexia and a specific deficit hypothesis. *Brain Language*. 1992; 42: 219–247.

Wolff PH. Impaired temporal resolution in developmental dyslexia [review]. *Ann NY Acad Sci*. 1993; 682: 87–103.

Wolff PH. In: Tallal P, Galaburda AM, Llinas RR, von Euler C, eds. *Temporal Information Processing in the Nervous System: Special Reference to Dyslexia and Dysphasia*. New York, NY: New York Academy of Sciences; 1993:87–103.

Wolff PH, Melngailis I, Kotwica K. Family patterns of developmental dyslexia, Part III: Spelling errors as behavioral phenotype. *Am J Med Genet*. 1996; 63: 378–386.

Wolff PH, Melngailis I, Obergon M, Bedrosian M. Family patterns of developmental dyslexia, Part II: Behavioral phenotypes. *Am J Med Genet*. 1995; 60: 494–505.

Wolff PH, Michel GF, Ovrut M, Drake C. Rate and timing precision of motor coordination in developmental dyslexia. *Dev Psychol*. 1990; 26: 349–359.

Woods RP, Zeffiro TA. Abnormal processing of visual motion in dyslexia revealed by functional brain imaging. *Nature*. 1996; 382: 66–69.

Y

Yamaden J. Developmental deep dyslexia in Japanese: a case study. *Brain Language*. 1995; 51(3): 444–457.

Yasutake D, Bryan T. The influence of affect on the achievement and behavior of students with learning disabilities. *J Learn Disabil*. 1995; 28: 329–334.

Ygge J, Lennerstrand G, Rydberg A, et al. Oculomotor functions in a Swedish population of dyslexic and normally reading children. *Acta Ophthalmolog (Copenh)*. 1993; 71: 10–21.

Yu AC, Margoliash D. Temporal hierarchical control of singing in birds. *Science*. 1996; 273: 1871–1875.

Z

Zago L, Pesenti M, Mellet E, Crivello F, Mazoyer B, Tzourio-Mazoyer N. Neural correlates of simple and complex mental calculation. *Neuroimage*. 2001; 13: 314–327.

Zamarian L, Ischebeck A, Delazer M. Neuroscience of learning arithmetic—evidence from brain imaging studies. *Neurosci Behav Rev*. 2009; 33: 909–925.

Zametkin AJ, Nordahl T, Gross M, et al. Cerebral glucose metabolism in adults with hyperactivity of childhood onset. *N Engl J Med*. 1990; 323: 1361–1366.

Zeffiro T, Eden G. The cerebellum and dyslexia: perpetrator or innocent bystander? [review]. *Trends Neurosci*. 2001; 24: 512–513.

Zigmond N. Models for delivery of special education services to students with learning disabilities in public school. *J Child Neurol*. 1995; (suppl 1): S86–S92.

Zhuo M, Hawkins RD. Long term depression: a learning related type of synaptic plasticityin the mammalian central nervous system. *Rev Neuroscience*. 1995; 6: 259–277.

Zorzi M, Houghton G, Butterworth B. Two routes or one in reading aloud? A connectionist dual-process model. *J Exp Psychol Hum Percept Perform*. 1998; 24: 1131–1161.

oculomoter abnormalities, 139–140
vision abnormalities, 139–140
visual magnocellular system abnormalities, 137–139
See also eyesight
Voeller, K.K.S., 189
volumetric studies, 84–88
voxel-based morphometry (VBM), 84–88

Warrington, E.K., 153, 157
water diffusion in the brain. *See* DTI (diffusion tensor imaging)
Wechsler Intelligence Scale for Children (WISC-IV), 217

Weintraub, S., 185, 187
"whole reading" method, 21
WISC-IV (Wechsler Intelligence Scale for Children), 217
WJ-R (Woodcock-Johnson Test of Achievement-Revised), 216
Wolf, M., 120
word blindness
precursor to SLD, 5, 7–8
See also SLD (Specific Learning Disabilities)
working memory, 46–47
WRAT-R (Wide Range Achievement Test-Revised), 216